# TREATMENT AND REHABILITATION OF SEVERE MENTAL ILLNESS

# Treatment and Rehabilitation of Severe Mental Illness

WILLIAM D. SPAULDING, *1950-*
MARY E. SULLIVAN, *1948-*
JEFFREY S. POLAND

THE GUILFORD PRESS
New York   London

© 2003 The Guilford Press
A Division of Guilford Publications, Inc.
72 Spring Street, New York, NY 10012
www.guilford.com

Printed in the United States of America

This book is printed on acid-free paper.

Last digit is print number:  9  8  7  6  5  4  3  2  1

**Library of Congress Cataloging-in-Publication Data**

Spaulding, William D. (William Delbert), 1950–
    Treatment and rehabilitation of severe mental illness / by William D.
Spaulding, Mary E. Sullivan, Jeffrey S. Poland.
        p.   cm.
Includes bibliographical references and index.
    ISBN 1-57230-841-9 (hardcover)
    1. Mental illness—Treatment. 2. Mentally ill—Rehabilitation. 3.
Mentally ill—Care. I. Sullivan, Mary E. (Mary Elizabeth), 1948–
II. Poland, Jeffrey S. III. Title.
RC480 .53 .S638   2003
616.89′1—dc21                                        2002152969

# About the Authors

**William D. Spaulding, PhD,** received his doctorate in clinical psychology at the University of Arizona in 1976. He completed a postdoctoral fellowship in mental health research and teaching at the University of Rochester School of Medicine and Dentistry. Dr. Spaulding is currently Professor of Psychology in the Clinical Psychology Training Program, Department of Psychology, University of Nebraska–Lincoln, and a Clinical Psychologist in the Community Transition Program, Lincoln Regional Center.

**Mary E. Sullivan, MSW,** received her master's in social work from Syracuse University in 1978. She also received a certificate in health studies from the Maxwell School of Citizenship and Public Affairs, Syracuse University, in 1978. She is currently Program Director of the Community Transition Program, Lincoln Regional Center, and Adjunct Clinical Assistant Professor in the Department of Psychology, University of Nebraska–Lincoln.

**Jeffrey S. Poland, PhD,** received an MA in clinical psychology from Southern Connecticut State University in 1982 and a doctorate in the philosophy of science from Massachusetts Institute of Technology in 1983. He has held positions at Colgate University and the University of Nebraska–Lincoln, and he currently teaches in the Department of History, Philosophy, and Social Science at the Rhode Island School of Design. Dr. Poland has published articles on topics such as the unity of science, psychiatric classification, and psychopathology. He is coauthor with William D. Spaulding of a forthcoming book, *Crisis and Revolution: Toward a Reconceptualization of Psychopathology*, to be published by MIT Press.

# Preface

*Treatment and Rehabilitation of Severe Mental Illness* presents a comprehensive, integrated approach to treatment and rehabilitation for people with disabling mental illness. Some of the elements of this approach (clinical assessment and treatment technologies) have not been comprehensively described in the literature; this book provides a detailed account of these technologies, their theoretical and scientific bases, and practical guidelines for application. In contrast, some of the elements in the integrated approach, such as psychopharmacology, social skills training, and maintaining a therapeutic milieu, are familiar to mental health and rehabilitation professionals; the role of these elements in our comprehensive and integrated approach is described and supplemented by references to original sources for more details on application.

The integrated approach presented here aspires to be more than a collection of assessment and treatment technologies, more than a formula for clinical practice. It incorporates a conceptualization of mental illness that is informed by current scientific findings and principles related to the problems and goals of rehabilitation. It guides data collection and decision making in the context of our currently incomplete understanding of mental illness and the reality that clinical practice involves, in large part, a management of uncertainty. Finally, the approach systematically addresses the personal perspectives and values of people with mental illness and their families, as these perspectives and values relate to the rehabilitation enterprise.

We make no claim to originality regarding any part of the integrated approach described here. At the same time, we believe that our approach brings together disparate elements that have not been integrated previously. Our approach is thus subject to criticism that it "contains nothing new" *and* that it includes revolutionary premises. Reasonable individuals may disagree about which of these seemingly incompatible criticisms is more applicable. Our position on this is a pragmatic one. Clinicians, academicians, advocates, and consumers who understand rehabilitation in a broad and conceptually coherent framework are expected to be more effective than those who are familiar with various technologies or principles but who do not systematically engage these elements in an integrated approach. Similarly, individuals whose awareness is limited to particular technical elements within the rehabilitation armamentarium (e.g., psychopharmacotherapy, behavior therapy, occupational therapy, etc.) are not expected to incorporate, in their daily practice, the social values and ethical principles that help define the rehabilitation enterprise. This book aspires to demonstrate the viability and accessibility of a broad, conceptually coherent, ethical, and clinically useful conceptual framework for rehabilitation.

Our pragmatic concerns have been stimulated by the history of mental health services over the last three decades of the 20th century. Despite scientific advances in the biology, psychology, and sociology of mental illness, treatment outcome has remained poor for many individuals. Despite increasing public concern and consumer activism, scientific advances have not necessarily led to changes in clinical practice or in availability of potentially beneficial services. By the 1990s, concern about this state of affairs prompted investment of federal research dollars to study it. By the end of that decade, findings of a large-scale project began to appear and confirmed suspicions that technologies of known effectiveness are under-used (Lehman, Steinwachs, Dixon, Goldman, et al., 1998; Lehman, Steinwachs, Dixon, Postrado, et al., 1998). The causes have not been fully analyzed, but the "usual suspects" include under-funding of public sector services, limited coverage for mental illness in private health insurance programs, bureaucratic inefficiency, lack of pertinent curricula in professional training programs, guild rivalry between disciplines, a disjunction between academic research practices and clinical realities, and widespread stigmatization of mental illness. These problems are certainly familiar to those who advocate for, and/or attempt to provide services to, people with severe and disabling mental illness.

Obviously, a new (or newly synthesized) clinical approach cannot resolve all these problems. However, an integrated approach is a good place to start. Clinicians and service recipients are in a position to experience directly the consequences of an integrated approach, in the form of increased rehabilitation success and recovery. In addition, a broad and conceptually coherent understanding of rehabilitation, in all its complexity, should equip those individuals to serve as more effective advocates for better services and social policy. Administrators, advocates, and consumers informed by an integrated conceptual framework become more sophisticated purchasers and managers of rehabilitation services, and more effective advocates for appropriate funding. An integrated approach also helps bridge the gap between clinic and laboratory. Scientific advances become clinical tools as their relevance to real human problems becomes understood. The absence of an integrated approach for treatment and rehabilitation of severe mental illness has impeded the process of relating new scientific findings to old clinical problems. Researchers, clinicians, administrators, policymakers, advocates, and consumers need to communicate more effectively about their respective needs and resources, and they need a common (and therefore comprehensive) conceptual framework to do that.

Our presentation of the integrated approach is organized into three sections. Part I, on key concepts, identifies the major elements of the approach and describes the concepts that provide integration. The first chapter introduces the unifying concept of a *paradigm* to demonstrate how the separate domains of science, social values, and clinical practice must be brought together in a rehabilitation framework. The second chapter describes how scientific psychopathology can be made accessible for clinical application. The third chapter focuses on the nature of assessment and treatment planning in an integrated approach. In all three chapters, the relationships between service recipients, consumers, providers, advocates, and other important figures are considered in the framework of the integrated approach.

Part II, on assessment and treatment techniques, describes specific clinical techniques of known effectiveness and their appropriate role in the rehabilitation of severe and disabling mental illness. Part III, on the organizational context of rehabilitation, describes the organizational, administrative, and managerial challenges that confront implementation of effective rehabilitation, and shows how the integrated approach guides successful provision of services.

# Acknowledgments

First and foremost, we acknowledge the many individuals whom we have joined in their recovery from disabling mental illness, as well as their family and friends. It is from them that we have learned the most, and to them we are most deeply indebted. Second, we acknowledge the clinician-scientists who are the giants of our time in the area of treatment and rehabilitation for severe mental illness: William Anthony, Alan Bellak, Hans D. Brenner, Gerard Hogarty, Robert Liberman, and Gordon Paul. They have had a profound effect not only on clinical technology but on our fundamental understanding of mental illness and the recovery process. Next, we pay personal homage to our teachers, mentors, and others who have provided special help along the way: Leona Bachrach, Morris Bell, Rue Cromwell, Jerry Fodor, George Hohmann, Ed Ryan, and John Strauss. We wish to express our appreciation and affection to the many colleagues who have worked alongside us and helped us grow, most especially Vicky Buchholz, Joan DeVries, Thad Eckman, Robert Heinssen, Steve Higgins, Richard Hunter, Timothy Kuehnel, William Merkle, Dorie Reed, Charles E. Richardson, A. Jocelyn Ritchie, Steven Silverstein, Barbara Von Eckardt, and Martin Weiler. To the many individuals who staffed the Community Transition Program in Lincoln, Nebraska, our appreciation and admiration for the job you have done. Our dozens of graduate students over the past 20 years have taught us much, and without them our work would not have been possible. To them all, we extend a special thanks. Finally, we wish to thank Rochelle Serwator and Margaret Ryan for their editorial skills, encouragement, support, and expert advice in the conception and production of this book.

# Contents

## PART III. THE ORGANIZATIONAL          249
## CONTEXT OF REHABILITATION

# Part I

# KEY CONCEPTS

To be truly integrative, a clinical approach must be more than a diverse collection of tools and techniques. It must include a set of concepts and related representations of how nature works, usually called a *model* in contemporary scientific discourse. Ideally, models used in clinical practice are logically consistent with what we know from the more basic sciences. More importantly, they should account for things that happen within the particular frame of reference of mental health. A model's value is determined by how well it helps us explain, predict, and influence events of interest within that frame of reference.

In addition to models of how nature works, an integrated clinical approach requires models that identify social problems and assign value to solutions. In mental health, these models complement our scientific understanding of *how* a problem works with an understanding of *why* it is a problem. This is a prerequisite to determining what are appropriate solutions. Ultimately, it is a prerequisite to validating the goals of the clinical approach.

The chapters in this first part present ideas from three separate domains—scientific psychopathology, rehabilitation, and clinical case formulation—that come together as the conceptual basis of contemporary treatment and rehabilitation of severe mental illness. The ideas generate the models by which we understand mental illness as a natural process, as a personal experience, as a clinical phenomenon, and as a social problem. Together, they represent an integrated *paradigm*. A more complete appreciation of the key concepts in this paradigm, on the part of clinicians and everyone else associated with the rehabilitation enterprise, leads to more systematic, consistent, humane, and effective pursuit of that enterprise.

# Chapter 1

# An Integrated Paradigm

## Origins in Psychopathology, Rehabilitation, and Clinical Practice

*Rehabilitation* is a familiar term with a variety of meanings. In common usage, its meanings range from general sets of assumptions, values, and goals, to very specific clinical techniques. The term "psychiatric rehabilitation" is used extensively to describe the rehabilitation of people with severe mental illness, but there are different schools of thought and technologies even within the psychiatric rehabilitation community. When it comes to actual clinical practice and the development and provision of mental health services, confusion and disagreement about what constitutes rehabilitation remain, especially as it is applied to the treatment of people with severe mental illness.

There are a number of reasons for this ambiguity concerning rehabilitation. Historically, its application to mental illness derives from earlier theoretical systems and technologies, especially the psychology of physical rehabilitation, but also clinical psychology, social learning theory, social psychiatry, occupational therapy, and others, plus more recent contributions from the biological and cognitive neurosciences. Application of rehabilitation to people with mental illness has evolved over several decades. Specific treatments and related technologies have been added to its armamentarium by various research groups at various times, and its underlying premises and values have been shaped by the involvement of advocates, consumers, recipients, and other constituencies. The recipient population is highly heterogeneous, and different subpopulations and individuals benefit from different combinations of specific treatments within the broader armamentarium. Different rehabilitation goals are suitable for different individuals—a situation that requires considerable tailoring of services and discourages a "universal standard" of specific technologies applicable to all recipients.

Today rehabilitation continues to take shape, not just in mental health, but in health care in general. New theoretical insights and technologies are assimilated as they become available. Changing social policy, the politics of health care, and theories of management also affect how rehabilitation is provided, and to whom. (For a current account of rehabilitation outside the mental health domain, see Brandt & Pope, 1997.) It is this multiplicity of factors that creates the vaguely defined and sometimes controversial enterprise of rehabilitation for severe and disabling mental illness.

The rehabilitation field is currently experiencing a recognizable stage of development, characterized by a cacophony of perspectives, that is also showing signs of consolidation and integration—harmony out of cacophony. A premise of this book is that, in the foreseeable future, progress in rehabilitation for mental illness will be characterized not by dramatic new breakthroughs in science and technology but by steady progress toward a more systematic, relational, and effective application of principles and techniques that presently lie in separate, often isolated, domains. For this systems-wide coherence to become a reality, the field of mental health rehabilitation needs a unifying conceptual framework in which all its disparate values, principles, and technologies coalesce to provide a workable, successful product: effective rehabilitation of people who live with disabling mental illness.

The first three chapters of this book construct such a framework, and the succeeding chapters amplify it with specific principles and technologies. In this first chapter, the construction project begins with reflections on the role served by unifying conceptual frameworks, or *paradigms*, in science, technology, and society. Next, several historical paradigms for understanding and treating mental illness are reviewed. To understand where we are going, it is helpful to take a look at where we have been. Finally, we introduce the three major sources of our rehabilitation paradigm: the social values of rehabilitation, the research findings in the field of psychopathology, and the techniques of clinical case formulation.

## REHABILITATION NEEDS A PARADIGM

A paradigm is a set of interrelated concepts, principles, and methods related to the successful pursuit of some overarching enterprise. In this case, the overarching enterprise is rehabilitation. The paradigm we are proposing to guide the rehabilitation of severe and disabling mental illness includes (1) a set of premises and principles concerning illness, disability, and the purposes of treatment; (2) a collection of interrelated scientific methods and observations; (3) specific clinical technologies; and (4) a systematic approach to providing services to people with disabling mental illness.

A paradigm gives logical coherence to its overarching enterprise and individual meaning to its specific elements—the concepts, methods, treatments, and so on—that the paradigm incorporates. A paradigm is especially important for rehabilitation and related human service enterprises because these enterprises incorporate such diverse elements as social values, behavioral technology, and neuropharmacology. Social values by themselves do not necessarily lead to technical solutions, and the biobehavioral sciences do not necessarily lead to social values. If rehabilitation is to be both socially responsible and clinically effective, it needs a paradigm that establishes logical, conceptual, and ethical continuity between its various elements.

To some, systematic discussion of an approach's underlying paradigm may seem like an abstract philosophical exercise, lacking significant or direct implications for practice. This would be a defensible view for pursuits wherein the logical and philosophical premises are so accepted, or the technologies on which they are based so unequivocal in operation, that the paradigm in which they operate is not subject to productive debate. Electronics is an example. Most would find it quite annoying if the initial chapter of the manual for their new computer were a philosophical discussion of number theory or quantum mechanics. Although those subjects address the most fundamental aspects of how computers work, current controversies over the ultimate meaning of "zero" are unlikely to influence use of computers in our everyday lives. Even when paradigms contain intrinsic contradictions, important applications may remain unaffected. For example, we continue to build both nuclear weapons and radios, even though the paradigms that guide those activities—relativity theory and quantum mechanics, respectively—are theoretically incompatible. (Greene's [1999] account of the development of string theory sheds considerable light on the relationship between paradigms and the progress of science.)

Nevertheless, in certain applications paradigmatic ambiguities create more serious and immediate limitations. For example, the paradigms of law and medicine reflect complex human enterprises and enjoy a good deal of consensus. Both highly value the preservation of human life and have evolved sophisticated praxes for doing so. However, neither law nor medicine has been able to resolve the issue of elective abortion. There are logical and scientific ambiguities about what constitutes "human life" and when it begins. As a result, neither paradigm provides resolution of the issue of what it means to abort a human fetus. Controversy persists at the level of political and religious belief. In the case of mental illness and rehabilitation, there is no paradigm that enjoys the degree of consensus found in electronics, or even medicine or law. As a result, there is pervasive ambiguity about what the goals of rehabilitation should be, who can benefit, or even what *rehabilitation* and *severe and disabling mental illness* really mean. As with elective abortion, mental health controversies engage political and religious belief as well as tenets of science, law, and technology.

In mental health services, the judgments of clinicians and the choices of service recipients, consumers, and advocates are all based on some underlying set of premises, often unique and idiosyncratic to the individual, in the absence of a commonly accepted paradigm. As a result, decisions and choices that make sense to one individual may make no sense to others. Equally important, without the moderating influence of broad consensus, many people may harbor premises that are simply false (although, of course, having a paradigm is no guarantee against being wrong). In a mental health service system without a paradigm, policy is driven too little by science, technology, and real social needs, and too much by politics and misconceptions. The success of the rehabilitation enterprise ultimately depends on a sound paradigm to guide the judgments and choices of both providers *and* recipients.

## THE EVOLUTION OF PARADIGMS

Paradigms are sociological phenomena, in that they represent the collective beliefs and conventions of a community. In scientific communities, paradigms are associated with philosopher and historian Thomas Kuhn. Kuhn (1962) constructed a now well-known analysis of the formation and change of paradigms in science. As a result, *paradigm* is often used in the sense of "paradigms as described by Kuhn." However, Kuhn included a number of distinct ideas under the rubric of *paradigms,* and his analysis has been criticized for being vague and overinclusive in this respect. Furthermore, Kuhn's analysis of paradigms focused on progress in astronomy, chemistry, and physics—barely comparable to the sciences that address mental illness and the enterprise of rehabilitation. In short, much of Kuhn's analysis has questionable relevance to the evolution of rehabilitation paradigms.

Nevertheless, one of Kuhn's most important insights is highly applicable to contemporary rehabilitation: *Communities generally tend to adhere to a single, dominant paradigm even while new, alternative paradigms evolve.* The new paradigms evolve in response to limitations in the explanatory or practical power of the dominant paradigm. Eventually, the value of the dominant paradigm becomes outweighed by an alternative, and the community undergoes a *paradigm shift.* The new paradigm brings fundamental changes in key premises and usually an expansion of explanatory and practical power. For example, emergence of the quantum mechanics paradigm provided new explanations of natural phenomena that cannot be explained by Newtonian physics (e.g., the behavior of electrons) and also stimulated invention of modern electronic devices. Old paradoxes are resolved or obviated. The scope of the paradigm itself may change. The cycle then repeats itself, as the new paradigm accumulates disconfirmatory data and its practical limitations become salient.

Kuhn also recognized that paradigm shifts occur in response to developments that are unrelated to competition between paradigms. For example, acceptance of a heliocentric solar system was influenced by European social and cultural evolution as much as by an accumulation of astronomical observations. Paradigms of mental health and illness were historically influenced by social movements (e.g., the French Revolution) and population shifts (e.g., immigration to the New World) as much as by scientific advances (see Magaro, Gripp, McDowell, & Miller, 1978).

The currently dominant paradigm for mental health and illness, in place for at least a century, is creaking under the weight of disconfirmatory data and practical limitations. Extrinsic factors, such as health care politics and consumer activism, are pressuring for change. Attractive alternative paradigms have been appearing for over three decades. If there is a "Kuhnian cycle" in the evolution of mental health paradigms, then the scientific and health care communities seem poised for a shift. A new paradigm is emerging. It incorporates older ones and extends their explanatory power and practical utility. It is recognizably a *rehabilitation* paradigm, but it incorporates many features that have not previously been included in rehabilitation paradigms.

## REHABILITATION PARADIGMS FOR MENTAL ILLNESS

Paradigms for understanding and treating disabling mental illness have been evolving for at least three centuries. "Moral therapy," which appeared in Europe in the 17th century, is an early example (see Grob, 1973, for a historical account of moral therapy in America); it represented a protoscientific paradigm, in that it had a rational conceptual structure that did not depend on supernatural or theological assumptions but did not incorporate a scientific experimental methodology. The term *moral* lacked the religious and ethical connotations it has today and was closer to our contemporary use of *psychological*. In the late 19th century the medical model emerged as the dominant paradigm, and remained so throughout the 20th century. (See Grob, 1983, for a historical account of these developments in America; see Bynum, Porter, & Shepherd, 1988, for a historical account of parallel developments in Europe.) The modern rehabilitation paradigms for mental illness that appeared in the late 20th century represented distinct alternatives to the medical model. It is therefore important to understand the relationship between the older medical model and newer rehabilitation paradigms.

## The Medical Model

*Medical model* is a term used in markedly different ways by different individuals. In the present context, it refers to a paradigm of treatment and service provision in which mental illness is held to be fundamentally and pervasively comparable to medical diseases, which have no psychological or behavioral sequelae. There is a strong connotation that medical treatments have primacy, and that the professionals who control these treatments should control all aspects of the related service system. The community most centrally associated with the medical model is the profession of psychiatry, with its associated guild organizations (the American Psychiatric Association in the United States) and academic institutions (psychiatry departments in medical schools). The medical model includes other professionals as caregivers, "allied health professionals," who collaborate with physicians in a subordinate capacity.

Although many people associate the medical model with biological theories of mental illness and biological treatment technology, the model is not really tied to any particular theoretical view or technology. In the first half of the 20th century American psychiatry was dominated by the theories and practice of psychoanalysis. The second half of the century saw a shift to biological theories and pharmacological treatment, but this shift was accomplished without changes in the key premises of the underlying medical model. (For further discussion of the relationship between medical and psychoanalytic models in the mid-20th century, see Ullman & Krasner, 1965, pp. 1–20.)

A core feature of the medical model is *psychiatric diagnosis*, the process of identifying specific mental illnesses or diseases in the context of clinical assessment. The German psychiatrist Emil Kraepelin is usually credited with the first codification of psychiatric diagnoses, which occurred in the 1880s (Kraepelin, 1896/1987). Over the first half of the 20th century Kraepelin's original diagnostic system was reshaped by the theoretical influence of psychoanalysis, especially in the United States. However, the concept of diagnosis as a process of identifying specific disease entities remained at the heart of the psychiatric medical model. At mid-century the American Psychiatric Association began publishing an official *Diagnostic and Statistical Manual of Mental Disorders*, now in its fourth edition (American Psychiatric Association, 1994).

By the 1950s the medical model of mental illness was strongly dominant. People with disabling mental illness mostly lived in long-term mental or psychiatric hospitals and were understood to have specific "diseases," mostly schizophrenia. The etiologies of schizophrenia and other diseases were (and remain) unknown, and the mainstream view was that these disabling mental diseases were generally incurable. Treatment, provided with faint expectations of success, constituted little more than attempts to palliate patients' distress and to make their behavior more manageable in an institutional environment.[1] This treatment involved a mixture of archaic naturopathic practices (e.g., various kinds of shock therapy, hot baths, cold packs), traditional psychoanalytic methods adapted for conditions of severe mental illness, and interpersonal psychodynamic therapies.[2]

The public hospitals, usually operated by state governments, generally degenerated into dehumanizing institutions and became targets of social criticism. The private hospitals tended to provide better living conditions, but eventually they too came under fire—first, because of mounting evidence that the psychoanalytic treatment that was the norm was ineffective or even harmful, and later because of economic inefficiency. Sociological analyses (e.g., Goffman, 1961) and experimental research (e.g., Braginsky, Braginsky, & Ring, 1969; Gelfand, Gelfand, & Dobson, 1967) fanned suspicions that many of the disabling characteristics of severe mental illness were actually *caused* by the conditions that prevailed in psychiatric institutions (for a later but complementary analysis, see Magaro et al., 1978). The medical model, closely associated with institutional practices, simultaneously came under attack.

## The Social-Community Paradigm

Criticism of the medical model and interest in the sociological origins and characteristics of disabling mental illness led to an alternative paradigm. For heuristic purposes we call it the social–community paradigm. Embedded in a zeitgeist that also saw the emergence of social psychiatry and community psychology, this paradigm presumes that social factors are so salient in mental illness that treatment should focus on bringing them under control for therapeutic purposes. Historical precedents were identified in

---

[1]The term *patient* is a derivative of the medical model. There have been many objections to this term over the years, for various reasons. In this book, *patients* is used when referring to the medical model understanding of people with mental illness, and other terms are used when referring to people with mental illness as understood in alternative paradigms.

[2]Modern electroconvulsive therapy (ECT) should not be confused with historical forms of shock therapy. The modern version is performed under safe and humane conditions (e.g., the patient is anesthetized), and there is some evidence of clinical effectiveness for some conditions. However, the development of modern ECT from historical forms is an effective example of how modern treatment approaches sometimes develop from more primitive, even harmful, practices. It is noteworthy in this regard that modern ECT remains somewhat controversial and is still condemned by some individuals within the mental health advocacy community.

the seemingly successful moral therapy of pre-Enlightenment Europe (this model survived well into the 20th century in some parts of Europe).

One tangible outcome of the social–community paradigm was the conception and creation of a "therapeutic community," pioneered by English psychiatrist Maxwell Jones (Jones, 1953). The therapeutic community engages patients in self-government and other social activities requiring personal responsibility and empowerment. The idea that personal responsibility and empowerment have anything to do with recovery from mental illness was antithetical to the medical model, especially as it was practiced at that time. (A patient's role was not to accept responsibility and exercise choice but to accept the physician's judgments and decisions, and exercise *patience* while waiting for treatment to exert its effects.) Furthermore, the therapeutic community required organizational and administrative characteristics that were somewhat incompatible with the medical model's physician-driven decision-making processes. Interestingly, the therapeutic community was originally developed as a treatment approach for drug addiction, not mental illness. Nevertheless, it was widely applied to disabling mental illness in traditional psychiatric hospitals (for a comprehensive discussion see Paul & Lentz, 1977, especially Chapter 2). However, the approach's incompatibilities with traditional medical decision making created tensions and made faithful application difficult in psychiatric hospitals.

A somewhat similar realization of the social–community paradigm is Soteria (Mosher & Menn, 1978), a comprehensive treatment approach, designed for people with severe mental illness, that emphasizes a therapeutic social environment. Considerations of the phenomenological experience of acute and chronic psychosis are central to the approach, which also shows the influence of interpersonal psychodynamic perspectives and the "antipsychiatry" views of the 1960s (e.g., Laing, 1969; Szasz, 1961). Advocates of Soteria have expressed special concern about potentially adverse effects of antipsychotic medication, preferring drug-free treatment whenever possible. Soteria offers a distinct alternative to traditional medical model treatment of disabling mental illness.

A number of treatment approaches and programs with characteristics similar to Soteria evolved during roughly the same period, including the Fountain House (Glasscote, 1971), Thresholds (Bond, Dincin, Setze, & Witheridge, 1984), and Fairweather (Fairweather, Sanders, Maynard, & Cressler, 1969) models. All shared an emphasis on community support and cohesion, acceptance of personal responsibility in return for community support, a tolerant attitude toward psychotic behavior, and de-emphasis of traditional professional involvement in treatment. All appeared to produce better outcomes than standard medical model treatment. The original models are still in use and have been replicated in many locales around the world (for a comprehensive overview, see Mosher & Burti, 1989).

## The Social Learning Paradigm

A second alternative that emerged in the 1960s, the social learning paradigm, evolved primarily from the experimental psychological research of the first half of the 20th century. The late 1950s and the 1960s saw the first clinical applications of this work, often with people who had severe and disabling mental illness. In the late 1950s a group of applied learning theorists set up the first *token economy* program at Anna State Hospital, a public psychiatric institution in southern Illinois (Ayllon & Azrin, 1968)—in essence, a learning theory version of the therapeutic community where the focus is on the relationship between behavior and environmental rewards and punishments instead of social–interpersonal processes. On the premise (strongly supported by experimental research) that institutional environments tend to reward dysfunctional behavior and punish normal behavior, token economies are designed to ensure that distinct, meaningful rewards are systematically provided, contingent on the person producing behavior associated with recovery. Participants earn tokens that can be redeemed for desired commodities or privileges. Using the learning technique of "successive approximation," normal behavior is gradually developed while abnormal behavior is extinguished. The early token economies produced dramatic improvements in the behavioral functioning of severely disabled, institutionalized people (reviewed by Kazdin & Bootsin, 1972).

Even as token economy programs were first demonstrating their effectiveness, paradigm shifts were underway in academic psychology, and these shifts led directly to rehabilitation paradigms. General learning theory gave rise to social learning theory, which applied the precision and specificity of learning theory to the full complexity of human behavior. Psychology also shifted from a behaviorist paradigm toward a cognitive-based one, because social learning theory used principles of cognitive functioning to articulate the mechanisms by which humans apprehend and evaluate their environments, acquire new behaviors, and formulate behavioral strategies (Bandura, 1969). The clinical application of these principles gave rise to cognitive-behavioral therapy and related techniques. Particularly important for the rehabilitation field was the practical application of these principles in the development of *social skills training*, a systematic approach to fostering effective social behavior through instruction, demonstration, practice, and systematic reward.

The most important implementation of the social learning paradigm in rehabilitation was a comprehensive treatment approach developed by psychologist Gordon Paul and his colleagues in the 1960s. In keeping with academic psychology's emphasis on procedural and observational precision, the Paul treatment program included an elaborate array of sophisticated behavioral assessment techniques and treatment procedures. Social skills training and token economy were the core of treatment. Using this technology, Paul and colleagues undertook a monumental 10-year study of rehabilitation outcome (Paul & Lentz, 1977). The study was a controlled experiment in which participants were randomly assigned to one of three treatment conditions: social learning, therapeutic community, or standard medical model. The results were unequivocal. The social learning program produced better outcomes than the medical model treatment on every dimension, with the therapeutic community coming in a distant second.

In the 1980s and 1990s the social learning paradigm was a key influence in the productions of the UCLA Center for Research on Rehabilitation of Schizophrenia. Under the leadership of psychiatrist Robert P. Liberman, the center provided auspices for a diversity of basic and applied research. Among the center's most important innovations was a series of highly operationalized social skills training modules, prepared and packaged for use in public sector rehabilitation settings. The modules were developed to cover a broad range of special skill areas, including symptom and medication management, leisure activities, and interpersonal problem solving. These and other center materials continue to be important tools in rehabilitation (for a practical compendium of this technology, see Kuehnel, Liberman, Storzbach, & Rose, 1990). The center was also the source of key clinical research studies that helped establish the effectiveness of skills training and other social learning techniques (e.g., Liberman, 1992; Wallace, Nelson, Liberman, 1980).

## The Shift to Psychopharmacology

While the early rehabilitation paradigms were appearing in the 1960s, there were other major developments in the mental health world. The discovery and subsequent widespread use of psychotropic drugs struck the final blow to psychoanalysis as the dominant paradigm in mental health. Already embattled by social critiques and a lack of supporting scientific evidence, psychoanalysis gave way to psychopharmacology as the principle technology of American psychiatry. Almost simultaneously, the deinstitutionalization movement began. Over the span of a decade, America's psychiatric institutions decreased in population by some 80%. The co-occurrence of these two developments was not pure coincidence. Deinstitutionalization was probably accelerated by the belief that antipsychotic drugs would enable virtually all hospital residents to live safely and comfortably outside the institution. However, deinstitutionalization was also the result of a decade of disparate developments in social policy and science (Hogarty, 1977; for updated analyses of deinstitutionalization, see Bachrach, 1983, 1999).

The shift from psychoanalysis to psychopharmacology may have saved psychiatry from extinction, and it probably helped restore some credibility to the medical model. What did *not* change in the course of that shift was the presumption of (1) comparability between physical and mental illness, (2) the importance of psychiatric diagnosis, (3) the role of physicians and other professionals in treatment and service provision, and (4) the role of the patient as passive recipient of prescribed treatment (whether psychotherapy or drugs). Psychopharmacology has more of the familiar trappings of general medical practice than psychoanalysis, and its biotechnology is traditionally the province of medical practitioners. With the clinical success of psychotropic drugs in the 1960s, biological views of mental illness gained ascendancy. The medical model was revived as the dominant paradigm in mental health, and psychiatric diagnosis was purged of psychoanalytic theory. The third edition of the American Psychiatric Association's *Diagnostic and Statistical Manual*, introduced in 1980, used highly operationalized criteria to determine discreet neo-Kraepelinian categories as an intended means of resolving past problems of reliability and validity in diagnosis. There was decreased interest in nonbiological aspects of mental illness and the alternative paradigms that addressed them.

Interest in alternative paradigms was renewed in the late 1970s, in the wake of widespread opinion that deinstitutionalization had failed (see Bachrach, 1999). Antipsychotic drugs had not totally solved the problem of psychosis; institutions still housed psychiatric patients, and former residents often led lives of squalor and desperation despite the drugs. In retrospect, the expectations seem naïve. Although drugs did control some symptoms, they could not instill basic skills of daily living, create interpersonal relationships, or find someone a job (May, Tuma, & Dixon, 1981). The key medical model concept of psychiatric diagnosis became implicated in the false expectations. The new drugs seemed effective in suppressing the *symptoms* of schizophrenia and other severe disorders—that is, the behavioral expressions on which psychiatric diagnosis is based—but they did not alleviate other characteristics of the disorders, irrelevant to diagnosis but critical for normal functioning. In an attempt to bring this reality into conformity with the medical model, a new class of disease expressions, *negative symptoms*, was invented and integrated into diagnostic practices (Crow, 1985). Along with hope that newer drugs would address negative symptoms was an expanded awareness of the need for more comprehensive treatment, especially in the psychological and social domains, to address problems untouched by the medical model.

## The Psychiatric Rehabilitation Paradigm

A third alternative paradigm emerged during the reflective, deinstitutionalizing 1970s. This one was recognizably a rehabilitation paradigm, as it derived from the principles and technologies of conventional rehabilitation psychology. Originally focused on helping patients overcome physical disabilities such as paralysis, rehabilitation psychology incorporated social learning theory, client-centered psychotherapy, and other psychosocial components as it evolved outside the mental health system. A parallel evolution took place in the developmental disability service system. The evolving view of severe mental illnesses as "disabilities to be overcome" rather than "diseases to be cured" was especially compatible with rehabilitation psychology. Treatment included palliative measures, such as drugs to suppress psychiatric symptoms, but the emphasis was on *functional recovery*—that is, overcoming disability and living as normal a life as possible. Most importantly, treatment included a process of evaluation and appraisal, in which the *client* (the "identified patient" in the medical model) was seen as the key participant. This process, still in use, identifies the client's desires and needs as well as those conditions or circumstances preventing their realization. A plan is then formulated, specifying a systematic acquisition of the new skills needed to overcoming the barriers, and the client acquires these skills in an educational, rather than clinical, format.

In its most extensive realization, this paradigm became known as *psychiatric rehabilitation*.[3] Its most well-known figure has been William Anthony, a rehabilitation psychologist who, with colleagues, reformulated rehabilitation for application to mental illness (Anthony, 1979). Because Anthony's group is headquartered in the Sargent School of Allied Health Professions at Boston University, their paradigm has become colloquially known as "the Boston model." This model continues to exert significant influence today in the rehabilitation for mental illness. However, the field of psychiatric rehabilitation has grown to include a broader range of models and technologies than those used in the Boston model. (For an inclusive survey of the psychiatric rehabilitation paradigm, see Liberman, 1992.)

Applying Kuhn's terms, the alternatives to the medical model that emerged in the 1960s and 1970s exhibited the expected characteristics of alternative or *preparadigmatic* challengers to a dominant paradigm. They were (and still are) varied with respect to scope, client population, theoretical orientation, and technology. Their explanatory and practical ranges tended to be relatively focused, emphasizing and detailing some aspects of treatment and rehabilitation while dismissing others or accepting them as "givens." For example, the community, social learning, and psychiatric rehabilitation models focus on psychological and social processes, with rela-

---

[3]The term *psychiatric rehabilitation* may be confused with *psychosocial* rehabilitation, and the two are sometimes used interchangeably. In practice, both are sometimes used as a contraction of *biopsychosocial* rehabilitation. However, psychosocial rehabilitation sometimes refers specifically to a particular type of program, associated with specific prototypes, such as Fountain House in New York and Thresholds in Chicago. For example, a recent set of practice guidelines (McEvoy, Scheifler, & Frances, 1999) explicitly distinguishes between psychiatric and psychosocial rehabilitation in this way.

tively little consideration given to the biobehavioral aspects of mental illness. In the short run, narrow scope is advantageous if it illuminates weaknesses in the dominant paradigm and helps generate disconfirmatory data. In the long run, however, narrowness is disadvantageous for a paradigm, as it reduces the chances of accommodating new discoveries within its circumscribed purview.

In the late 20th century experimental demonstrations that the alternative paradigms could produce better outcomes once again began to undermine the dominance of the medical model, or at least certain interpretations of it. Ironically, advancing biological views of schizophrenia and other severe mental illnesses further dampened expectations for a "miracle drug," as it became increasingly evident that the origins of mental illness involve developmental processes that begin as early as the second trimester of gestation, causing structural abnormalities in the brain that conventional drug therapy in adulthood probably cannot reverse.

Dissatisfaction with the medical model in the late 20th century was not driven solely by discontentment with clinical outcome but also by increasing difficulties in reconciling research findings with psychiatric diagnoses, especially schizophrenia. The highly operationalized DSM-III criteria did not resolve the validity problems, as had been expected. A consensus gradually grew that (1) schizophrenia is a heterogeneous "family" of disorders (ironically, this view had been introduced by Bleuler early in the 20th century), (2) there are multiple etiological pathways that interact over decades of human development, and (3) each person who meets the diagnostic criteria has a unique constellation of problems. In the literature, calls for new diagnostic subtypes (e.g., Knoll et al., 1999; Strauss, Carpenter, & Bartko, 1974) were joined by criticisms of the basic concept of symptom-based diagnosis (Cromwell, 1984; Cromwell, Elkins, McCarthy, & O'Neil, 1994; McHugh, 1992; Poland, VonEckardt, & Spaulding, 1994; Sorenson, Paul, & Mariotto, 1988; Wakefield, 1992; Yudofsky, 1991). Ironically, the lack of association between diagnosis and psychotropic drug response contributes to disaffection with the neo-Kraepelinian diagnostic system (Ban, 2001). Today, the future of neo-Kraepelinian diagnosis appears doubtful. It may not even survive revolutions within the community that currently adheres most closely to the medical model.[4]

---

[4]An anthropological analysis of conflict within contemporary psychiatry is provided by Luhrmann (2000). Although her analysis does identify conflict over diagnosis as one component, it emphasizes the historical conflict between psychoanalysis and biological reductionism and gives little attention to the paradigmatic alternatives represented by biosystemic and rehabilitation paradigms. Perhaps this is to be expected of an analysis of conflicts within psychiatry, but it reflects an incomplete analysis of contemporary thought in the larger mental health and psychopathology communities.

## EMERGENCE OF THE INTEGRATED REHABILITATION PARADIGM

Today there is a growing sense in the mental health community that a new paradigm is needed to account for what is now known about the nature and origins of disabling mental illness and illness-specific (or not) response to treatment and rehabilitation. Similarly, the structures of clinical decision making (and service administration) associated with the conventional medical model are under attack by constituencies ranging from managed health care administrators and practitioners to consumer activists. These are conditions in which a paradigm shift is likely to occur. Nevertheless, it is unlikely that the medical model will be overthrown in a Kuhnian scientific revolution and replaced by a competing alternative paradigm. We will probably never see anything in mental health as dramatic as the triumph of relativity and quantum mechanics (although abandoning neo-Kraepelinian diagnosis may be fairly dramatic). Unlike Newtonian physics, the construct of the medical model is not specific enough that experiments could definitively support or contradict its theoretical premises. Indeed, this lack of scientific specificity has allowed it to remain intact despite the shift from psychoanalysis to psychopharmacology. Furthermore, existing alternative paradigms have their own limitations, in their ability to incorporate and use new findings in neurobiology and the cognitive and behavioral sciences—this in turn limits their clinical effectiveness.

Not all aspects of the medical model are incompatible with rehabilitation paradigms. Certain areas where rehabilitation paradigms conflict with standard praxis under the medical model are due to a conflict between guilds and interests within the mental health community, not between competing scientific theories. Over time, economic, political, and sociological pressures have instigated a process of gradual change within the medical model. Clinical research is slowly sorting out what is effective treatment and what is not, and basic research is producing new theories to account for treatment effects, in all their complexity. Instead of a competing alternative paradigm for rehabilitation in mental health, a new, inclusive *integrated* paradigm is evolving.

The approach described in this book can be thought of as a prototype of the integrated paradigm that is evolving today. For heuristic purposes, the approach is called the *integrated paradigm for rehabilitation of disabling mental illness*, or the integrated paradigm, for short. This new paradigm is the product of key ideas and methods from three sources, woven into a new whole: (1) the principles and values of *rehabilitation*, as applied to disabling mental illness, (2) the findings from research in *experimental psychopathology*, as it is informed by neuroscience and the cognitive and behavioral sciences, and (3) *hypothetico-deductive models of case formulation* in mental health clinical practice and service provision. These ideas are

**TABLE 1.1. Comparison of Historical Paradigms for Assessing and Treating Severe and Disabling Mental Illness**

| | Medical Model* | Therapeutic Community | Social Learning | Psychiatric Rehabilitation |
|---|---|---|---|---|
| Conceptual understanding of "mental illness" | Mental illness is a medical disease, reducible to specific but unknown biological abnormalities; all aspects of mental illness are consequences or complications of the biological abnormalities. | The most important expressions of mental illness are observable in social and interpersonal functioning; mental illness compromises the person's ability to participate in normal community life. | Mental illness impairs a person's ability to acquire and use essential skills, and to respond appropriately to the routine, environmental demands of life. | Mental illness is a disability to be overcome, not a disease to be cured; the salient expressions of the illness are those that obstruct normal functioning. |
| Purpose and goal of treatment | If the disease cannot be cured, the symptoms must be controlled as well as possible. | The purpose of treatment is to enable the person to participate meaningfully and effectively in community life. | The purpose of treatment is to enable the person to acquire skills, engage in adaptive behavior, and refrain from maladaptive behavior. | Rehabilitation is unlike treatment; the purpose is to overcome disabilities that are barriers toward realizing one's own wishes and aspirations. |
| Role of person receiving services | The patient's role is to follow the directions of the doctor (psychiatrist). | The role of people in treatment is to participate in the therapeutic community as best they can. | The role of people in treatment is to acquire skills and change their behavior. | The role of all participants is to identify goals and work toward them. |
| Methods of assessment and intervention | Psychiatric diagnosis is the key to treatment; once the disease is diagnosed, its causes and symptoms are the targets of medical treatment. | The role of assessment is to determine specific problems that prevent a person from participating in the social community; the problems are overcome by designing the social environment so as to enhance effective participation. | Assessment identifies specific skills deficits and maladaptive behaviors; skills are acquired through training and an environment designed to provide appropriate incentives and disincentives. | Assessment identifies the person's desires and aspirations and relevant barriers to achieving them; rehabilitation imparts the means to overcome the barriers. |
| Organizational principles and decision-making practices | Services are directed by the doctor (psychiatrist), who makes all key decisions about what treatment will be provided and how. | The key organizational principles are those that define the therapeutic community and its processes; key decisions are made by the community as much as possible. | Decisions are driven by functional analysis of behavior and its environmental concomitants; services are organized to enhance collection of behavioral and environmental data. | Services are organized around the rehabilitation client; decisions are driven by the client's choices. |

*Note.* The medical model, as described here, is that of biological psychiatry in the later 20th century. It shares most of its key characteristics with the psychoanalytic version that dominated psychiatry earlier in the 20th century, with the exception of the assumption that mental illness is reducible to specific but unknown biological causes.

represented to varying degrees in the conventional medical model and in the alternative paradigms that appeared in the late 20th century. Ultimately, the question of which aspects of the integrated paradigm come from the medical model and what parts come from the alternative paradigms is more an academic than a utilitarian one. Table 1.1 provides an overview of the historical paradigms influencing the field of mental health rehabilitation.

## The Principles and Values of Rehabilitation in the Integrated Paradigm

Applications of rehabilitation for disabling mental illness generally share a number of specific values and principles that contribute key precepts to the integrated paradigm:

Purposes and goals of rehabilitation:

1. The purposes of treatment and rehabilitation are ultimately determined by the needs and desires of individual recipients (clients), in all their unique complexity.
2. The recipient has a central operational role in determining how rehabilitation is to be accomplished, and toward which objectives and goals.
3. The goal of rehabilitation is *recovery*, meaning that the recipient has overcome disabilities associated with mental illness, to the maximum possible degree.
4. Outcome is judged on the balance of goal attainment as identified by the recipient, symptom control, neutralization of disability, degree of independent and autonomous functioning, subjective sense of well-being, and objective quality of life.

Mental illness:

5. When an illness cannot be "cured" (which is the case for most severe and disabling psychiatric conditions), the goal of treatment is to neutralize disability and maximize independent functioning.
6. When disability cannot be neutralized, various forms of prosthesis (artificial physical, psychological, or environmental supports such as artificial limbs, eyeglasses [physical prostheses]; date books [a memory prosthesis]; self-affirmation or religious calendars and notepads [emotional prostheses]; wheelchair ramps [physical environmental prostheses]; support groups [social environmental prostheses]) are used.

Clinical assessment:

7. Clinical assessment includes articulation of the functional nature of the disabilities and how the disabilities interact with other characteristics of the person and his or her environment.

Clinical processes:

8. Treatment is planned, implemented, coordinated, and evaluated by an interdisciplinary team.
9. The recipient is a participating member of the treatment team, to the degree allowed by functional capacity and legal status.
10. Family members are included as much as possible in relation to rehabilitation goals.
11. Treatment addresses as many of the expressions, diatheses (vulnerabilities), and disabilities of the illness as possible.
12. Treatment of each expression, diathesis, or disability proceeds as an iterative hypothetico-deductive trial-and-test process, until success occurs or treatment options are exhausted.

Context of service provision:

13. Successful rehabilitation requires coordination of a multiplicity of services, which requires, in turn, careful attention to basic management principles for effective and cost-efficient service provision.

The following chapters illustrate how these principles provide a coherent set of standards and guidelines for enacting a comprehensive program of rehabilitation for people with disabling mental illness.

## Psychopathology in the Integrated Paradigm

The second key contributor to the integrated paradigm is experimental psychopathology, a group of different but overlapping scientific disciplines that address biological, psychological, and sociological processes that produce or influence abnormal behavior. The principles of experimental psychopathology most pertinent to the integrated paradigm include:

1. People can be usefully understood as complex self-regulating biological systems, operating in specific physical and social environments.

2. Disabling mental illness can be usefully understood as the result of failures in biobehavioral regulation, interacting with environmental failures to compensate for the dysregulation or otherwise neutralize its effects on the person's functioning.

3. The "causes" of system failure are seldom simple, linear, or unidirectional; rather, reciprocal influences and feedback loops are ubiquitous.

4. Treatment has suboptimal effectiveness when it presumes linear causes and seeks to disrupt falsely assumed linear cascades of system failure, because problems tend to be pervasive, functionally autonomous, to varying degrees, and influenced by multiple contributing factors.

5. Optimal treatment effects can be expected when treatment addresses multiple contributors to system failure, both inside and outside the person.

6. The methods, principles, and findings of research in psychopathology provide important clues to the precise nature of system failures involving individuals; these clues can be pursued, through systematic observation and treatment, toward the goal of gaining a comprehensive, scientifically credible and utilitarian understanding of a person's strengths and disabilities.

The following chapters illustrate how these principles provide crucial conceptual links between clinical assessment, selection of treatment, and evaluation of progress.

## Hypothetico-Deductive Models in the Integrated Paradigm

The third key contributor to the integrated paradigm, hypothetico-deductive models of clinical practice in mental health, conceptualizes clinical practice as a "trial-and-test" process, wherein "diagnoses" are experimental hypotheses, informed by scientific principles and findings, and treatment is a controlled experiment designed to test the hypotheses. Hypothetico-deductive models of clinical practice evolved over the second half of the 20th century. Historical origins are debatable, but the clearest line of development begins in the 1950s with the early applications of the experimental methods of behavioral science to clinical behavior problems (see Ullman & Krasner, 1965, pp. 20–59). Evolution proceeded through the "cognitive revolution" in psychology, the formulation of social learning theory, and the maturation of cognitive-behavioral therapy. Two major clinical assessment paradigms, *functional assessment* and *functional analysis of behavior*, are central to the models' evolution. These are discussed in detail in later chapters of this book.

Experimental design methodology also inspired the formulation of this approach. Given the early realization that pristine experimental designs are usually impractical in clinical situations, the concept of clinical intervention as a completely controlled experiment remained a theoretical ideal. However, the 1950s and 1960s saw a proliferation of less than ideal but still scientifically credible methods, collectively known as *quasi-experimental designs*. As the name implies, these designs have some of the features that characterize true experimental designs but not so many that they are clinically impractical. There is an inherent trade-off between the practicality of a quasi-experimental design and the certainty with which one can interpret its data. Well-designed and implemented quasi-experiments can significantly reduce uncertainty about the effectiveness of a clinical intervention, short of the standards of theoretical science, but sufficient to draw rational, if tentative, conclusions about individual cases (for a comprehensive treatment of this subject, see Kazdin, 1980).

For the purposes of rehabilitation, the most important concept from quasi-experimental design procedures is that of *multiple baselines*. In a multiple baseline design, several independent measurements are made repeatedly while interventions are performed at specific points in time. By observing which measures change and which do not, tentative but informative inferences can be made about which interventions produce which changes. Confidence in the results is bolstered when the experimenters formulate specific and accurate predictions about what changes will occur when, based on their preliminary hypotheses about factors controlling behavioral functioning in a particular case. Thus quasi-experimental designs, in general, and multiple baseline designs, in particular, are well suited to a hypothetico-deductive approach to clinical practice.

In the 1980s and 1990s hypothetico-deductive models and quasi-experimental designs were incorporated into integrated the *case formulation* approaches to clinical practice (e.g., Eells, 1997; Gambrill, 1990). The case formulation approach enjoys substantial scientific credibility in the mental health community, and it has proved capable of accommodating new clinical technologies as they evolve (e.g., clinical neuropsychology and cognitive-behavioral therapy). Furthermore, the case formulation approach is especially well suited to the current level of technological development in mental health treatment. There are many treatment modalities that have statistically established efficacy in large recipient populations, but less is known about which members of a population will optimally respond to which treatment. The case formulation approach is essentially a systematic way of finding which treatment is optimal for a particular recipient.

Starting in the 1960s, a similar model of clinical practice evolved, somewhat parallel to the evolution of hypothetico-deductive models. It was, in part, a response to the need for practical clinical problem solving and documentation of clinical activities. In hospital settings, it became known as *problem-oriented medical information systems*, or PROMIS (Phillips, 1972). With the rise of nationally organized health care accreditation, the principles and conventions of PROMIS were integrated into standards of practice. In the medical world, they appear as standards of hospital accreditation promulgated by the Joint Commission on Accreditation of Healthcare Organizations (JCAHO; Cesare-Murphy, McMahill, & Schyve, 1997; Fauman, 1990). In the rehabilitation world, similar principles and conventions appear in the standards of the Commission on Accreditation of Rehabilitation Facilities (CARF; Mazmanian, Kreutzer, Devany, & Martin, 1994; Wilkerson, Migas, & Slaven, 2000). Today most organizations that provide services to people with disabling mental illness are accredited by JCAHO or CARF, or both.

The following chapters illustrate how a hypothetico-deductive approach organizes the processes of assessment, treatment planning, and progress evaluation in a way that permits optimal use of theory and scientific findings, while maximizing the ability to tailor the rehabilitation enterprise to individual recipients.

Taken together, the key ideas from the arenas of rehabilitation, psychopathology research, and hypothetico-deductive case formulation form the premises that give conceptual coherence to rehabilitation as it is applied to people with disabling mental illness. The next step in construction of the integrated paradigm is to develop a working understanding of disabling mental illness that is consistent with the paradigm's premises. That is the role of psychopathology research, and the topic of the next chapter.

# Chapter 2

# The Psychopathology of
# Severe Mental Illness

Rehabilitation is, among other things, a technological enterprise. *Technology*, in this context, refers to the systematic manipulation of natural states and processes for a specific purpose. Effective technology requires a reliable scientific understanding of those states and processes, which, in turn, gives conceptual coherence regarding choice of treatment and other decisions made in the course of rehabilitation. A scientific understanding of mental illness is provided by psychopathology research. This chapter shows how a psychopathological perspective on disabling mental illness gives conceptual coherence to rehabilitation, and guides the application of its technologies.

## EVOLUTION OF THE PSYCHOPATHOLOGY PARADIGM

Psychopathology is defined as the study of the causes, conditions, and processes of mental illnesses. This definition is problematic, however, to the degree that it depends on the meaning of "mental illness"—which currently carries conceptual, emotional, and political baggage that has been accumulating for two centuries. (For historical accounts of the paradigms of mental illness and psychopathology, see Bynum et al., 1988; Grob, 1983; Willerman & Cohen, 1990). Unfortunately, this baggage creates misconceptions and ineffective practices among scientists, clinicians, service recipients, advocates, and mental health administrators. Optimal application of what is learned through psychopathology in rehabilitation contexts requires that at least some of the old baggage be jettisoned and replaced by modern concepts and principles.

When the term *psychopathology* appeared in the first quarter of the 20th century, it was associated with psychoanalysis. The term's subsequent importance derived, in part, from the differences it connoted between psychoanalysis and the psychiatric paradigm associated with Kraepelin. In the psychoanalytic view, or, more broadly, in *psychodynamic* views, the conditions commonly known as mental illnesses are states of distress that result from complex interactions between person and environment over the course of decades of individual development. Psychodynamic taxonomy is a taxonomy of hypothetical psychological processes and functions—for example, the id, ego, and superego, defense mechanisms, repression, sublimation, and so on—with emphasis on those whose maldevelopment is related to clinical problems. Although these processes are biological, to the degree that they reflect biological activity and are a product of human evolution, their maturation toward effective adult functioning is shaped primarily by environment and experience. Clinical signs and symptoms are symbolic expressions of the process dysfunctions associated with mental illness. Treatment is a process of enhancing or restarting developmental processes so that effective adult psychological functioning becomes possible.

As discussed in Chapter 1, a core characteristic of Kraepelinian psychiatry is its emphasis on categorization through diagnosis; its taxonomy is one of diseases or disease-like conditions. This focus was inspired by a century of discovery and revolution in medicine, wherein scientific understanding of such historic human maladies as cholera and typhoid fever was associated with the systematic clinical description and categorization of the signs and symptom patterns of those diseases. It was generally expected that application of descriptive–categorical methods to the identified symptoms of mental illness would yield comparable insights.[1] Around the turn of the century, discovery of the disease processes of *general paresis* (psychiatric illness consequent to the tertiary stage of syphilis) and *pellegra* (psychiatric illness consequent to a nutritional deficiency) enhanced confidence that comparable biological processes—ones causing other Kraepelinian "diseases" such as schizophrenia—would soon be discovered.

By the 1920s the mental health community had become somewhat polarized on these issues, especially the nature–nurture question: how important were environmental and experiential factors versus heredity and disease-like biological processes (e.g., metabolism and infection of the brain). Although psychodynamic theories are very different from those of scientific psychology, the terms *psychological* and *psychosocial* came to connote the psychodynamic pole, in contrast to the implicitly biological Kraepelinian pole. Psychodynamic or psychological views of mental illness tended to re-

---

[1]Strictly speaking, a *sign* is an objectively observable abnormality, whereas a *symptom* is a subjective complaint by the patient. Psychiatric diagnosis incorporates both signs (e.g., . bizarre motor acts) and symptoms (e.g., reports of depressed mood), but in common parlance "symptoms" covers both categories.

ject the importance of heredity or disease-like biological processes. In this atmosphere, the rubric of *psychopathology* was given to the corpus of psychodynamic theories, in contrast to the disease-oriented Kraepelinian paradigm. Use of the term *psychopathology* became associated with the psychological side of a feud between "psychological" and "biological" views of mental illness.

A caveat: The term *Kraepelinian* is used for convenience. It does not necessarily refer to views held by Kraepelin himself. Kraepelin is generally regarded as a brilliant scientist and clinician, whose ideas had a pervasive and enduring influence on the fields of mental health and psychopathology, the most important being his categorical nosology. All the details of what he actually believed would certainly be voluminous. Scholars (e.g., Green, 1998) have recently pointed out that Kraepelin had prescient ideas about the role of neurocognition, but, in contrast to the nosology, it was to be 100 years before this insight was explored in the experimental research. Admittedly, the association between diagnosis and biological etiology was less important to Kraepelin than to some of his successors. The term *Kraepelinian* is used here to refer to the theoretical association between diagnostic categories and biological etiology, as it played out over the 20th century. Later in this book, the term *neo-Kraepelinian* is used to refer to particular developments in the late 20th century.

Neither psychoanalysis nor Kraepelinian psychiatry was successful at demonstrating the scientific validity of its respective assumptions. Indeed, psychoanalysis eschewed the methods of experimental science, rendering experimental verification of theories unimportant to its proponents. Biological research has illuminated some of the processes that may contribute to mental illness, but that research is not supportive of the Kraepelinian assumption that diagnostic categories reflect unitary disease processes. The Kraepelinians were probably right in assuming that mental illness can be influenced or even produced by biological processes, but the psychoanalysts were probably right in assuming that mental illness reflects complex combinations of biological and psychological factors and does not fall into neat categories defined by specific signs and symptoms.

## Hybridization of Psychoanalysis and Kraepelinian Psychiatry

Despite their logical incompatibilities, the two psychiatric paradigms of the late 19th and early 20th century hybridized within the medical model. The psychiatric community adopted Kraepelin's approach to classification and the assumption of its primacy in theory and clinical practice. However, the classification system in general use by mid-20th century included diagnostic categories based on psychodynamic concepts and principles, in addition to

Kraepelin's original categories. Psychodynamic explanations of mental illness predominated, and *psychopathology* was the discipline that generated these explanations. Psychodynamic psychotherapy was the most common form of treatment. Nevertheless, the "mental illnesses" being addressed by psychopathology and treated by psychodynamic therapists were, to a significant degree, Kraepelinian diagnostic categories.

By the middle of the 20th century, experimental psychologists had begun to study mental illness, bringing a perspective that contrasted with both the Kreapelinian and the psychodynamic views. Unlike psychoanalysis, experimental psychology adhered rigorously to the empirical scientific premise that the most reliable route to "truth" is through a process of testing specific hypotheses under carefully controlled conditions. Unlike Kraepelinian psychiatrists, experimental psychologists were distrustful of categorical schemes for understanding behavior. Because psychology had gone through a period of unproductive theorizing about "types" of people and personalities earlier in the century, the psychodynamic emphasis on understanding psychological *processes* had more appeal than the Kraepelinian emphasis on *types* of persons or diseases.

Psychology had also gone through a *behaviorist* revolution, which included rejecting biological explanations of behavior. In the middle of the 20th century, behaviorism and psychoanalysis represented opposite poles of belief in the mental health community, mostly because of their different positions regarding scientific method, but, ironically, they agreed on the irrelevance of biology for a complete understanding of human behavior. Psychoanalysis was the predominant paradigm of psychiatry, and behaviorism was the predominant paradigm of the academic psychology community, where many of the challenges to the legitimacy of psychoanalytic psychiatry and the medical model originated. This common position on the irrelevance of biology was later rejected within the medical model community, and elsewhere, as too radical and as perpetuating a silly debate (comparable to the debate between the psychoanalysts and the Kraepelinians) about whether nature or nurture is the determinant of human behavior. (For a historical account and analysis of this debate in psychology, see Baars, 1986.) At the same time, the psychological community was optimistic that an extensive scientific understanding of behavior could be achieved without a complete account of its biological underpinnings. This optimism was born of necessity, for at that time, technology for observing or measuring biological processes relevant to behavior was extremely limited. On the other hand, progress in biology had shown that much could be learned at that level of analysis without a full understanding of its "most molecular" underpinnings (e.g., quantum physics). Accordingly, there was confidence that scientific psychology could proceed without a complete biology. Psychological research focused on observable behavior and its environmental determinants, with the understanding that research on biological factors was not being rejected, just postponed. In fact, it was expected that better technology for measuring behavior and psychological processes would eventually complement research on the biology of that behavior.

Psychoanalysis had generated many ideas about mental illness which, with some revision, could be translated into testable experimental hypotheses. In addition, the burgeoning experimental research on perception, memory, learning, psychophysiology, and motivation was a rich source of entirely new hypotheses. Thus did *experimental psychopathology* evolve into a systematic means of studying mental illness. Experimental psychopathologists tended to make no assumptions about whether the "causes" of mental illness are essentially biological or psychological. The expectation was that biological, psychological, and environmental factors would sort themselves out as research progressed. (For a textbook account of experimental psychopathology at mid-20th century, see Maher, 1966.)

In the second half of the 20th century, the biological, psychological, and environmental factors in mental illness did indeed begin to sort themselves out. As discussed in Chapter 1, the 1950s saw convincing demonstrations that mental illness is shaped by social and environmental factors. The 1960s saw the widespread use of psychotropic drugs, demonstrating the importance of understanding behavior at its biological levels. Research on the genetics of mental illness over 5 decades supported both biological and psychological views. The evidence for genetic contributions became overwhelming, but it also became clear that genetic factors interact with other variables over the course of a person's development to produce the actual illness. Longitudinal studies of *vulnerability* to mental illness began to trace the contributing nature–nurture interactions as well as the impact of individuals' lifelong styles of coping. Research on the effects of stress on brain development established a measurable link between biological and environmental agents. Experimental research on learning, memory, and other basic psychological processes produced much data on the roles of these processes in mental illness. (For a representative collection of articles on later-20th century experimental psychopathology applied to severe mental illness, including biological, psychological, and social levels of analysis, see Spaulding & Cole, 1984.)

Meanwhile, psychology went through yet another revolution, this time rejecting the remaining influence of radical behaviorism in favor of the *cognitive* paradigm (Baars, 1986; Gardner, 1987). Cognitive psychology provided a vast new array of possibilities for understanding mental illness. As noted in Chapter 1, learning theory gave rise to *social* learning theory, bringing together behavioral and cognitive principles in a powerful technology for assessing and changing behavior. (For a collection of representative articles on cognitive paradigms at the end of the 20th century, see

Spaulding, 1994.) The new discipline of neuropsychology, initially a clinical application of cognitive psychology, became a bridge between the behavioral and biological sciences. Cognitive science and cognitive neuroscience became areas of intense interdisciplinary research. Psychopathology absorbed these developments, retained its more traditionally psychological paradigms, expanded, merged on some fronts with other disciplines such as neuropharmacology and neurophysiology, and became a large, diverse scientific community.

Today it is clear that biology and psychology occupy neighboring points on a continuum of levels at which life can be studied scientifically. We have psychological measures that inform us about biological states, and biological measures that inform us about psychological states. We can manipulate psychological states with biological means, and we can manipulate biological states with psychological means. Psychopathology incorporates methods and principles from a range of disciplines and levels of analysis, from molecular genetics to social psychology. The old debate about whether biological or psychological factors "cause" mental illness is now as antiquated and irrelevant as the nature–nurture controversy.

## EMERGENCE OF THE CONTEMPORARY PARADIGM OF PSYCHOPATHOLOGY

The growth and diversification of psychopathology was accompanied by a need for overarching, unifying conceptual schemes—or *paradigms*—to articulate the relationships between its various biological, psychological, and sociological components. Around mid-century *general systems theory* was introduced to the mental health community (von Bertalanffy, 1965, 1966). Originally developed as an approach to understanding complex biological processes, general systems theory was better suited than psychoanalysis to the task of integrating biological, psychological, and sociological perspectives. In the context of psychopathology, general systems theory conceptualizes people as complex self-regulating biological systems, or *biosystems*. Mental illness became understood as the result of complex, often idiosyncratic, failures in systemic regulation, potentially involving biological, psychological, and socioenvironmental components. The diverse developments across the various biological and behavioral sciences in the second half of the century made the biosystemic view appealing as a unifying and integrating concept (see, e.g., Buckley, 1967). Complementary developments in computer science, cybernetics, cognitive and social psychology, sociology, and the neurosciences helped general systems theory evolve into a broader biosystemic paradigm for both theory and clinical practice (see, e.g., Andreae, 1996; Masterpasqua & Perna, 1997; Sameroff, 1995).

Psychopathologists have been constructing theoretical models of disabling mental illness using biosystemic principles at least since the 1970s. Probably the most complete example is a complex model of schizophrenia devised by Nuechterlein and colleagues (Green & Nuechterlein, 1999; Nuechterlein et al., 1992). Although subject to the problems associated with schizophrenia as a neo-Kraepelinian diagnostic category, the model successfully demonstrates how a multiplicity of biological and social factors interrelate to produce the various expressions of mental illness. Equally important, the model is constructed from rigorously collected experimental data, showing that it is feasible to evaluate empirically even complex etiological hypotheses about mental illness.

As psychopathology was incorporating strains from the biological and behavioral sciences and unifying into a biosystems theory, the Kraepelinian paradigm was following its own course of development. Its marriage to the psychodynamic paradigm ended in the 1970s with the rise of the *neo-Kraepelinians*, a community of academic psychiatrists who advocated reform of the diagnostic system. The DSM-III, published in 1980, reflected these reforms. (For a detailed account of the development of the DSM-III and its successors, see Kirk & Kutchins, 1993.) Diagnostic categories based on psychodynamic theory were eliminated or replaced with categories defined purely by behavioral characteristics (i.e., symptoms). In fact, the neo-Kraepelinians sought to remove *all* theoretical implications from the diagnostic system, thus obviating the old issue of whether the origins of mental illness are biological or psychological. Nevertheless, like Kraepelin himself, the neo-Kraepelinians showed a distinct preference for implicitly biological, disease-like accounts of mental illness. They were closely associated with *biological psychiatrists*, an enclave within psychiatry that advocated understanding and treating mental illnesses as essentially biological conditions. They expected that the greater reliability of the new diagnostic system, which was a product of objective behavioral criteria, would hasten discovery of the biological processes that "cause" the diseases being diagnosed. (For a detailed historical account and analysis of the neo-Kraepelinian movement, see Kutchins & Kirk, 1997.) Table 2.1 summarizes the "neo-Kraepelinian credo."

Biological psychiatry was not the only scientific community to put so much faith in Kraepelinian diagnosis. In the late 20th century cognitive-behavioral accounts of anxiety disorders, depression, and other clinical problems adhered to Kraepelinian principles and produced effective new assessment and treatment technology. However, as of this writing, the importance of Kraepelinian distinctions is a subject of serious reconsideration. Despite substantial methodological attention to diagnosis, neither causal processes nor effective treatment seem to respect diagnostic distinctions. Interestingly, the failure of psychosocial treatments (such as cognitive-

TABLE 2.1. The Neo-Kraepelinian Credo

1. Psychiatry is a branch of medicine.
2. Psychiatry should utilize modern scientific methodologies and base its practice on scientific knowledge.
3. Psychiatry treats people who are sick and who require treatment for mental illness.
4. There is a boundary between the normal and the sick.
5. There are discrete mental illnesses. Mental illnesses are not myths. There is not one but many mental illnesses. It is the task of scientific psychiatry, as of other medical specialties, to investigate the causes, diagnosis and treatment of these mental illnesses.
6. The focus of psychiatric physicians should be particularly in the biological aspects of mental illness.
7. There should be an explicit and intentional concern with diagnosis and classification.
8. Diagnostic criteria should be codified, and a legitimate and valued area of research should be to validate such criteria by various techniques. Further, departments of psychiatry in medical schools should teach these criteria and not deprecate them, as has been the case for many years.
9. In research efforts directed at improving the reliability and validity of diagnosis and classification, statistical techniques should be utilized.

Note. From Klerman (1978, pp. 104–105). Copyright 1978 by Harvard University Press. Reprinted by permission.

behavioral therapy) to show diagnosis-specific effects disappointed the neo-Kraepelinians in the psychology community much as the failure of drug treatments to show diagnosis-specific effects disappointed the neo-Kraepelinian biological psychiatrists.

Kraepelinian diagnostic categories were never particularly helpful to experimental psychopathologists. Early on, it was noted that when diagnosis is used as an independent variable in experimental designs, groupings of subjects show significant within-group variability, compared to between-group variability, suggesting that there are differences between individuals within the group that are at least as important as differences between the groups.[2] Some individuals were clearly more impaired than others in basic psychological functions, but impairments did not appear exclusively within any particular group. In the language of experimental psychology, Kraepelinian diagnosis did not achieve *construct validity*. That is, diagnostic categories are not systematically related to other variables of interest to

[2]In scientific terminology an *independent variable* is one that is taken as a "given" (e.g., a natural grouping) or manipulated by the experimenter (e.g., treatment vs. no treatment), to distinguish different conditions or groups. In the present context, psychiatric diagnosis is the independent variable in experiments where groups with different diagnoses are compared on some other set of measures.

researchers—for example, cognitive impairments, developmental characteristics, and clinical course. Researchers experimented with alternative kinds of independent variables in the hopes of finding more interpretable results; this experimentation eventually led to the sophisticated developmental neurocognitive models that dominate psychopathology research today.

A good example of alternative independent variables from the mid-20th century research was the *process–reactive dimension* identified in schizophrenia studies (Cromwell, 1975). Inspired by a psychodynamic perspective, the process–reactive dimension was originally thought to represent a categorical distinction between two "types" of schizophrenia. Later, it was understood to be a continuous dimension, reflecting the overall severity of developmental compromise. The process pole of the dimension was associated with earlier age of onset, poorer premorbid social functioning, more hereditary involvement, a less differentiated symptom pattern, more cognitive impairment, more baseline deficits in personal and social functioning, poorer response to treatment, and a more malignant course. The relationships among these various characteristics were consistently stronger than with Kraepelinian categories or the symptom criteria that defined them.

Ironically, criticisms of the neo-Kraepelinian diagnostic system have more recently come from within the biologically-oriented part of the psychopathology community (as well as other quarters). There is growing concern about whether a diagnostic system can or should be "atheoretical." Although biological research has identified many mechanisms of potential relevance to mental illness, they are not closely related to diagnosis, and it is unclear that diagnosis plays a helpful role in organizing or directing the research. If research *assumes* that diagnoses represent meaningful categories of disease, then research cannot *test the hypothesis* that the categories are meaningful. The importance of newly discovered neurophysiological and neuropsychological processes is not their association with DSM categories but with specific impairments in personal and social functioning. Although the DSM will probably remain the accepted standard for categorizing mental illness in the immediate future, it is unclear whether it or the Kraepelinian paradigm will have much impact on the future of psychopathology.

Nevertheless, the neo-Kraepelinian reform was an influential movement within the powerful medical model-based mental health industry, and its influence pervaded the scientific community as well. As a result, most of the research in psychopathology is organized within a diagnostic frame of reference. For example, "schizophrenia research" is an identifiable area of scientific endeavor, ostensibly distinct from "bipolar disorder research" or "psychosis not otherwise specified" research. Neo-Kraepelinian concepts do not prevent valid research, but they do make it less efficient. For example, one can draw valid conclusions about the particular nature of neuro-physiological or cognitive processes "in people with schizophrenia," but the arbitrary nature of the schizophrenia diagnosis prevents valid conclusions about what such processes have to do with "schizophrenia," or whether they are unique to "schizophrenia." As a result, the psychopathology literature yields much value in understanding disabling mental illnesses, including those labeled "schizophrenia," but much caution is required in interpreting results that purport to be specific to or even relevant to neo-Kraepelinian diagnosis. The discussion in this book draws heavily on psychopathology, but aspires to great caution in making unwarranted assumptions about diagnosis. Unfortunately, this is still a departure from convention, even as concern about the neo-Kraepelinian model mounts in all quarters of the psychopathology community.

The prospects for psychodynamic paradigms playing a predominant integrating role in psychopathology ended in the 1970s. The prospects for the Kraepelinian diagnostic paradigm filling that role appear to be ending "as we speak." Biosystems theory has been evolving toward that role for 50 years, and it is emerging as the best candidate for helping us achieve a unified understanding of mental illness, in all its biological, psychological, and sociological complexity. The remainder of this chapter discusses biosystemic psychopathology as it is applied to the rehabilitation of people with disabling mental illness. This is a paradigm within the broader integrated paradigm that provides scientific coherence to the rehabilitation enterprise.

## A BIOSYSTEMIC PARADIGM FOR PSYCHOPATHOLOGY

A useful contemporary psychopathology of disabling mental illness begins with an understanding of people as complex self-regulating biological systems, or *biosystems*. We (and other biological organisms) are "systems" in the sense that we consist of many distinct processes and mechanisms that perform functions that are different yet highly interrelated, unified by the common purpose of maintaining biological and behavioral functioning. "People-systems" are self-regulating in the sense that their various processes and mechanisms control each other so as to maintain functional stability or *homeostasis*. Homeostasis is a familiar term in biology, where it usually connotes physiological equilibrium—for example, a balance between anabolism and catabolism, energy consumption and expenditure, maintenance of optimal blood acidity and body temperature, etc. Less familiar, but equally important, are regulation and equilibrium at the molar level of behavior—for example, balancing energetic activity against resting, aggression against accommodation, pursuit of individual needs against respect for social conventions, work against leisure, avoidance against confrontation, social activities against solitary activities, etc.

It is increasingly evident that self-regulation occurs in the domain of cognition as well. Focused attention is balanced against diffuse attention, conventional thought against creative thought, problem solving against role performance. In the course of adapting to complex, changing environments, an individual's various biosystemic components and mechanisms continually interact, adjust, and regulate each other—like a thermostat and a furnace interact to maintain a house's temperature—but many times more complex.

A caveat: Ultimately, it is arbitrary to distinguish "person-systems" from the socioenvironmental systems in which they function. It would be more strictly correct to speak of "person–environment systems." However, the individual has a special status in rehabilitation that must be protected against dehumanizing tendencies that pervade the mental health industry. De-emphasizing the integrity of the individual carries a risk. There is no conceptual compromise for rehabilitation in regarding the person as a system, as long as socioenvironmental factors are systematically analyzed, understood and manipulated (when needed) in pursuit of rehabilitation goals.

## The Organizational Dimensions of Biobehavioral Functioning

Biosystems have two key structural dimensions: level of organization and component organization.

*Level of organization* refers to the complexity level of biobehavioral activity, ranging from the most elemental to the most complex. The most elemental level of biosystemic organization pertinent to psychopathology is the neurophysiological level. In the nervous system and elsewhere, biochemical processes operate to maintain the optimal medium for processing information necessary to monitor the environment (through sensation and perception), recognize objects and situations (learning and memory), and select and execute behavioral responses (executive functioning). The most complex level of organization in humans is society and culture. Our behavior is constrained and guided by traditions, customs, and laws as much as by our biological substrate. A complete understanding of human nature must incorporate both of these levels of organization as well as the many intervening levels of intermediate complexity.

Throughout the following discussion, the terms *molecular* and *molar* are used to denote the poles of this dimension. These terms are derived from distinctions that appeared in experimental psychology beginning in the early 20th century. In our context, *molecular* refers to a relatively elemental or "micro" level of organization, and *molar* to a relatively more complex level. Hence, for example, memory processes are more molar than the neurophysiological processes that support memory, and more molecular than the higher cognitive functions that manipulate information stored in memory.

Science has developed a range of methods to study specific processes at these various levels. The disciplines of physiology, psychology, and sociology roughly reflect these gross levels; in addition, there are many subdisciplines, corresponding to more specific *levels of analysis*, within those larger levels. For heuristic purposes, in the integrated paradigm the psychopathology of disabling mental illness can be understood to span five levels of analysis, or levels of biosystemic functioning: neurophysiological, neurocognitive, sociocognitive, sociobehavioral and socioenvironmental.

Although heuristically useful, such categories are ultimately arbitrary, as their boundaries are not distinct. More importantly, each level is associated with particular research methods and findings. Each level can be addressed in terms of processes within an organism, plus external or environmental processes with which organismic processes interact. Future scientific developments will require continuous revision of specific aspects of the various levels, but for the foreseeable future such multilevel heuristics provide a reasonable approximation of the organizational levels of human biobehavioral functioning, at least for the purposes of psychopathology and rehabilitation. Accordingly, these five levels provide the rubrics for the various chapters on rehabilitation technologies that follow.

The term *component organization* refers to the way biosystems are organized across multiple levels of complexity to accomplish specifiable functions or tasks. Human behavior involves processes at all levels of organization, from neurophysiological to socioenvironmental, working in concert. Many, though not all, of these functions can be understood as accomplished by *modules*: assemblies of processes linked together by a common function (Fodor, 1983, 2000). In some views, modules are the result of evolution (Barkow, Cosmides, & Tooby, 1992). Modular organization and evolutionary development are promising ideas in psychopathology, although the integrated paradigm does not necessarily include the premise that mental illness reflects the failure of evolved biobehavioral modules. (For a recent discussion of the relevance of modular organization and evolution to severe mental illness, see Penn, Corrigan, Bentall, & Racenstein, 1997.) It is sufficient to identify specific, functionally significant processes involved in mental illness, without resolving whether they constitute "modules."

The impairments of mental illness can be identified and studied with reference to the failure of specific modules or other component processes, and to abnormalities at specific levels of organization. Such impairments are rarely isolated, however, and usually contribute to problems in other modules, or in processes at other levels of organization, that are otherwise operating normally. In addition, external or environmental factors may interact with the impairments. A complete understanding of the specific conditions that "cause" mental illness requires a comprehensive account of all of these impairments, abnormalities, and environmental influences. Achieving such a thorough account is a particular challenge for the psychopathology of severe, disabling mental illness, because impairments tend to be *pervasively distributed* across functional modules and across levels of systemic organization. That is, abnormality or impairment of some kind can be found practically wherever one looks in the biosystems of people with severe mental illness.

The biological and behavioral sciences have evolved subdisciplines that combine specific levels of analysis for specific purposes, and these subdisciplines are important features in the psychopathology landscape. They do not compete with a biosystemic paradigm but highlight areas of emphasis or focus within that broader paradigm. Examples of subdisciplines that represent a span of specific levels of analysis are psychophysics, psychopharmacology, psychophysiology, neuropsychology, and social psychology. *Psychophysics* relates the physical dimensions of environmental stimuli (a very molecular level of analysis, such as examining the amplitude and frequency of light and sound waves) to the perceptual and cognitive experience of those stimuli (a more molar level of analysis). Experiments in psychophysics have been helpful to psychopathology research primarily by providing laboratory measures that reflect neurophysiological or other abnormalities (e.g., abnormal amplification or attenuation of sensory input). *Psychopharmacology* relates activity at the subcellular level (e.g., interactions between biochemicals and structural features of neurons) to the consequences of that activity in sensation, perception, emotion, and higher cognitive functions. Studies in this area have had a pervasive impact on psychopathology. *Psychophysiology* relates relatively molecular physiological processes, such as autonomic arousal, to environmental events and to higher cognitive processes (e.g., achieving a level of arousal appropriate to a particular problem or situation). Psychophysiology has increased our understanding of failures in autonomic regulation and its relationships to cognitive and behavioral functioning. *Neuropsychology* relates the activity of anatomical regions and neurophysiological mechanisms of the brain to more molar behavioral abilities, including sensation, perception, learning, and higher-level cognition. The last 10 years have seen an explosion of neuropsychological research in psychopathology. This research has revealed much about the central role of impaired cognition in mental illness and has generated important clues about the brain abnormalities associated with these impairments. *Social psychology* relates molar-level cognitive processes to even more molar social behavior and the social environment. This research shows how complex social behavior is supported by specific cognitive processes and provides clues about how cognitive impairments lead to problems in social functioning. Experimental models from this subdiscipline provide clues about how people manage or fail to manage vulnerabilites and failures in their biosystems, and how social factors may impinge on those vulnerabilities and failures.

These subdisciplines provide important insights into the roles of specific functional components that are embedded in the complete biosystem, at various levels of its organization. Failures in the operation or regulation of these system components can be exacerbating factors in disabling mental illness. Furthermore, a broad, integrated consideration of such components amplifies our understanding of how biosystems fail. Together, these insights lead not only to better scientific understanding but also to more effective clinical technology and greater success for those recovering from disabling mental illness.

## Causal Relationships in the Biosystems Paradigm

Much of the old baggage in theories of mental illness contain outmoded hypotheses or, worse, assumptions about the "cause" of illness. The biosystems paradigm includes unconventional concepts of cause that avoid the old conundrums and provide a more useful way of conceptualizing how mental illness occurs.

In Western thought there is a pervasive tendency to adopt a *reductionistic* view of causation in biobehavioral functioning, wherein more elemental processes determine the activity of more complex ones. That is, socioenvironmental processes are seen as the direct result of sociobehavioral processes, which, in turn, are seen as the direct result of sociocognitive processes, and on down the ladder to neurophysiology (and eventually subatomic physics). Ultimately, we humans are, after all, complex "bags of chemicals." However, it is also true that human behavior is affected by innumerable factors across all levels of functioning, and more complex biosystemic processes can causally affect the activity of more elemental processes. The biosystemic view asserts that causation can occur in all directions, between processes at any and all levels of organization. Any causal principle is valid only to the degree that it is restricted to particular processes in a multicausal system.

This development in Western scientific thinking brings it into greater conformity with principles of some Eastern naturalistic and philosophical traditions. A lesson from Buddhism, popularly retold by the philosopher Alan Watts, invites consideration of a person looking through a narrow slit in a fence. On the other side of the fence, a cat walks by. The viewer sees first the cat's head, then its body, then its tail. The viewer would be misled to conclude that cats' heads cause cats' tails. From a perspective different from the viewer's, it is easy to see that the "causal" relationship is restricted to a particular context, and that it depends on a much more complex set of systemic relationships, that is, the cat. A related lesson is conveyed in the familiar story, generally attributed to the Islamic Sufi tradition, of the blind scholars who, after their encounter with an elephant, debated about whether an elephant is shaped like the particular appendage that each had encountered. This allegory is especially reminiscent of historical disputes between psychoanalysts, radical behaviorists, and biological reductionists.

The biosystemic perspective suggests another important consideration regarding the so-called causes of impairments and other problems. There are two essential types of relationship that can occur between discrete problems in a system: a *cascade* and a *stable dysfunctional cycle*. In a cascade, one problem causes another in a direct and linear way, eventually producing a catastrophic outcome. In a stable dysfunctional cycle, problems interact with each other in circular and causally reciprocal ways. This interactive pattern produces general dysfunction of the system but not necessarily a catastrophe. The cascade process is ubiquitous in traditional medicine, whereas stable dysfunctional cycles predominate in modern psychopathology. In understanding the role of a particular impairment in disabling mental illness, it is important to consider whether the impairment is part of a cascade or a cycle. For example, specific symptoms of acute psychosis, such as hallucinations, may be understood as steps in a linear sequence (cascade) of events, beginning with overactive dopaminergic pathways, proceeding to compromise of specific sensory and perceptual mechanisms, and resulting in the person's anomalous perception of disembodied voices. However, the abnormal dopaminergic activity itself may be part of a cyclic process of episodic neurophysiological dysregulation, breakdown of social functioning, inability to manage stress, and inadvertent creation of an increasingly stressful environment.

A dysfunctional cycle can be quite stable, maintaining its suboptimal status, or it can take the pattern of a downward spiral. In the latter case, various components of the system gradually lose functioning, and the cumulative consequences of these failures are distributed throughout the system. As the downward spiral progresses, component failure may, at times, give rise to cascades, producing a more rapid deterioration. In the example above, the linear *cascade* producing acute symptoms occurs because the *cycle* of social impairment and high stress creates a low threshold for the neurophysiological events that start the cascade. The dysregulated cycle makes the person more vulnerable to the cascade.

Because of these complexities, use of the term *cause* can be problematic when discussing the problems of mental illness. It is usually preferable to use the term *etiology*, which does not presume simple, linear pathways of causation between expressions of illness. The term *proximal cause* is sometimes useful to refer to specific linear causal relationships, without implying that there are not other, equally important, causal relationships elsewhere in the system. These terms are used instead of *cause* throughout this book.

## AN APPLICATION OF BIOSYSTEMIC ANALYSIS

The following hypothetical case example illustrates how a biosystemic analysis that includes multiple levels of organization and functional components and uses principles of reciprocal causation is necessary to fully understand the etiology of mental illness. Many will recognize the first part of this case as a fairly typical picture of the onset of disabling mental illness, informed and embellished by current psychopathological theory and research. The second part is a hopeful and optimistic (but not unrealistic) account of rehabilitation and recovery.

> Joe's mother underwent a series of personal catastrophies when Joe was in his second trimester of gestation. The stress she was under was so extreme and prolonged that the levels of cortisol, the stress hormone, in her blood exceeded the threshold that normally insulates a fetus from its toxic effects. The cortisol elevation produced a slight disruption in Joe's fetal brain development. Expert observation of Joe's motor behavior and cognitive functioning in early childhood would have revealed subtle abnormalities, but they were not evident enough to warrant attention. Joe's development was otherwise fairly normal. He finished high school and went to college. All seemed well.
>
> In college, Joe's cognitive functioning began to deviate subtly from that of his peers'. While his friends were developing the adult levels of social judgment and problem solving that normally appear in late adolescence, Joe's functioning in these domains remained in the early adolescent phase. He began experimenting with drugs, although initially no more than most of his friends. He became socially withdrawn and his school performance deteriorated. He began experiencing auditory hallucinations and intense, unexplainable emotional arousal and anxiety. He developed a belief that classmates were persecuting him, and these beliefs became increasingly bizarre, incorporating ideas about the CIA and mind-reading machines. His family and friends became alarmed and urged him to seek treatment, but he denied that anything was wrong with him. He dropped out of school and disappeared.
>
> Many months later he surfaced in a psychiatric hospital, having been civilly committed following an altercation. His diagnosis was schizophrenia, paranoid type. He was incoherent, disheveled, belliger-

ent, and aggressive. He had been living as a street person, occasionally taking jobs but not holding them, using whatever street drugs he could obtain. While hospitalized, he agreed to take antipsychotic medication but continued to deny that he had an illness. Once stabilized on the medication, he became less incoherent and reported that his hallucinations were muted. However, conversation with him quickly revealed that he still held his bizarre beliefs. Upon discharge he resumed frequent use of street drugs, took his prescribed medications sporadically, and dropped out of outpatient treatment. He was repeatedly hospitalized over a period of 2 years. His aggressive behavior sometimes landed him in locked seclusion to prevent injury. Eventually, this pattern of recurring relapse and dangerousness lead to long-term inpatient treatment and rehabilitation.

After several months in the inpatient rehabilitation program, Joe continued to have severe difficulty, despite the program's structured milieu and assured adherence to medication and abstinence from other drugs, attending to the demands of following a daily routine, including grooming and self-care. On neuropsychological tests he performed like a person with extensive frontal head injury. He was unable to avoid or resolve interpersonal conflicts, even over the most trivial matters. Although he expressed interest in making money, he was unable to attend to work tasks, even in the hospital's sheltered workshop. Furthermore, his interpersonal conflicts with supervisors and coworkers often got him expelled from the workshop.

In the course of his treatment and rehabilitation, Joe slowly regained an ability to think and talk about himself and his life. Doing so was extremely painful for him, as he came to realize how terribly shattered his life had become. His youthful aspirations for a fulfilling life, productive work, and meaningful relationships seemed forever out of reach. His impulse to escape from this reality through drugs and psychosis seemed overwhelming. He became demoralized and depressed, as anyone would in such circumstances. At times he became suicidal.

In the midst of this turmoil, however, he began to notice small changes that he himself was making. He had begun to earn ward privileges consistently by attending to self-care and a daily routine. He found he could avoid being aggressive by using self-control techniques. He noticed that his feelings and desires were acknowledged and respected by his care providers, and he increased his participation in treatment decisions. It occurred to him that perhaps he had more control over his situation than he had previously believed. He noticed that he was increasingly able to concentrate on work tasks, evidenced by larger paychecks from the workshop. At one point he decided to try to resolve an ongoing conflict between himself and another patient, and was successful. He gradually developed the idea that he was challenged by a condition that would not go away—but one that he could manage. He began to think of himself as a student, learning the special techniques needed to overcome the disabilities that fate had inflicted upon him. He learned all he could about his condition, its unique symptoms, its episodic course, the role of stress, the medications and their effects and side effects, the nature of his neuropsychological impairment, and the importance of daily routine and supportive relationships. He began to think about his future. Instead of a cloud of chaos and painful memories, his image of the future began to take shape as a series of steps toward better health, personal effectiveness, greater freedom, and a more fulfilling life.

Joe made the crucial decisions required to construct and follow his step-by-step plan. He negotiated with his caregivers and the mental health commitment board about his living situation and his treatment. He continues to progress through the steps of his plan, taking on new challenges as his recovery allows.

The "origin" of Joe's illness in the prenatal transference of environmental stress, via neuroendocrine effects on his fetal brain, illustrates how pervasively biological and environmental factors can interact to create a vulnerability to mental illness in adulthood. The vulnerability likely arises from the abnormality in brain structure produced by toxic levels of a stress hormone, and possibly the genetics that make Joe's family vulnerable to stress and the consequent maldevelopment. However, to understand how the vulnerability leads to the illness, in this case, requires an account of how the brain's neurochemical self-regulation is compromised by the structural abnormality, how drugs may precipitate or exacerbate the self-regulation failure, and ultimately, why Joe put himself at risk by using drugs. (Obviously, drugs are not always implicated in the onset of psychosis or mental illness. The biological vulnerability may be so severe in some individuals that the normal stresses of life are sufficient to precipitate onset. However, it is also clear that drug abuse can be a factor, and in this example it serves to show how the causal relationships between neurophysiology and molar behavior [taking drugs] can be reciprocal.)

The path from high cortisol level to structural abnormality is a linear cascade, and Joe's vulnerability to psychosis is the result of that cascade. However, the episodic pattern of Joe's psychosis is part of a stable but dysfunctional cycle that includes his biological vulnerability, his psychotic episodes, his drug-taking behavior, neurocognitive functioning, social judgment, emotional functioning, and values and attitudes. Each component of the cycle influences the other components. Despite the short-term stability of the dysfunctional cycle, over time, the overall severity of dysfunction worsens in a (relatively) slow downward spiral. Even Joe's biological vulnerability to recurring psychotic episodes, a seemingly immutable condition determined by his brain anatomy, can be exacerbated by the cumulative effects of poor self-care, drug abuse, and protracted psychotic episodes. Once his threshold vulnerability is exceeded, a linear cascade—beginning with the neurophysiological dysregulation of acute psychosis—interrupts his functioning until it regains a stable, but even more dysfunctional, stasis.

Joe's descent into the lifestyle of a "chronic mental patient" exemplifies the point that in a stable but dysfunctional cycle, correcting just one component of the biosystem is usually insufficient. Antipsychotic medication and abstinence from drug abuse could control the biochemical chaos that produced the acute psychosis, but without the continuing environmental structure of the hospital, the other components quickly returned his biosystem to its stable but dysfunctional state. In contrast, some individuals with biological vulnerabilities have such strong assets in other aspects of their personal and social functioning, and such reliable social support, that intervention at the neurophysiological level is sufficient for them to regain an optimal state of biosystemic homeostasis. Similarly, some individuals may have biological vulnerabilities so slight that adjustments in behavioral functioning are sufficient to prevent psychosis without protective medications. These individuals may benefit from the approach described in this book, although they may not typically be identified as having a *disabling* mental illness. Joe's recovery required changes in multiple components of the vicious cycle that had commandeered his biosystem. A consistent therapeutic environment helped him to reorganize his thinking. Graduated progress and experiences of success helped him recover from his depressed, demoralized emotional state. Anger self-control techniques helped him eliminate a serious behavior problem. Education and self-study helped him reach an adaptive understanding of his condition, and the social support inherent in the rehabilitation enterprise helped him find reasons to struggle on for a better life. Without these additional levels of improvement, the temporary relief from neurophysiological dysregulation he experienced had too little meaning, and the modest mental clarity only brought self-confrontation with his failures and his dismal future.

## Causal Processes and Their Implications for Treatment Strategy

Joe's case—and indeed everyone's "case"—has unique characteristics. The particular components that interact in a stable but dysfunctional cycle vary considerably from one person to the next, and the broadest expanse of contemporary psychopathology, from neurophysiology to social support, is required to even begin to appreciate and understand the many processes that may be involved. Nevertheless, most cases of disabling mental illness involve some variation of a stable but dysfunctional cycle and require multiple treatment targets and rehabilitation goals. The integrated paradigm of rehabilitation formulated in this book diverges from traditional models of psychiatric treatment most fundamentally on this point. The conceptual differences are graphically represented in Figures 2.1 and 2.2.

The diagram in Figure 2.1 represents the underlying assumptions associated with a traditional medical model, which presumes that illness is caused by a linear cascade of events beginning at molecular (biological) levels and then impinging upon molar (psychological and behavioral) levels of experience. When diseases conform to this picture (and many do, especially infectious diseases), the best treatment strategy is to correct the problem at its origin. Doing so reverses the cascade and brings about desired change at the more molar levels as well. Direct treatment of the more molar expressions of the illness can only be palliative rather than curative and therefore only has value when the more molecular-level treatment is not available. The overriding strategy is to find the one treatment that resolves the most molecular-level cause of the illness.

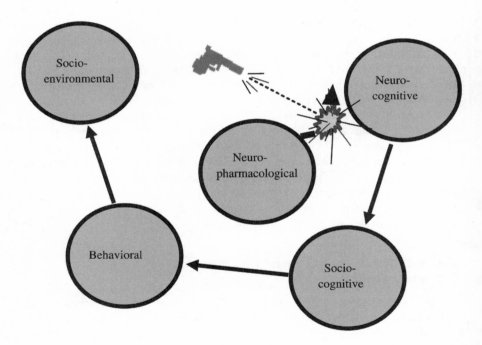

**FIGURE 2.1.** A cascade model of dysfunction and treatment. Problems originate within a single, molecular level of functioning and cascade to more molar levels. The arrows represent the direction of causal influences that produce the cascade. The ideal treatment approach is to disrupt the cascade at its most molecular level, thereby preventing the cascade. This intervention paradigm invokes the imagery of "the magic bullet," the ultimate achievement in allopathic medicine.

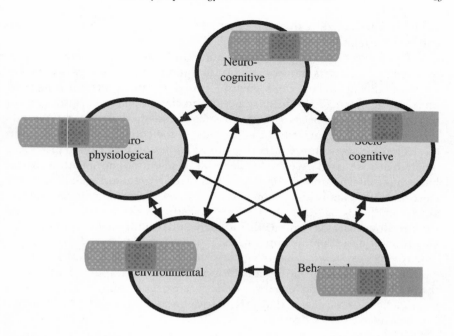

**FIGURE 2.2.** A stable dysfunctional cycle undergoing rehabilitation. Problems are the product of reciprocal causal influences among various levels of functioning. Interruption of only one level of these influences is unlikely to stabilize the others and bring about optimal functioning. The Band-Aid imagery, so often used to disparage a systemic or naturopathic approach, accurately connotes the harsh realities and challenges of severe mental illness and rehabilitation. Allopathic magic bullets are fine when they solve everything—which is the case with disabling mental illness, wherein optimal systemic functioning is usually regained through more modest effects distributed throughout the system.

The diagram in Figure 2.2 represents the characteristics of an integrated rehabilitation paradigm based on biosystemic psychopathology. The prevailing condition is not a cascade (though there may be cascades at various points in development of the illness) but a stable dysfunctional cycle, involving multiple components at multiple levels of organization interacting in a reciprocal manner. The "bad news" in this model is that there is no one original cause, no single target for treatment whose resolution will reverse the entire illness process. The "good news" is that because of the distributed pattern of reciprocal causation, any treatment benefit accruing to any component of the biosystem will be distributed throughout the system, at least to some degree. Thus the overriding treatment strategy is not to focus solely on the "original cause" but to apply as many specific treatments to as many of the systemic components as possible. Success in this model is determined by the total effect of all the individual treatments, distributed throughout the biosystem.

These two models reflect two distinct traditions in medicine. The systemic model reflects a naturopathic tradition, in which diseases are understood as imbalances between regulatory processes, and treatment is focused on restoring balance. This idea is traceable to classical Greece. Naturopathic treatment tends to consist of "natural" substances—herbal preparations, administered in large quantities to compensate for deficiencies. The cascade model represents the more recently evolved *allopathic* tradition in medicine, wherein diseases are viewed to be the result of an interloping agent, such as a bacterium, and treatment consists of eliminating the interloper. Allopathic treatments are usually highly potent synthetic substances, administered in relatively small doses ("drugs"). The superior efficacy of allopathic treatment for infectious diseases in the 19th and early 20th century led to a general devaluation of naturopathic approaches. However, in the later 20th century a rediscovery of *systemic diseases*—that is, conditions not attributable to a single causal agent—led to a reevaluation of naturopathic approaches. Today the two traditions are no longer seen as separate or competing in general medical practice. To the degree that psychiatric conditions such as schizophrenia can be understood as diseases at all, they are systemic diseases (Claridge, 1990). Nevertheless, these realizations have not led to a greater appreciation of the naturopathic perspective in medical model psychiatry, where the search continues for "magic bullet" drugs to disrupt the cascades that are believed to cause mental illness. This search has certainly produced highly potent and sometimes useful medications, but their effects on personal and social functioning, and their clinical use, conform more to a naturopathic than an allopathic model of illness and treatment.

The biosystemic paradigm of psychopathology thus reveals a need for two distinct types of knowledge and skill in rehabilitation. The first type involves identification of specific processes and functional modules whose malfunctions are contributing to a person's disabilities. To achieve this step requires an understanding of how those processes normally operate, within and across their various levels of organization. As our understanding becomes more specific and mechanistic, our ability to apply technology to individual problems improves. For example, as we learn more about the biochemical and neurophysiological mechanisms of drug action, we are able to develop more effective medications and employ them more usefully in treatment and rehabilitation. Similarly, as we learn more about the cognitive underpinnings of social competence, we can design more effective techniques for social skills training.

The second type of knowledge and skill involves identification of the causal relationships among these various process and components, as they play themselves out, in linear cascades or stable but dysfunctional cycles, in individuals. A complete account of systemic relationships in an individual case helps ensure that all the contributors to disability are identified and addressed. If the first kind of knowledge and skill informs the *tactics* of rehabilitation, the second kind informs the *strategy*. A successful campaign requires careful attention to both. The overarching principles of psychopathology—systemic organization and causality—provide basic guidelines for formulating rehabilitation strategy; detailed, mechanistic understanding of specific processes and functional modules provide the tactics of treatment.

The next chapter describes a *case formulation* method for constructing and maintaining an individualized *strategy* for rehabilitation. The remaining chapters then explore the *tactics* of rehabilitation associated with the various levels of organization and functional components of human biosystems.

# Chapter 3

# The Structure of Clinical Assessment, Formulation, and Rehabilitation Planning

In the integrated paradigm the purpose of clinical assessment is to inform and facilitate pursuit of *rehabilitation goals*. These goals are the product of common understandings between members of the *rehabilitation team*, which is comprised of the person undergoing rehabilitation and recovery, his or her family and friends, professional providers of rehabilitation services, and other stakeholders in the rehabilitation enterprise. A *stakeholder* in this context means a person who has some investment or interest in the person undergoing rehabilitation. Stakeholders vary from one case to the next, and may include relatives, friends, advocates, or even representatives of the public interest. Composing the treatment team in a way that best serves the interests and desires of the person undergoing rehabilitation, while acknowledging the legitimacy of other interests, is itself an important and sometimes difficult task (this is discussed in more detail in later chapters).

Clinical assessment, conducted by the members of the rehabilitation team, is a process of gathering information about the recovering person's values and desires, how these relate to the values and desires of the recovering person's family, friends, and community, the nature of the barriers that must be overcome in order to establish better personal and social functioning, the skills and abilities necessary to achieve the rehabilitation goals, strengths and assets that can serve rehabilitative purposes, and environmental conditions that may help or hinder rehabilitation and recovery.

The rehabilitation team uses the information gathered in clinical assessment to construct a *rehabilitation plan*—a procedural map or blueprint that guides provision of specific services and other aspects of rehabilitation and recovery, toward achievement of the rehabilitation goals. In this plan, the barriers to achieving the goals are defined as specific *problems*. Each

46

problem is associated with its own *long-term goal* whose resolution serves the purposes of the broader rehabilitation goals. Each problem is also associated with a set of *short-term goals* that identify specific, measurable steps toward the long-term goal. Finally, each problem is associated with a set of *interventions*—the specific services and other activities expected to directly contribute to problem resolution. Rehabilitation is accomplished by applying the services, as planned, and measuring progress toward achievement of the goals.

The complete process—identifying rehabilitation goals, conducting clinical assessment, conceptualizing problems, constructing a rehabilitation plan, implementing the plan, and achieving the goals—does not follow a linear sequence. Clinical assessment informs identification of rehabilitation goals, and those goals may change over time as rehabilitation progresses and barriers yield or persist. The team may reconceptualize problems as more information becomes available. The membership of the rehabilitation team may change, its only invariable member being the recovering person. Although the course of rehabilitation is punctuated by key events, such as comprehensive assessments, inauguration of rehabilitation plans, and achievement of goals, it is ultimately a cyclic process of renewing and revising the goals, the problem conceptualizations, and the solutions. The recovery cycle reflects a reversal of the downward spiral of a stable but dysregulated system described in the previous chapter. Just as poorly functioning components contribute to the failure of other components in the system, the benefits of recovered components are distributed in a similar manner. As the functioning of the various components improves, the functioning of the entire system improves.

Assessment and rehabilitation planning are *unifying* processes intended to bring together the perspectives of the recovering person and the various other members of the rehabilitation team. The personal values of the people involved, their shared community values, scientific knowledge (especially in psychopathology), and clinical technology are integrated toward a common purpose. In conventional clinical parlance, unification of assessment data, scientific perspective, and service planning is the process of *case formulation*. This view of assessment and rehabilitation planning (or treatment planning) is consistent with principles that pervade the entire mental health community (and even, to a significant extent, the broader health care community) and reflects an idealized, but broadly shared, vision of how health care *should* be viewed. This process has been discussed in the literature from the perspectives of behavior therapy (Nezu, Nezu, Friedman, & Haynes, 1998), psychodynamic psychotherapy (Horowitz, 1999), cognitive therapy (Mumma, 1998), the medical model (Stoudemire, 1990), and cognitive-behavioral therapy (Bruch, 1998). (For an extensive bibliography on case formulation and related aspects of clinical judgement, see

Waddington, 1997.) Some contributions to this discussion are specifically pertinent to issues of severe mental illness (e.g., Haddock & Tarrier, 1998; Hunter, 2000; Morrison, 1998).

The key concepts in case formulation are codified in regulations and standards for health care services, from federal regulations for developmental disability services to hospital accreditation standards promulgated by the Joint Commission on Accreditation of Healthcare Organizations (JCAHO), to standards for rehabilitation services promulgated by the Commission on Accreditation of Rehabilitation Facilities (CARF), to federal health care regulations promulgated by the Centers for Medicare and Medicaid Services, formerly the Health Care Finance Administration (HCFA). Among other things, accreditation rules stipulate the structure of treatment and rehabilitation plans, the roles of team members, the role of assessment in treatment planning, and rules for defining specific problems and solutions.

Clinical assessment and treatment planning in the integrated paradigm involves detailed elaboration of key elements, most notably *problems,* and the assessment technology required to measure and characterize them. In addition, certain practical realities, such as the complexity of rehabilitation services and the time frame in which rehabilitation-related changes sometimes occur, require new and specialized components in the assessment and planning process. The result is an elaborate but unified model that uses sound psychopathological principles and all currently available clinical technology, but that still applies the scientific method to clinical practice and adheres to the basic concepts and practices codified in health care regulations and accreditation standards.

## THE EVOLUTION OF KEY CONCEPTS
## IN ASSESSMENT AND REHABILITATION PLANNING

### The Salience of the Client's Perspective

The integrated paradigm's emphasis on the recovering person's values and desires has roots in the development of nondirective psychotherapy, an approach that emphasized clarification of clients' personal goals and desires. In fact, it was this emphasis that inspired use of the term *client,* implying active collaboration in treatment, instead of *patient,* implying a passive recipient of treatment. As early as the 1950s, research showed that therapists' use of specific techniques to facilitate the clarification process, including a nonjudgmental, empathetic, and unconditionally supportive manner, leads to better psychotherapy outcomes. (For a historical account and analysis of psychotherapy research relevant to this point, see Frank & Frank, 1991.) Nondirective therapy is not generally considered to be an appropriate treatment, by itself, for disabling mental illness, but its techniques for supportively clarifying personal values are highly applicable to rehabilitation.

The influence of nondirective psychotherapy is evident in the rehabilitation counseling techniques associated with the Boston Model of psychiatric rehabilitation in the 1970s (discussed in Chapter 1). The rehabilitation psychology paradigm, which the Boston Model transformed for mental illness, recognized that acknowledging the client's values and goals is a prerequisite to engaging him or her in the rehabilitation enterprise. Clarifying personal values and goals is often difficult enough, without the complications that disabling mental illness can bring. It was evident, early on, that vigorous application of nondirective techniques would often be important in integrating the client's perspective into assessment and rehabilitation planning. The Boston Model's rehabilitation counseling techniques gave providers and their clients a useful tool for doing that work.

The other alternative paradigms of the mid-20th century (also discussed in Chapter 1) paid attention to the client's perspective as well. The social–community paradigm relied on group processes, rather than dyadic therapist–client processes, to develop shared understandings of individuals' perspectives. Activities such as self-government, which promotes recognition of, and respect for, individual perceptions, beliefs, and values, were seen as important components of treatment. In social learning theory, individuals are motivated by rewards whose meaning lies in those individuals' personal expectations and associations. It is therefore of paramount importance to assess what those expectations and associations are, in each individual case.

This attention to the client's perspective in the alternative paradigms contrasted with the medical model in the mid-20th century. The dehumanizing qualities of psychiatric institutions, the authoritarian tone of many psychoanalytic practitioners, and later the impersonal and reductionistic implications of drug treatment were associated by many with the medical model's neglect of the client's (or "patient's," in medical terms) perspective in diagnosis and treatment. (For an incisive critique of these aspects of medical model psychiatry, from within the psychiatric community, see Breggin, 1991.) Psychiatry's increasing focus on drug treatment provided no new impetus for concern about the patient's perspective, other than interest in phenomenological descriptions of the symptoms that would be targets for treatment. The medical model did not incorporate patients' attitudes and values into its psychopathology, nor did it develop special techniques or technologies for evoking and clarifying them. However, a reexamination by medical model psychiatry of patients' perspective has been motivated, in large part, by high levels of nonadherence to drug regimens. Similarly, the unexpected finding that drug-induced symptom reduction may be only weakly correlated with overall outcome is inspiring some reconceptualization. Research evidence today suggests that patients have mixed and heterogeneous views about the value of drug effects. More research is required to articulate this picture sufficiently to be of use in clinical practice. Until recently, funding priorities in the mental health research community were not conducive to such research. (It is regrettable that antipsychotic drugs were in use for 40 years before patients' perspectives on them were given systematic scientific attention, but hopefully current trends will continue and bear fruit.) As with the general dismissal of psychosocial treatment as "social welfare," it was assumed that any necessary understanding of the patient's perspective would be achieved through the "common human decency" of the psychiatrist. The science and technology of human attitudes, values, and beliefs were not part of the medical model.

As the alternative rehabilitation models evolved in the 1970s and 1980s, their emphasis on the recovering person's goals and desires complemented the increasing involvement of consumer and advocacy organizations in public mental health policy and services. However, issues regarding client perspectives became more complex. As the cognitive impairments of mental illness came to be better understood, questions arose as to whether those impairments must be taken into account in ascertaining a person's values, beliefs, and desires (which, after all, are cognitive phenomena). The problem of involuntary treatment became more complex as the mental health system itself became more complex. (For a detailed, recent analysis of involuntary treatment, focused on issues pertinent to disabling mental illness, see Dennis & Monahan, 1996.) Balancing the recovering person's desires and prerogatives against the rights and prerogatives of family and community became a focal concern.

Today there is broad agreement that historically, the recovering person's perspectives (and that of family as well) have been neglected, and that contemporary mental health services must do a better job of addressing them. (For an enlightening empirical analysis of client perspectives on contemporary rehabilitation, see Bachrach, 1994.) However, there is substantially less agreement about the limits of including the recovering person's perspective in treatment planning and other clinical decision making, and the degree to which family and community can or should intervene. Standards and regulations can "require" that treatment plans systematically include the recovering person's perspective, but it is unknown whether such standards really do work. From a scientific and technological perspective, it is even unclear what must be done to ensure that a particular recovering person's participation in treatment planning occurs in an optimal manner for that individual. Management of these complexities requires continuing reappraisal of law and social policy, as well as new science and technology for ascertaining and working with the recovering person's perceptions, beliefs, and desires. The rehabilitation counseling techniques of the Boston

Model are useful, but they are insufficient for some individuals under some circumstances. Recent developments in cognitive psychology, neuropsychology, cognitive therapy, mental health policy, and legal scholarship provide more tools for assessing the recovering person's perspective and putting that assessment to use in rehabilitation. These will be discussed in detail in later chapters.

## Measurable Goals

The concept of identifying and pursuing rehabilitation goals has a number of progenitors in the mid-20th century. The very abstract and general goals of psychoanalysis ("to love and work") gradually gave way to the less general but still somewhat abstract language of psychotherapy (to "self-actualize," to achieve "congruence"). Within psychoanalysis, there was increasing attention to specific "ego functions," whose strengthening was expected to produce more specific improvements in personal and social functioning; hence strengthening ego functions became a goal of treatment. The interpersonal model, originating with George Meade and clinically applied by Harry Stack Sullivan and others, identified more specific aspects of social functioning as targets for treatment. The infusion of behavioral psychology into mental health introduced the use of highly specific, measurable behaviors as treatment goals. The subsequent evolution of behaviorism into social learning theory, and of behavior modification into cognitive-behavioral therapy, gave rise to a sophisticated technology for engaging the client in the process of identifying goals and evaluating progress toward their achievement.

Cognitive-behavioral approaches were also influential in rehabilitation psychology, where stepwise approximations to measurable goals were applied to overcome physical disabilities. Psychiatric rehabilitation translated the very functional language of goal setting pertinent to physical disabilities into language relevant to disabling mental illness. The practice of *comprehensive functional assessment*, central to psychiatric rehabilitation, involves an exhaustive accounting of a person's strengths and weaknesses in relation to achieving pragmatic goals.

The advent of psychopharmacotherapy also encouraged the specification of treatment goals, because psychotropic drugs have relatively specific and measurable effects. This is not to say that drug effects constitute legitimate treatment goals. This legitimacy depends on the meaning and importance of the effects to the recovering person. Recent research suggests that the most evident, specific, and measurable psychiatric drug effects are less pertinent to individuals' personal and social functioning and quality of life than had been assumed. However, the technology that evolved for assessing drug effects does provide opportunities for scientific precision in measuring important aspects of rehabilitation, such as reduction of psychotic symptoms.

Identification and pursuit of goals have been the subjects of considerable research in social and cognitive psychology and related areas, and this research has benefited assessment and treatment planning in rehabilitation. One important program of research produced a technological tool, "goal attainment scaling" (GAS; Heavlin, Lee-Merrow, & Lewis, 1982), still used in various mental health and rehabilitation contexts today. GAS is a systematic procedure for defining goals that can be stated in either behavioral or subjective/experiential terms, and measuring progress toward those goals. It serves to evaluate the outcome of treatment interventions (e.g., Austin, Liberman, King, & DeRisi, 1976; Beidel, 1983; Lewis, Spencer, Haas, & DiVittis, 1987; Malec, 1999) as well as the performance of service programs (Cline, Rouzer, & Bransford, 1973; Kiresuk, Stelmachers, & Schultz, 1982; Ottenbacher & Cusick, 1990). Using GAS procedures, treatment teams can transform the recovering person's (and other team members') subjective and objective desires into measurable rehabilitation goals. Progress rating scales are then constructed, where varying scores on the scale reflect varying degrees of progress toward the goal. One of GAS's most appealing features is that it allows the use of laboratory measures, functional criteria, and subjective reports in constructing and using its rating scales. These scales can then be used to evaluate progress toward rehabilitation goals, which, in turn, guides personal and clinical decisions involved in rehabilitation.

GAS methods evolved over approximately the same time period as PROMIS and related treatment planning concepts, and there was considerable reciprocal influence. Contemporary treatment planning standards reflect some of the key concepts of the GAS model. However, formal GAS is not typically used in clinical mental health settings and certainly is not required by health care standards. There is concern about its ecological validity—that is, the degree to which formally identified goals really are meaningful, reflect treatable problems, and correspond to the recovering person's subjective and objective quality of life (Calsyn & Davidson, 1978; Cytrynbaum, Ginath, Birdwell, & Brandt, 1979; Sheldon & Elliot, 1998). Inevitably, a rehabilitation team's goals reflect the *abilities and limitations of the people on the team at that time*; GAS arguably has inadequate safeguards against the impact of provider limitations on formulation of goals and progress criteria. Validity aside, GAS is a somewhat ponderous, labor-intensive procedure requiring considerable specialized training and supervision. If it were to be practical in rehabilitation, GAS would have to be streamlined and tailored to mental health rehabilitation circumstances, and it would have to demonstrate ecological validity.

Fortunately, achieving these two conditions turns out not to be a difficult problem. The integrated paradigm provides a conceptual and procedural framework in which the most important aspects of GAS could be applied meaningfully. This ease of fit between GAS and the integrated paradigm derives in large part from the way the *clinical problems* in the rehabilitation plan are conceptualized and defined. We will return to the issue of setting goals and evaluating progress after reviewing the evolution of the concept of clinical problems.

## The Concept of Clinical Problems

The *clinical problem* is a core concept in contemporary health care documentation practices. Standards and regulations generally require that the identified patient's treatment plan be organized around a set of specifically defined problems—circumstances or conditions that impair the patient's functioning in domains relevant to the service provider. The nature of the problems must be determined by formal clinical assessment. To qualify as a legitimate part of treatment, a service must address one or more of the documented problems. Similarly, treatment goals must reflect resolution, or progress toward resolution, of a specific problem. Progress toward resolution of these identified problems must be evaluated through formal clinical assessment. The collection of specific problems in a treatment plan, the "problem list," thus represents an overarching summary of the reasons the patient needs treatment, the entire array of treatment to be provided, and the criteria by which progress and success will be evaluated. The problem list is the organizational backbone of the treatment plan.

Contemporary use of the clinical problem concept had its clearest origins in PROMIS—problem-oriented medical information systems. However, problem-oriented models evolved amid a broader interest in how people make decisions (D'Zurilla & Nezu, 1982). The idea of teaching systematic problem-solving skills appeared in a range of applications, from business administration to medical education and nursing practice, to models of human creativity. An entire approach to cognitive-behavioral therapy sought to teach problem-solving skills to improve the personal and social functioning of people with disabling mental illness, as well as less disabling conditions (D'Zurilla, 1986, 1988). All of these developments reinforced the centrality of the clinical problem in assessment and treatment planning. As the health care accreditation industry grew, and standards for treatment planning became increasingly salient to accreditation processes, it became increasingly important for clinicians to be able to think and plan in terms of clinical problems and their solutions.

The medical model concept of psychiatric diagnosis maintained a peripheral role in the evolution of the clinical problem concept. Much of the early impetus for identifying those problems was the limited practical utility of diagnostic categorization. In nonpsychiatric health care settings, medical diagnoses could be linked to relatively specific sets of services, giving rise to the concept of *diagnosis-related groups* (DRGs; for a historical account and analysis of DRGs in general health care, see Geist & Hardesty, 1992). DRGs are administrative categorizations that reliably indicate what kinds of services a patient is expected to need, based on that patient's diagnosis. In the mental health field, DRGs were found to be infeasible because psychiatric diagnoses do not reliably indicate service needs (Ashcraft, Fries, Nerenz, & Falcon, 1989; Choca, Peterson, & Shanley, 1987; English, 1986; Holcomb & Thompson, 1988; Horn, Chambers, Sharkey, & Horn, 1989; Taube, Eun, & Forthofer, 1984). Neo-Kraepelinians hoped the operationalized diagnostic criteria of the DSM-III and subsequent editions would make DRGs possible in psychiatry and mental health. However, the efficacy of specific pharmacological and psychosocial treatments do not correspond closely enough to DSM categories to justify DRGs. This infeasibility of applying DRGs further reinforced the importance of clinical problems as the basic unit of analysis in mental health service administration.

The robust presence of problem-oriented treatment planning in standards and regulations, at least since the 1970s, suggests that it is useful in some sense. It provides a relatively straightforward organizational structure for individual service planning documents and therefore facilitates regulatory enforcement practices, such as review of medical records by accreditation referees. Arguably, it is a helpful factor in promoting clinical accountability. Logic would predict that an agency that can document its services with reference to problems that are reliably identifiable is providing better, more cost-efficient services than one that cannot. However, logic would not predict that the exact problem-oriented model optimal for, say, a surgery service, would also be optimal for rehabilitation of mental illness. It must be expected that a generic problem-oriented model will be applied in different ways in different settings. A generic model may broaden the accreditation industry's market, but it sets limits on the degree to which that model can be optimized for any particular setting.

Paradoxically, the success of problem-oriented assessment and treatment planning in the health care accreditation industry is due, in large part, to its separation of practical clinical needs from the need for logical coherence. It is one thing to explain why a condition exists, and another to translate that explanation into helpful interventions. Of course, both are important, but they must be addressed in rather different ways. Logical coherence in etiological formulations can be pursued through science or other theoretical paradigms (e.g., psychoanalysis). In the mental health field, theories that have provided compelling explanations of conditions have not necessarily been informative about practical treatment needs (and vice versa).

Psychiatric diagnosis aspired to serve as a scientific classification system *and* a useful prescriptive guide—but largely failed at both. The problem-oriented approach, as it evolved in the late 20th century, emphasizes specification and documentation of practical clinical needs and solutions but does *not* specify the logical (scientific or otherwise) framework in which needs are identified and solutions chosen. The problems identified on a treatment plan are whatever the treatment team deems them to be, the only parameter being that of measurability. The logic by which certain conditions become identified problems, and the logic by which particular solutions (treatments, etc.) are chosen, are left to the team (which may be a surgical team, or a rehabilitation team, or an individual practitioner) to determine.

This does not mean that achieving logical coherence is beyond the scope of problem-oriented standards and accreditation processes. Agency policy documents are expected to provide rationales for the nature and scope of the problems that the agency addresses. Service providers are expected to provide rationales for their assessments and treatment choices in their narrative assessment reports and progress notes. However, it is not an uncommon criticism from accreditation referees that although an agency's documentation adheres to standards for defining and measuring problems and interventions, there is insufficient logical coherence in the treatment plans. Nevertheless, the demand for logical coherence is difficult to enforce, and conversely, criticisms are difficult to refute, because the standards do not specify what kind of logic may be used. Disputes over logical coherence thus can devolve into arguments over the validity of competing theoretical assumptions.

This ambiguity concerning the logical coherence of problem-oriented assessment and treatment planning gives accreditation referees some latitude in evaluating how well an agency's documentation complements that agency's particular mission and function. Similarly, it allows referees to use their clinical experience and judgment beyond the constraints of formal rules and regulations. In other words, a diversity of agencies and institutions can be evaluated under a single set of standards, creating a broader market for purveyors of accreditation services (this may be an advantage for the purveyors of accreditation services but for nobody else). The disadvantage, for administrative purposes, is the problem with judging the logical coherence of treatment plans. This is an even bigger disadvantage when attempting to assess treatment effectiveness. Presumably, in the long run, the most effective treatment plans are those that are maximally informed by a logical and scientific understanding of the identified problems. It is scientific understanding of a problem, in relation to social values, that guides application of available technology. The lack of connection between identification of a problem and understanding it scientifically, as in the problem-oriented approach, thus represents a serious limit in the degree to which technological applications (i.e., treatment and rehabilitation) can be systematically informed by psychopathology. The solution is to conceptualize identified problems as representing an *intersection* of practical, scientific, and technological considerations.

Characterizing a problem in terms of both etiology and technological solution leads to violation of a key principle of psychiatric diagnosis: that "treatment response" is not a legitimate criterion for diagnosis. This principle is sound in some contexts, but it is not applicable here because of the differences between problem-oriented assessment in the integrated paradigm and in psychiatric diagnosis. The practical reality is that with mental illness, all assessments are somewhat conjectural, and treatment response is often an important source of data for validating an assessment. Differential treatment response may be the best indication that a particular set of circumstances represent more than a single problem. Hence, there are key advantages to using treatment response as part of the criteria for particular problems. This approach is also more compatible with a complete view of science and technology as two reciprocally interactive endeavors, rather than a lockstep progression from theory to application. Especially in contemporary mental health, basic science is as much informed by the outcome of technological applications as vice versa (see Figure 3.1).

There is a sense in which the concept of "a problem" is incompatible with science. The universe works according to immutable natural laws. Living things come into existence as a consequence of those laws, and the same laws determine their demise. People are born, live, become sick, and die, quite naturally. No problem. This assertion of the naturalness of all life forms and their myriad processes often seems counterintuitive to people from Western cultures, perhaps evidenced by the salience of the idea to Westerners encountering it as a fundamental principle of Eastern traditions of thought, especially Taoism and Buddhism. The centrality of human purpose and meaning in Western thought may be advantageous for technology, but it may distract us from the ultimate amorality of science. It is human social circumstances that give meaning to "problems." Rivers may be following all the natural laws of physics and geology, but they still present us with the "problem" of getting across them. Sickness may be a perfectly natural condition, but it often obstructs our plans and intentions. When someone's death is identified as occurring "not from natural causes," sociobehavioral causes (e.g., foul play), not supernatural causes, are the implication. Nevertheless, we have a cultural tendency to think of molecular process as "natural," but more complex processes as due to something else. Perhaps this bias arose because our culture was initially most successful at recognizing natural laws in "molecular-type" processes (falling objects, in-

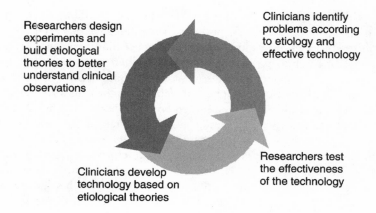

**FIGURE 3.1.** March of science or *pas de deux*? Science and technology progress as reciprocally interactive enterprises. Scientific theory inspires development of technology, and the outcome of technological application inspires new theory.

teracting chemicals), whereas reliable laws describing more complex processes (quantum mechanics, chaos theory) came later.

The usual pathway from science to technology begins with a circumstantial delimitation of the scientific issues—that is, identification of a social *problem* and the scientific principles that bear upon it. For example, the highly scientific and technological enterprise of bridge building begins with the highly social (even political) circumstance that a river must be crossed at a particular place. Universal natural laws come into play later, and certainly are never violated, but only certain natural laws are relevant (relativity theory, for example, usually does not figure in bridge design). Also, bridge building requires particular, even unique applications, reflecting the geography of the site, available building materials, the composition of the substrate, anticipated user traffic, and so on. These complex considerations tend to create *classes* of solutions, so that, for example, we recognize different *types* of bridges. However, we do not mistake these solution classes as expressions of the properties of the rivers. We recognize that they emerge from complex interactions between natural laws (involving gravity, hydrodynamics, tensile strength, etc.) and the various circumstances (geographical and social) that bridge building encounters. Similarly, we do not justify ignoring the laws of physics by invoking the social need for a bridge.

We *do* make such mistakes in the mental health industry, for the reasons discussed in the previous chapters. The key error in neo-Kraepelinian diagnosis is to mistake complex circumstances for the results of unitary lawful processes. If this error were applied to bridge building, we would believe that rivers cause bridges, perhaps even that different types of rivers cause different types of bridges. We would expect that the characteristics of any bridge, including its location, are determined solely by the physical properties of the bridge site. Of course, we do not make this mistake in bridge building, because we know that people build bridges for social reasons. With mental illness we encounter bridges we did not build, and we need to understand why they are there as well as their physical properties.

At the opposite extreme from the Kraepelinian error is the key limitation in problem-oriented assessment and treatment planning: its failure to identify systematically, or even theorize about, the lawful processes that may be operating in a complex circumstance (perhaps this lacuna is the product of an overreaction to the flaws in neo-Kraepelinian diagnosis). If this limitation were applied to bridge building, we would attempt to build bridges solely on the basis of social determinants, disregarding physics, and engineering would become a political activity. In mental health care, *neither* psychiatric diagnosis *nor* problem-oriented assessment provides a conceptual link between problems, scientific understanding of problems, and technological solutions.

The following section describes the "upgrades" that must be made in traditional problem-oriented assessment and treatment planning to make them fully operational in the integrated paradigm. These include: (1) definition of a comprehensive set of the identified problems addressed in rehabilitation of mental illness; (2) integration of etiological hypotheses in problem selection; (3) prioritization of problems according to etiological hypotheses; and (4) a cyclic process of assessment, progress evaluation and treatment plan revision. These upgrades require a particular conceptualization of the rehabilitation enterprise that is accomplished by the integrated paradigm. At the same time, at more concrete levels, the upgrades translate into a number of procedural conventions in the assessment, formulation, planning, and progress evaluation process.

## PROBLEM-ORIENTED ASSESSMENT AND REHABILITATION PLANNING IN THE INTEGRATED PARADIGM

Optimal problem-oriented assessment and rehabilitation planning must combine circumstantial problem identification with logical and scientific analysis of the factors relevant to defined problems. This endeavor might constitute an impossibly difficult task at the level of health care regulations and accreditation standards, because of the large diversity of circumstances and processes that would have to be addressed. However, within *particular* health care settings, the variability of problem-defining circumstances can be manageable, though still large. This is indeed the case in the particular health care settings where rehabilitation services are provided to people with disabling mental illness. In the integrated paradigm, the scope of clinical circumstances together with scientific models of mental illness and rehabilitation technology permit a marriage of problem-oriented assessment and rehabilitation planning based on scientific rationality.

Assessment and rehabilitation planning in the integrated paradigm rests on a key premise:

> *At our current stage of scientific and technological progress, it is possible to identify a manageable number of clinical circumstances, which: (1) represent barriers to personal and social functioning; (2) collectively represent all the barriers associated with disabling mental illness; (3) are at least partially understood through existing models of psychopathology; and (4) can be assessed and manipulated with existing technology.*

The key implication of this premise is that it is possible to construct an exhaustive list, with definitions, of the identifiable problems a rehabilitation team can address in its assessments and include in its rehabilitation plan. These are not the problems identified on any particular individual plan, but *all* problems that could be identified on *any* plan—in other words, a list of *allowable* problems. To avoid confusion with the problem lists of individual treatment plans, the group of allowable problems is termed the *problem set*. For policy and administrative purposes, the problem set defines the universe of problems addressable by the provider. In effect, the problem set also identifies the recipients of the provider's services (i.e., people who have problems defined in the provider's problem set). In a clinical and scientific context, the problem set defines the paradigm in which the provider operates *and* the technological resources at the provider's disposal. As with types of bridges, the nature of the problem is intimately associated with the nature of the solution.

## A Prototype Problem Set

Appendix 1 contains a sample problem set for rehabilitation of disabling mental illness. Note that each entry in the set has two elements: the *problem title* and the *problem definition*. (Readers are encouraged to study Appendix 1 before continuing with this section.) The problem definition describes the problem with respect to four key dimensions: (1) the way in which the problem represents a barrier to personal and social functioning, (2) how the problem is understood in terms of psychopathology, (3) how the problem is typically identified and assessed, and (4) how the problem is typically treated or otherwise resolved. The problem title uses a single phrase that incorporates the major categories cited in the definition. The information will guide the rehabilitation team as they select the problems from the set that apply to individual rehabilitation plans. Table 3.1 provides an overview of the elements contained in the prototype.

The problem set contained in Appendix 1 evolved over a 15-year period, during which we gradually made revisions in response to clinical experience and developments in science and technology. Throughout that period, we also repeatedly tailored it to conform to health care accreditation criteria. Three different settings serving people with disabling mental illness have contributed to its development: a comprehensive, intensive rehabilitation program housed in a state hospital, a community-based residential rehabilitation program, and a program for providing vocational rehabilitation services. The prototype reflects a diversity of circumstances within the general area of rehabilitation for people with disabling mental illness. It should not be expected that this particular problem set would serve optimally in any and all such settings. In fact, a provider's problem set is ex-

TABLE 3.1. Problem Titles in the Prototype Problem Set

| Neurophysiological | Neurocognitive |
|---|---|
| Episodic CNS dysregulation | Post-acute neurocognitive impairment |
| Tonic CNS dysregulation | Residual neurocognitive impairment |

| Sociocognitive | Sociobehavioral—psychophysiological |
|---|---|
| Social problem-solving insufficiency | Dysregulation of behavioral activation |
| Symptom-linked attribution problem | Dysregulation of mood |
| Achievement-linked attribution problem | Dysregulation of anger/aggression |
| Mood-linked attribution problem | Dysregulation of fear/anxiety |
| | Dysregulation of appetitive behavior |
| | Dysregulation of sexual behavior |

| Sociobehavioral—skills deficits | Sociobehavioral—other |
|---|---|
| Self-care skill deficit | Substance abuse |
| Independent living skill deficit | |
| Disorder management skill deficit | |
| Leisure/recreational skill deficit | |
| Occupational skill deficit | |
| Interpersonal skill deficit | |

Socioenvironmental

Rehabilitation nonadherence
Socialized psychiatric symptoms
Socially unacceptable behavior
Social–environmental conflict
Restrictive legal status
Unstable living conditions

pected to portray the role and mission of *that provider* within the larger mental health system. It should be somewhat individualized, if not unique.

On the other hand, the general boundaries set by science and technology (as opposed to clinical circumstance) are fairly universal. This universality militates for greater commonality across settings. Different providers may use *subsets* of the complete problem set, reflecting various degrees of specialization and interagency collaboration. The march of science is expected to be the main influence on the particular composition of problem sets. Our conceptualizations of problems, and hence optimal problem sets for rehabilitation, will change in response to advances in psychopathology and new technological solutions. All things considered, then, the problem set presented in Appendix 1 is expected to be optimal, or close to optimal, for most providers of rehabilitation for disabling mental illness, in 2002. This is the sense in which it can be considered a prototype: as a terminological convention known to be workable in rehabilitation for mental illness but expected to evolve over time.

The prototype problem set also serves as an organizational framework for the integrated paradigm, and more concretely, for this book. The psychopathology and the technology of rehabilitation for mental illness are organized in conformance with the elements of the problem set. This should not be surprising, considering that psychopathology and technology figure in the identification and definition of problems. The problem set is the organizational basis of the next seven chapters, sorted into the more general domains of neurophysiological, neurocognitive, sociocognitive, sociobehavioral, and socioenvironmental functioning. These chapters discuss assessing and solving the specific problems identified in the prototype.

## Constructing a Rehabilitation Plan

In the integrated paradigm, the outcome of the team's clinical assessments is reflected in their selection of problems for an individual rehabilitation plan. Provided the assessments are appropriate and the problem set is optimized for the particular setting, the team members should be able to recognize the presence of problems obstructing the recovering person's functioning. As the treatment plan is constructed, these problems become the targets of treatment and rehabilitation.

The first conceptual issue the team confronts in the problem selection process is whether a particular clinical presentation—for example, episodes of acute psychosis, persistent auditory hallucinations and aggression—is comprised of one or more than one problem. This question cannot be answered by the clinical presentation itself, because different problems may have similar or overlapping clinical presentations. The reality in mental health is that seemingly identical behaviors may have multiple etiologies and/or different etiologies in different individuals. When problems are defined by nonoverlapping clinical presentations, any given problem may have an unspecified etiology and therefore unspecified solutions. This ambiguity is a flaw in psychiatric diagnosis *and* traditional problem-oriented assessment, both of which avoid links to etiology, which, in turn, invites the criticism that particular treatment choices are illogical or insufficiently justified. It is better to identify problems with discrete etiologies and treatment responses but potentially similar clinical presentations, than to identify problems with discrete clinical presentations but unspecified etiologies and treatment responses.

The integrated paradigm requires that the treatment team incorporate hypotheses about etiology and treatment response in selecting problems. These hypotheses determine which clinical circumstances are included under which problem. For example, if the team hypothesizes that the recovering person's episodic psychosis, hallucinations, and aggression are all part of a single linear cascade, beginning with dopaminergic CNS dysregulation, and that resolution of the dysregulation will eliminate all three symptoms, then there is a single problem. Alternatively, if the team hypothesizes that the psychotic episodes and auditory hallucinations are closely linked, but that the aggression occurs independently, and that aggression will not be eliminated by successful treatment of psychosis, then there are two problems.

Separation of problems based on hypothesized etiology and treatment response, rather than clinical presentation, requires specification of the features of the clinical presentation that (hypothetically) express the etiology. This is the *problem description*. As each problem is selected for inclusion in the rehabilitation plan, its clinical features are described, as they manifest themselves in the individual case. In traditional problem-oriented treatment planning, this description is often used as the problem itself, but without etiological or treatment response implications. The integrated paradigm requires that the problem description be consistent with the known (or at least putative) psychopathology of its problem title, and subject to objective measurement, while acknowledging that any etiology may have idiosyncratic expressions.

Deriving long-term and short-term goals based on the problems is the next step in constructing a rehabilitation plan. Here the integrated paradigm uses the convention of traditional problem-oriented treatment planning, in which a single long-term goal describes resolution of the problem, while the short-term goals describe incremental steps toward the long-term goal. The long-term goal is described in the same functional language as the problem definition, tailored to the particular features enumerated in the problem description, so that the goal's relevance to the recovering person's functioning is clear to everyone. It must be operationally defined, to the degree that the team can determine unambiguously whether the goal has been achieved. An operational definition fills two different but complementary roles. First, *processes and conditions* can be operationally defined in terms of quantitative measures. For example, the severity of auditory hallucinations can be operationally defined in terms of numeric values on a structured interview scale. Second, *goal achievement* can be operationalized in terms of degrees or changes in scale values. For example, a long-term goal of eliminating auditory hallucinations could be operationally defined as a score of zero on a structured interview scale, and a short-term goal of reducing their severity could be defined as a change of two points on that scale.

Short-term goals are of two types: proximal and component goals. *Proximal goals* describe sequences that progress toward success in a systematic manner. For example, if the long-term goal is to perform reliably 100% of a daily schedule without assistance, proximal short-term goals might include performing 25%, 50%, and 75%. *Component goals* describe specific components of a long-term goal that are expected to be achieved separately. For example, if the long-term goal is to have a circle of friends, component short-term goals might include developing better social skills, cultivating interests conducive to social interaction, and participating in social opportunities in the community. Short-term goals can be a mixture of component and proximal goals, reflecting the nature of the long-term goal and the recovering person's circumstances. The particular technologies to be applied toward problem resolution can also influence configuration of the short-term goals (selection of problem solutions, which includes selection of technology, is the next step in construction of the rehabilitation plan). Short-term goals can be revised or refined as solution strategies and tactics are formulated.

The integrated paradigm requires that long-term goals have an established ecological validity—that is, any reasonable person would acknowledge the relevance of achieving the goal to a person's functioning. Short-term goals must have obvious relevance to the long-term goal. In addition, short-term goals must be defined in a way that permits quantitative measurement of progress toward their achievement.

In traditional problem-oriented treatment planning, solutions to problems are variously termed "approaches," "interventions," or "treatments." *Interventions* is the best choice for the integrated paradigm; *approaches* is overly broad and *treatments* is overly narrow. Selection of interventions follows directly from selection of problems, because the etiology of the problem suggests the preferred solution. In addition to a specific operational description of the intervention modality,[1] the integrated paradigm requires that all interventions include objective, quantitative measures of relevant

---

[1]*Modality* is a broad term that incorporates all treatments, education, skills training, therapy, social interventions, and so on.

dimensions of the specific intervention modality. Such quantitative measures would include the administration regimen (e.g., hours and times of social skills training, dosage and schedule of medication), whether administration occurred as planned, and the nature of the recovering person's participation in, and response to, the modality. These details are termed *intervention parameters*.

Once a problem is identified and described, its short- and long-term goals articulated, and interventions selected, particular clinical instruments suggest themselves as useful indicators of relevant dimensions of the problem. For example, problems whose descriptions include behaviors associated with psychosis can be assessed usefully with structured interviews and/or behavioral–observational scales. Problems whose descriptions include interpersonal functioning can be usefully assessed with role-play–based measures of social competence. The integrated paradigm requires that for every problem, the team identify one or more *key indicators*, objective measures that will be used to evaluate changes in relevant dimensions of the problem.

The next step in the construction of the plan is to prioritize the problems for resolution. In our usage *prioritization* means determining the sequence in which problems are to be addressed, and the sequence in which progress and resolution are expected. Prioritization does *not* refer to the "importance" of different problems, because all problems are equally important, in that they all constitute significant barriers to personal and social functioning. However, it is the nature of mental illness that certain problems sometimes affect intervention choices for other problems. For example, if the recovering person is currently suffering from acute psychosis and participation in some rehabilitation activities may not be beneficial, or even harmful, then some resolution of the acute psychosis may be stipulated as a prerequisite to those activities. The integrated paradigm requires the rehabilitation plan to document such relationships between problems. A four-category coding system can be used for this purpose:

*Priority 1:* The problem is accessible for treatment, and no other problems are expected to interfere with intervention and solution.

*Priority 2:* There is another problem that is expected to interfere with intervention and/or solution, so that progress is not expected to be optimal, but due to circumstantial reasons, intervention will proceed anyway. Circumstantial reasons for intervention might include the following rationales: (1) the potential benefits of intervention outweigh the cost, even when response is suboptimal; (2) intervention must be provided for safety, legal, or humanitarian reasons, whether optimal response is expected or not; or (3) intervention produces valuable clinical data that would not otherwise be available.

*Priority 3:* There is a problem that is expected to interfere with intervention and/or solution, such that intervention is not justified until the preemptive problem is resolved to some degree.

*Priority 4:* Further resolution of the problem is neither necessary nor expected. Intervention is either discontinued altogether, or continued with the expectation that it will maintain the status quo rather than produce further changes (e.g., use of maintenance medication regimens to prevent recurrence of acute psychosis).

Prioritization of the problems in this manner clarifies the team's hypotheses about relationships between problems, clarifies expectations about intervention response, helps justify selection, timing, and sequencing of specific interventions, and serves as a guide for later evaluations of progress and success.

It is noteworthy that the integrated paradigm's prioritization procedure solves a dilemma in which treatment teams sometimes find themselves. On the one hand, mental illness sometimes presents problems that cannot all be addressed at one time. If the treatment team attempts to address too many problems at once, they are subject to the criticism (usually from accreditation referees) that they are being unrealistic and overly ambitious. On the other hand, if they do not address evident problems, or, more commonly, attempt to lump problems that can be addressed immediately with problems that require preliminary resolution of other problems, they are subject to the criticism that they are neglecting important aspects of the clinical presentation. The integrated paradigm allows the team to identify all relevant problems, while specifying the strategy by which those problems will be addressed.

As the problems are prioritized and assigned interventions, a time frame for rehabilitation emerges. The final step in the initial construction of the rehabilitation plan is to assign *target dates* to start the interventions and achieve the goals of all priority-1 and priority-2 problems. Together, the various goal definitions, key indicators, priorities, intervention choices, and target dates reflect the team's collective expectation about how rehabilitation will progress. Expectations in this context are complex and influenced by countless exigencies. Nevertheless, it is necessary to establish reasonably specific expectations in order to evaluate progress and success. The concept of goal attainment scaling provides a bridge between the complexity of expectations, indirectly expressed by various elements of the formulation and rehabilitation plan, and the need to determine whether the plan is proceeding toward success.

Once the rehabilitation plan is complete, a narrative account of the team's thinking and expectations must be formulated. Such an account is usually required by health care documentation standards. Its most important function is to facilitate a comprehensive understanding of the plan by all team members. To complement the particular, operational structure of the problems and their subordinate elements, the narrative account should describe the plan in plain English (or whatever language applies). This does not prohibit the use of technical terminology, which is sometimes necessary for rhetorical precision and efficiency. However, technical terms should be carefully explained and their meaning and significance made clear. The narrative account, or *narrative formulation,* becomes a companion document to the completed plan.

## Evaluating and Revising the Rehabilitation Plan

The hypothetical nature of problem identification necessitates a hypothetico-deductive approach to treatment, meaning that identification of a problem is, in an important sense, an *experimental hypothesis,* proposed by the team and tested by the recovering person's response to intervention. Although the integrated paradigm explicitly acknowledges and manages this reality, it did not create it. Psychiatric diagnosis and traditional problem-oriented models presume too much about the reliability and validity of initial assessments of mental illness. In mental health and rehabilitation, it is necessary to formalize the process of validating initial assessments, especially in terms of response to interventions. Although many would argue that a hypothetico-deductive process always underlies clinical practice, the reality remains that neither psychiatric diagnosis nor traditional problem-oriented models systematize the testing of assessments with interventions. The familiar clinical picture of institutionalized people on massive, complex regimens of psychiatric medications that have no detectable benefits is a troubling and all-too-frequent manifestation of this shortcoming (see Hunter, 2000). Administering these drug regimens "across the board" results from initial hypotheses that recovering individuals will benefit from drug treatment, but those hypotheses are never tested or challenged with data that indicate lack of response or a negative response.

Of course, sound experimental designs are difficult to implement, even in laboratory environments. True experiments, wherein all intervening variables are carefully controlled or counterbalanced, are seldom feasible in clinical settings. Nevertheless, uncertainty about the true nature of the recovering person's problems and which solutions will be effective can be reduced significantly by using as much experimental logic and systematization as is feasible in any given situation.

The key elements in experimentally validating hypotheses, in ascending order of difficulty, include:

1. Clarity and measurability (i.e., the degree of operationalization, which is the degree to which a hypothesis can be stated in objectively measurable terms)
2. Specificity in defining the intervention
3. Repeated measurement of the variables that operationally define the hypothesis, in an appropriate time frame
4. Implementation of the intervention in such a way that its effects will not be confounded by other interventions or changing circumstances.

Traditional problem-oriented models encourage clarity and measurability of problems and goals, and they encourage specificity in defining interventions to some degree. However, generally biomedical interventions (drugs) are highly specified, but psychosocial interventions (skills training, counseling, occupational therapy) are only vaguely defined. Traditional problem-oriented models require that treatment plans be evaluated for progress at regular intervals but otherwise do not encourage systematic analysis of repeated measurements in those evaluations—and they do nothing to encourage controlling interventions to minimize confounding effects.

The integrated paradigm encourages sound hypothesis testing by (1) linking problems to specific etiological and intervention implications, (2) using goal-setting procedures (as in traditional problem-oriented models), (3) requiring specific key indicators to operationally define changes predicted by the hypothesis, and (4) requiring that problems be prioritized according to etiological hypotheses (thus reducing the risk of confounding interventions). Quantitative changes on key indicators and achievement of specific goals constitute operational expressions of the team's hypotheses about the nature of the problem and its most effective solution. In addition, the integrated paradigm includes a formal procedure of progress evaluation to be conducted by the team, at the regular intervals prescribed by accreditation standards. This procedure, which is an adaptation of goal attainment scaling, takes advantage of the high degree of specification and measurement already built into the rehabilitation plan. For each problem, the team reviews all data on provision of intervention modalities, the recovering person's participation and response, attainment of short-term goals, key indicators, and anecdotal reports, and translates this information into a single quantitative characterization of progress toward the long-term goal and remaining short-term goals.

A seven-point scale is sufficient to characterize a team's appraisal of progress toward long- and short-term goals. On the scale, a value of zero indicates that the team can discern no progress, or "no change," since the previous evaluation (or the initial assessment). Positive numbers reflect progress toward the goal. A value of two means that the recovering person has made "expected progress" toward the goal. A value of one means that some progress is discerned—that is, the scale value is not zero, but the degree of progress falls short of expectation. A value of three means that progress has exceeded expectation. Negative numbers mean negative progress, or "backsliding," and the scale values reflect degrees of severity: minimal, marked, or severe.

In the conventional use of goal attainment scaling, operational definitions would be constructed for each of the scale values, so that, for example, a "two" would be defined in terms of a specific degree of change on a particular instrument. However, in rehabilitation, progress toward meaningful goals can seldom be represented credibly by a single operational measure. It is usually advantageous to include several independent measures to characterize a problem and its associated rehabilitation goals. In addition, unanticipated information that has significant implications for progress evaluation may become available. To accommodate these realities, the integrated paradigm requires the team to use all available data to determine the progress rating for each goal.

Thus, as a progress review is completed, the team assigns a progress rating value to each long-term goal and to short-term goals not yet achieved. This collection of ratings then assists the team in making an overall determination about whether the rehabilitation plan is working according to expectation. A preponderance of "minimal progress" and "no change" ratings suggests that something is wrong. A rehabilitation plan may not yield expected progress for a number of reasons:

1. The particular intervention modalities selected for addressing problems have been ineffectively implemented.
2. The problems themselves are mischaracterized (i.e., the team's etiological hypotheses are incorrect).
3. The team has overlooked a preemptive problem (i.e., one that is compromising the effectiveness of the intervention modalities).
4. The key indicators are not accurate indicators of progress.
5. The goals generally reflect unrealistic expectations.

It is necessary for the team to assess all such possibilities and revise the rehabilitation plan accordingly. Revision may constitute anything from minor adjustments in the parameters of intervention modalities to a complete overhaul of the team's formulation.

It bears repeating that progress evaluation is an extension and continuation of assessment. The planned use of specific measurements for progress evaluation purposes is guided by hypotheses constructed in response to initial assessment data. The progress evaluation is the last step in implementing the rehabilitation plan but the first step in updating or revising the plan. Rehabilitation is a continuous cycle. Like science itself, rehabilitation proceeds as a formal discipline of hypothesis construction, testing, and revision. Also like science, the formal discipline is accompanied by human valuation and creativity, and by a shifting and evolving understanding of human nature and the universe. The cycle of assessment, planning, and progress evaluation brings all these processes together, as they play themselves out in the work of rehabilitation teams. In the integrated paradigm, the progress rating procedure plays a key role in coordinating the scientific, technological, and social processes that drive the rehabilitation cycle. A summative, consensual interpretation of all available information, operationally defined as the progress rating, is central to this role.

## Integration of Technological and Social Processes

In the integrated paradigm, assessment and rehabilitation planning are unifying processes that require a degree of scientific precision in defining and measuring the problems, goals, and solutions. However, identifying problems and goals and interpreting progress data are not lockstep processes that occur "automatically" when the scientific and technological conditions are optimal. Human social processes are involved at every stage. Rehabilitation is inevitably a collaborative enterprise, involving individuals working together in different roles. A given individual may even perform different roles at different times. The members of the treatment team must interact to ensure that goals are meaningful as well as measurable. Each team member's personal perspective helps define what is meaningful, but a person's beliefs and desires cannot change scientific realities. In constructing hypotheses about the etiology of problems, team members must make "educated guesses," and some guesses will be better than others. It is *expected* that initial hypotheses will be unsupported by data occasionally, that interventions will fail or be only partially effective, that problems will have to be redefined, that plans will have to be reformulated. In evaluating progress, the effectiveness of interventions, and, ultimately, the validity of their formulation, the team must consider variables that are too numerous and complex to anticipate fully, and they must arrive at a social consensus about what it all means. Procedural conventions, such as those described in this chapter, provide guidance and structure as teams struggle with the complexities of rehabilitation, but no conventions can replace the judgments and decisions that emerge from the totality of human experience. The integrated paradigm requires that team members not only follow the conventions of assessment, formulation, planning, and progress evaluation, but also that they perform their various roles—as recovering person, consumer, mental health professional, scientist, technologist, therapist, and human being—as circumstances demand.

The next seven chapters focus on the scientific and technological particulars of rehabilitating people with disabling mental illness. Some of these particulars are helpful in elucidating relevant human values as well as suggesting solutions to problems. Chapters 9 and 10 focus on the social processes that must occur within a team, and within a mental health service agency, to bring together human values, scientific understanding, and technological solutions into unitary, effective rehabilitation plans. The assessment, formulation, planning, and progress evaluation conventions described in this chapter provide an organizational framework for these social processes. To provide a working appreciation of the role of the integrated paradigm's procedural conventions in the larger rehabilitation enterprise, an annotated rehabilitation plan is included in Appendix 2. The plan shows how the rehabilitation team formulated the case of Joe, our fictional recovering person introduced in Chapter 2. Readers are invited to study Appendix 2 now for its overall organizational framework, and to return to it periodically to observe how the technological particulars of the following chapters are represented in it.

# Part II

# ASSESSMENT AND TREATMENT TECHNIQUES

The seven chapters of Part II describe the clinical technologies relevant to the rehabilitation of people with disabling mental illness. In keeping with the concept that technology represents the convergence of social problems and science, the chapters discuss distinct types of problems encountered in this field; in keeping with principles of contemporary psychopathology, the chapters also utilize heuristic divisions that reflect levels of biosystemic organization: neurophysiological, neurocognitive, sociocognitive, sociobehavioral, and socioenvironmental. Chapter content progresses from the most molecular level of functioning pertinent to rehabilitation, the neurophysiological level, to the most molar, the socioenvironmental level. Each chapter includes an account of the aspects of mental illness that are associated with the respective levels of analysis, a description of the technologies that derive from this understanding, and a discussion of the systematic use of those technologies within the integrated paradigm.

# Chapter 4

# The Neurophysiological
# Level of Functioning

The neurophysiological level of functioning includes all biochemical activity and its interactions with cellular structures in nerve tissue. The neurophysiological functioning of the central nervous system (CNS) is of primary importance in rehabilitation. However, the neurophysiology of peripheral sensory and motor nerves and the autonomic nervous system is not generally thought to be relevant to mental illness. Although dysfunctions in the peripheral and autonomic nervous systems certainly occur in mental illness, these are generally attributable to problems in CNS physiology or more molar levels of organization (e.g., psychophysiological processes) discussed in Chapter 9. Recent findings regarding the role of humoral factors in mental illness suggest that interactions between the endocrine system and the CNS should be included as neurophysiological factors relevant to rehabilitation.

## EVOLUTION OF NEUROPHYSIOLOGICAL
## MODELS FOR MENTAL ILLNESS

Our scientific understanding of the role of neurophysiology in mental illness comes from numerous sources. The first important contributions of our contemporary era came from the experimental psychopathology laboratories of the 1930s, in the form of paradigms for measuring sensory, psychomotor, and autonomic processes that are closely linked to neurophysiology (for historical accounts, see Green, 1998; Maher, 1966). Abnormalities in such molecular psychological processes as reaction time, flicker fusion (the time frame in which two brief light flashes are seen as one), and habituation of the orienting reflex were difficult to explain with psychoana-

73

lytic or sociological theories of mental illness. Other experimental paradigms of this period showed abnormalities at more molar levels of cognitive functioning as well, such as in concept manipulation, but these had credible (at the time) accounts in psychodynamic theories. Neurophysiology was implicated only indirectly, but for several decades this implication was the strongest scientific evidence available for biological factors in mental illness. Later, these paradigms provided important clues about the nature of biological vulnerability to mental illness as well as the neurophysiology of the illness itself.

There had been widespread suspicion for over a century that mental illness "runs in families." Heredity must be expressed in some kind of physiological process, so evidence for a genetic factor in mental illness would be evidence, though still indirect, of neurophysiological factors. In the 1960s credible evidence of a genetic factor in mental illness began to appear. Scientific detection of a genetic factor was not so much a conceptual breakthrough as a methodological feat. Separating purely biological (genetic) factors from social and psychological factors in family environments required study of people with identical genes (identical or monozygotic twins) raised in different environments. Gradually this logistical challenge was met, and the preponderance of evidence indicated there are genetic factors in mental illness, separate from environmental factors (Gottesman, Shields, & Hanson, 1982).

By the end of the 20th century it was broadly accepted that severe mental illness has a significant genetic component, but the research had also revealed unexpected complexities. Specific diagnoses do not "breed true"; that is, a family history of schizophrenia does not appear to produce only schizophrenia. The genetic evidence is strongest when a range of diagnoses is included. The term "schizophrenia spectrum" was used to characterize this range, which included severe affective disorders and sometimes even alcoholism. The genetic factors, and presumably the neurophysiological factors that reflect them, appear to represent a broad *vulnerability* to severe mental illness, not to a specific disease. The vulnerability concept was quickly assimilated into theories of psychopathology. In the last two decades of the 20th century, much research was conducted on individuals with genetic vulnerabilities to mental illness, not only to articulate the nature of these vulnerabilities but to discover possible protective factors that would keep vulnerable individuals from developing the illness (e.g., Carter & Flesher, 1995; Kern, Green, & Goldstein, 1995; Liberman, 1986; Nuechterlein et al., 1992; Zubin & Spring, 1977). Theorists began constructing models of mental illness (including neurophysiological models) that were consistent (or at least, not inconsistent) with the concept of vulnerability.

In the 1960s, contemporary psychiatric drugs came into widespread use.[1] Rigorous clinical studies confirmed that antipsychotic drugs dramatically suppress psychotic symptoms in 70–80% of the individuals who report them (reviewed by Marder, 1998). This was more direct and clinically important evidence for the role of neurophysiology in mental illness than the early findings of the experimental psychopathologists or even the genetic evidence. Antipsychotics generally perform dual roles in treatment: They act to resolve acute psychosis, and they prevent or postpone recurrence of psychosis.

Research on the mechanisms of antipsychotic drug action provided important clues about the neurophysiology of mental illness. Early on, the neurotransmitter dopamine appeared to play a central role in antipsychotic drug effects and therefore was suspected of playing a central role in mental illness. For a short time, it appeared that drug action might correspond to specific diagnoses, as expected by the neo-Kraepelinians. The dramatic effects of lithium salts on cycles of severe depression and mania, associated with the diagnosis of bipolar disorder, were especially suggestive of simple, straightforward relationships between diagnostic category, neurophysiological etiology, and drug action. Even genetics appeared to be linked to the effectiveness of drug treatment. However, the picture became more complicated as new drugs were introduced and more research was conducted. The actions of antipsychotic drugs turned out to be enormously complex and are not fully understood to this day. Dopamine continues to be a focus of attention, but the mechanisms of psychosis and antipsychotic drug action are also thought to involve a large number of neurotransmitters and possibly other types of biochemicals. By the end of the 20th century there were antipsychotic drugs whose properties and mechanisms of action were so diverse, they were labeled "atypical antipsychotics." The atypical antipsychotics appear to be more effective than typicals in controlling symptoms associated with schizophrenia, and they may also be helpful with affective and psychophysiological problems (Meltzer & Fatemi, 1998). Bipolar disorder is increasingly treated with drugs other than lithium, such as atypical antipsychotics and anticonvulsants (Bowden, 1998). Some antidepressants are effective in suppressing obsessive–compulsive symptoms and social phobia, classified in DSM-IV as types of anxiety disorders (Taylor, 1998). Current research on drug effects increasingly includes neuropsychological and behavioral functioning as well as "symptom suppression." This research focuses on effects of drugs on specific domains of functioning,

---

[1]The term *psychiatric* is used here to distinguish the subset of drugs having broadly recognized clinical uses from the larger set of "psychotropic" drugs that has significant psychological and/or behavioral effects. *Contemporary* distinguishes these drugs from those used in psychiatry before the 1960s (e.g., barbiturates and reserpine), whose effects lacked both the efficacy and the specificity of contemporary drugs.

from neurophysiological to cognitive to behavioral, and psychiatric diagnosis is a secondary consideration, at best.

The late 20th century saw scientific progress in many areas that contributed to an understanding of the neurophysiological substratum in mental illness (reviewed by Knable, Kleinman, & Weinberger, 1998). Electrophysiological paradigms provided important clues about the links between neurophysiology and cognition and about individual differences in neurophysiological functioning among people with mental illness. For example, deficits in attention and vigilance were found to correspond to low amplitudes of brain waves evoked by experimental stimuli. Radioimaging techniques made it possible to study neurophysiological activity in living, working brains, both healthy and ill. Advanced methods for behavioral observation and assessment provided a clearer picture of the course of illness and the nature of its symptoms—considerations that must be taken into account in neurophysiological models. Examples include the Nurses Observational Scale for Inpatient Evaluation (NOSIE; Honigfeld, Gillis, & Klett, 1966) and the Brief Psychiatric Rating Scale (BPRS; Ventura, Green, Shaner, & Liberman, 1993), both still in common use. Although data produced by these instruments tend to undermine rather than support the validity of diagnostic categories, they provide an unprecedented level of precision and accuracy in the measurement of abnormal behavior as it changes over time. Neuropsychology made it possible to extend assessment of drug effects to an entirely new domain, neurocognitive functioning (e.g., Green & Nuechterlein, 1999; Meltzer, Thompson, Lee, & Ranjan, 1996). The cumulative understanding of mental illness that these scientific enterprises have produced fills volumes, and many believe the most important discoveries are yet to come.

As with drug effects, much work has been invested in determining which neurophysiological abnormalities are unique to specific diagnostic categories. Differences are often found between one or another categories, but these are generally overshadowed by the heterogeneity within categories and overlapping distributions. We understand quite a lot about neurophysiological abnormalities in mental illness, but what we understand is only loosely linked to diagnostic categories. Nevertheless, there is still a tendency in the psychopathology community to think about, organize, and discuss the neurophysiology of mental illness in terms of diagnostic categories. Hence there are neurophysiological theories about the etiology of schizophrenia, and so on. However, such theories are actually explanatory models of specific processes or characteristics associated with, but not unique to nor required for, diagnosis. Recognition of this separation between what we know and our theories and categories *about* that knowledge is central to the growing separation of theoretical psychopathology (including the neurophysiological level of analysis) from the neo-Kraepelinian diagnostic system.

There is a corresponding trend in the main branch that applies the findings of neurophysiological research: *psychopharmacotherapy*.[2] As drug treatment of mental illness evolves, it is increasingly clear that drug effects do not respect diagnostic boundaries. As a result, diagnosis has limited usefulness when making decisions about pharmacotherapy. Nevertheless, as a central tenet of the medical model, Kraepelinian and neo-Kraepelinian diagnostic categories are deeply entrenched in the psychiatric community. Standards of psychiatric practice are organized according to diagnostic groups, which means that clinicians are compelled to consider diagnosis in their clinical decision making. It is noteworthy that there are no standards of practice for people who almost, but not quite, meet diagnostic criteria for schizophrenia—for those who receive a diagnosis of "psychosis not otherwise specified." Also, it is never clear how standards of practice should be applied in cases of comorbidity. Standards of practice do not have to be organized around diagnoses, and such standards generally recommend treating specifically targeted problems anyway. We really do not know very much about how clinicians make decisions about psychopharmacotherapy, and the contrast between different kinds of standards of practice (e.g., accreditation of health care documentation requirements vs. clinicians' standards of practice) presents a paradoxical picture. If current trends continue, however, clinical decision making in psychopharmacotherapy is expected to focus increasingly on targeting specific functional problems in specific domains, with decreasing consideration of neo-Kraepelinian diagnosis. This shift may necessitate a fundamental change in how standards of practice are organized and articulated.

## CONTEMPORARY MODELS OF NEUROPHYSIOLOGICAL DYSREGULATION IN MENTAL ILLNESS

For the purposes of rehabilitation, a few key concepts emerge from the neurophysiology of mental illness. A biosystemic paradigm of psychopathology is helpful in organizing these concepts.

### Neurophysiological Dysregulation in the CNS

In the brain's biosystem there are a number of relatively distinct subsystems, defined by combinations of anatomical structures and biochemical

---

[2]*Psychopharmacotherapy*, the use of psychotropic drugs for therapeutic purposes, is to be distinguished from *psychopharmacology*, which is the broader scientific discipline that studies the psychological and behavioral effects of drugs.

constituents. Normally these subsystems interact to maintain optimal neurophysiological conditions for processing information. The interactions are essentially regulatory in nature, in the sense that homeostasis is maintained in a biosystem through the mutually regulatory actions of the system components upon each other. Suboptimal operation of these regulatory mechanisms, or *dysregulation*, produces suboptimal information processing, which in turn produces suboptimal functioning at multiple levels and in multiple functional components of the complete biosystem.

One type of dysregulation, arguably that most associated with the diagnosis of schizophrenia, is thought to involve interactions between the brain's limbic system (including the basal ganglia) and the frontal cortex (Weinberger, 1994; Weinberger & Lipska, 1995). The limbic system includes a number of subcortical structures and phylogenically primitive parts of the cortex. The frontal cortex is the most recently evolved part of the human brain and appears to mediate the most complex aspects of human behavior. There is normally a regulatory relationship between these components, such that lower structures monitor sensory input for potentially alarming information and activate higher structures accordingly ("higher" and "lower" are used as a rhetorical convenience in this context to distinguish between phylogenically primitive brain areas, generally deeper in the brain, and more recently evolved areas, generally closer to the brain's outer surfaces).

Activation of higher cortical activity produces a negative feedback signal to the lower components, moderating their activity, and shutting off the alarm signals. Presumably, this regulatory process is a mechanism for activating those subsystems that formulate complex behavioral responses, when environmental conditions indicate such responses may be needed. In mental illness, this regulatory relationship is compromised, so that limbic activation fails to activate higher cortical activity (Weinberger, 1987). Two proximal effects result: First, the higher-level cortical activity is insufficient to cope with environmental exigencies; second, without the negative feedback from higher cortical areas, the lower structures remain in a highly active "alarm status." The lower structures cannot maintain neurophysiological stability under these conditions for very long. At some point, a cascade of neurophysiological events occurs that compromises the functioning of a number of brain mechanisms, including those responsible for the basic organization of sensory input, emotional regulation, and organization of complex behavior.

The limbic–cortical model accounts for a number of characteristics of severe mental illness, especially those associated with the Kraepelinian diagnosis of schizophrenia. However, there is no reason to believe the mechanisms described in the model do not apply to individuals with other diagnoses that share these characteristics. Abnormal development of limbic and cortical neural structures and pathways could produce the faulty activating mechanism. Such abnormal development could be caused by a variety of factors, ranging from birth-related brain injury to prenatal viral infection to high levels of prenatal stress (resulting in toxic levels of the stress hormone cortisol) to genetic anomalies. This multiplicity of potentially causal agents would account for the multiplicity of genetic and perinatal factors that appear to be involved in etiology. In addition, various anatomical, histological, and radioimaging studies have shown structural abnormalities, possibly the result of abnormal development, in limbic and cortical areas of the brains of people diagnosed with schizophrenia. The higher cortical structures in the model do not mature until adolescence (Casey, Giedd, & Thomas, 2000; Davies & Rose, 1999), suggesting an explanation for the adolescent onset of mental illness. Indeed, in adolescents who meet diagnostic criteria for schizophrenia, frontal functioning has been found to be impaired shortly after the onset of their illness (Karp et al., 2001). The compromised activation system represents a *vulnerability* that results in overt illness through interaction with stress (i.e., the conditions that trigger the limbic alarm). The model also accounts for the distinction between positive and negative symptoms of psychosis. Negative symptoms reflect insufficient activation of higher cortical functions, while positive symptoms reflect the sensory, cognitive, and behavioral organization associated with limbic overactivation. The episodic nature of limbic overactivation may correspond to the episodic pattern of psychosis observed in many individuals.

Of course, it will take considerably more research to flesh out the details of the limbic–cortical dysregulation, but it is now well enough supported to allow reasonable expectation that some such model will eventually provide a good account of a particular kind of CNS dysregulation in severe mental illness. Indeed, given the current rate of progress, we might expect that a fairly complete account is almost within reach. On the other hand, research has revealed an unexpected degree of complexity in the neurophysiology of mental illness, so a complete account may be more distant than it appears.

Antipsychotic drugs are thought to act upon various components of a dysregulated limbic–cortical system. The first generations of antipsychotic drugs, the neuroleptics, generally appear to act upon the D2 dopamine receptor, which is probably crucial to the limbic activating process. The most recent generation of antipsychotics, the atypicals, have a number of actions that do not involve the D2 receptor.

The scientific evidence suggests that there are at least four other types of neurophysiological CNS dysregulation that can operate independent of the limbic–cortical connection, and all are potentially relevant to severe mental illness:

- Depression-related dysregulation
- Mania-related dysregulation
- Excitation-related dysregulation
- Anxiety-related dysregulation

## Depression-Related Dysregulation

The first of these is associated with the clinical picture of depression (Musselman et al., 1998). It appears to involve a widely distributed neurophysiological subsystem, with at least two important neurotransmitters, noradrenalin (NA, also known as norepinephrine, NE) and serotonin (5-hydroxytryptamine, 5-HT). The antidepressant drugs alter the activity of these neurotransmitters by blocking their *postsynaptic reuptake*, the process by which neurotransmitters are retrieved, after release into the synapse, by the neuron that released them. The fact that severe depression can exist without any psychotic symptoms, and that antipsychotic drugs usually are not helpful with depression, indicates that neurophysiological dysregulation of this type can operate independent of the limbic–cortical axis. However, this is not to say that it *always* operates independently. Severe depression is sometimes accompanied by psychosis, psychosis is often accompanied by affective symptoms, and depression is often a warning sign of an impending psychotic episode (Herz & Melville, 1980). A clinical picture of mixed depressive and psychotic symptoms may respond best to antidepressants, antipsychotics, or some combination. Atypical antipsychotics appear to have significant effects on serotonin regulation, to which some of their effects on affective (as well as psychotic) symptoms may be attributable. It is reasonable to expect that, under some conditions and in some individuals, there is sufficient interaction between the limbic–cortical and depression-related systems that dysregulation of one could be closely associated with dysregulation of the other.

Ambiguities about the relationship between "psychotic" and "affective" disorders pervade psychopathology. These ambiguities correspond to the ambiguity about relationships between limbic–cortical dysregulation and dysregulations from other pathways. Neo-Kraepelinian diagnosis requires a rather subjective judgment about whether "schizophrenic" or "affective" symptoms "predominate" in a clinical picture. A diagnostic distinction between schizophrenia and depression may rest on whether the patient's delusions are "mood congruent"—also a subjective judgment, to some degree. Research on depression and schizophrenia generally does not include diagnostically ambiguous cases, making it difficult to draw conclusions about relationships between different types of underlying CNS dysregulation. At the more molecular level, it is certainly possible to construct plausible theories about how dopaminergic, noradrenergic, and serotenergic systems could be interlinked. However, diagnostic categories are not a key concept in such theories.

It is important to note that depression is an expected reaction to protracted adverse circumstances. In this context, there is nothing "abnormal" about a person with disabling mental illness being depressed. Although depression may have a neurophysiological component, this does not mean that the best solution is always pharmacotherapy. Chronic depression (in less severe forms, diagnosed as dysthymia) often reflects a complex constellation of cognitive and behavioral processes that contribute to the neurophysiological level of the problem. Psychosocial treatment is at least as effective as psychopharmacotherapy for many individuals with depression (reviewed by Schmidt, Koselka, & Woolaway-Bickel, 2001), and there is no reason to believe this is less true for people who also have severe mental illness. In the integrated paradigm, the concept of mood-related psychophysiological dysregulation (discussed in Chapter 9) represents an alternative that rehabilitation teams should always consider when assessing depression. In some cases, psychosocial interventions may be a better choice than drug treatment. (For a detailed discussion of balancing psychopharmacotherapy with psychosocial interventions in depression, see Pettit, Voelz, & Joiner, 2001.)

## Mania-Related Dysregulation

Another type of dysregulation is that associated with mania (Musselman et al., 1998). It is generally accepted that mania is the polar opposite of depression, produced by dysregulation of the same system but in the opposite direction. Antidepressant drugs can sometimes produce mania and related symptoms in people with depression who have never experienced those symptoms before. However, the neo-Kraepelinian distinction between unipolar and bipolar affective disorder implies two separate factors. It remains unknown whether the depression that accompanies mania in a cycling bipolar picture is different from depression in a unipolar picture. Neither the one-factor nor two-factor theory of mania–depression enjoys a preponderance of support in the psychopathology community. Like depression, mania often occurs in the absence of other symptoms, and mania and related symptoms often appear along with other psychotic symptoms. Whether there is a separate dysregulation associated with mania, or whether it is a variation of the depression-related dysregulation, it is reasonable to expect that it could be closely linked to limbic–cortical dysregulation in some people. Optimal drug treatment for a mixed presentation of schizophrenic and manic symptoms may prove to be an antipsychotic, lithium, an anticonvulsant, or some combination. An antidepressant may also contribute in some cases.

## Excitation-Related Dysregulation

A third type of dysregulation is associated with excitability, irritability, impulsiveness, and explosiveness, and with a reduction of these behaviors in response to drug intervention (Buchanan, 1995; Menditto et al., 1996; Yudofsky, Silver, & Hales, 1998). This type of dysregulation is the least understood of the types considered here. Although the behavioral characteristics occur in people who do not meet diagnostic criteria for bipolar disorder or schizophrenia, many of those who do meet criteria also show these characteristics. A wide variety of drugs may be beneficial, including anticonvulsants, anxiolytics, adrenergic beta-blockers, and atypical antipsychotics. This type of problem probably reflects broadly generalized cortical dysregulation, which can either exist independently or in association with the other types.

Behaviors associated with this type of dysregulation often cause a disproportionate amount of concern when they include socially unacceptable or aggressive features. However, such behaviors are not uncommon in settings that serve people with severe mental illness, and they are not always eliminated through neurophysiological intervention. Nevertheless, there is often strong pressure on providers to "do something" to control the behaviors. In medical model settings, where there is little or no use of psychosocial interventions, there is a tendency to persist with ineffective drug approaches, sometimes leading to complex regimens and/or excessive doses. Especially in institutional settings, people who exhibit persistent aggressive or otherwise unacceptable behavior often receive large amounts of ineffective drugs—while the behavior continues (Hunter, 2000). A neurophysiological hypothesis about this type of behavior is sometimes well supported by drug response data, but often not. The rehabilitation team must always be prepared to entertain an alternative hypothesis—that the behavior represents cognitive, sociobehavioral, and/or socioenvironmental problems, and use psychosocial interventions accordingly (discussed in Chapters 8, 9, and 10). (For discussions of choosing between psychopharmacological and psychosocial interventions for aggressive behavior, see Hunter, 2000; Yudofsky, Silver, & Hales, 1995. Interestingly, Yudofsky and colleagues' chapter in the 1998 edition of the American Psychiatric Association's *Textbook of Psychopharmacology* includes no mention of any psychosocial alternatives for addressing aggression, in contrast to the extensive discussion provided in the 1995 edition.)

## Anxiety-Related Dysregulation

The clinical expressions of a fourth type of dysregulation roughly fall under the neo-Kraepelinian rubric of anxiety disorders (Stein & Uhde, 1998; Taylor, 1998). However, this is another case where Kraepelinian categories fit neither clinical expression nor response to types of drugs (see especially Ban, 2001). In neo-Kraepelinian terms, anxiety disorders have high levels of comorbidity with depression and psychotic disorders. In the terms of the integrated paradigm, people with severe mental illness often have difficulty regulating their anxiety response. In clinical practice, people with severe mental illness are often prescribed anxiolytic (anxiety-suppressing) drugs for anxiety-related problems, and these drugs may indeed suppress anxiety (Sirota, Epstein, Benatov, Sousnostzky, & Kindler, 2001). Often, anxiolytic drugs (or other drugs chosen for their sedating or hypnotic effects) are used to treat insomnia, especially when it appears to be associated with anxiety. Interestingly, psychosocial interventions (especially cognitive-behavioral psychotherapy) are seldom used for anxiety problems in severe mental illness, even though their effectiveness in treating anxiety disorders is at least as good as psychopharmacotherapy (reviewed by Pettit, Voelz, & Joiner, 2001). There are several possible reasons for this lacuna, although they are not necessarily supportable or justifiable reasons. For one, clinicians may maintain a belief (that has no empirical support) that the characteristics of severe mental illness (e.g., cognitive impairments) render people less able to respond to psychotherapy. For another, resources for providing effective cognitive-behavioral psychotherapy in public settings may be scarce, especially compared to the expedience of drug treatment. Recently, many researchers have noted that people with severe mental illness sometimes have distinct patterns of anxiety dysregulation that do not simply cascade from their schizophrenia or other severe condition (Banchard, Mueser, & Bellack, 1998; Cosoff & Hafner, 1998; Halperin, Nathan, Drummond, & Castle, 2000; Penn, Hope, Spaulding, & Kucera, 1994). Hopefully, systematic research that uses interventions with known effectiveness for anxiety disorders will be conducted with people who also have a severe mental illness.

Clinical anxiety is associated with a fairly specific brain mechanism whose activity mediates passive avoidance learning in lower mammals and the subjective experience of fear and anxiety in humans. The mechanism appears to be regulated by a specific neurotransmitter, gamma-amino butyric acid (GABA), and the actions of anxiolytic drugs appear to involve a GABA receptor. However, serotonin also plays an important part, and serotonergic drugs have become the drugs of choice for anxiety disorders. It is not clear whether clinical anxiety represents an actual dysregulation of GABA or serotonin mechanisms, or, indeed, whether GABA and serotonin represent two discreet mechanisms or two components of a single mechanism. Fear and anxiety are complex psychological processes that involve learning and conditioning. Anxiety "disorders" may represent "normal" neurophysiological processes operating in the context of "abnormal" learning and conditioning. The dual role of serotonergic drugs in the treatment of both anxiety and depression disorders raises questions about whether these disorders represent the same neurophysiological etiologies.

Drug intervention for anxiety-related dysregulation may actually compromise psychosocial treatment effects, probably by interfering with learning and conditioning. The humanitarian intent to give a person relief from distressing anxiety must be carefully weighed against possible countertherapeutic effects. In addition to interfering with psychosocial treatment, there is a potentially harmful implication that drugs are a desirable antidote to the normal anxieties and stresses of everyday life. As with depression, rehabilitation teams working in the integrated paradigm should always consider a hypothesis that anxiety responses are normal responses to extraordinary stress, and/or a failure of psychophysiological self-regulation skills (discussed in Chapter 9), before resorting to pharmacological interventions. (For detailed discussions of balancing psychopharmacotherapeutic and psychosocial interventions for anxiety problems, see Antony & Swinson, 2001; Morin, 2001; Schmidt, Koselka, & Woolaway-Bickel, 2001.) Similarly, teams should carefully consider whether anxiety and depression represent two different problems or a single problem, whether expressed at the neurophysiological, cognitive, or behavioral levels.

## Tonic and Episodic Dysregulation

The clinical picture most closely associated with CNS dysregulation in severe mental illness is that of *episodic psychosis*. This is a pattern in which relatively severe psychotic symptoms emerge during the episode, or "acute psychosis," interspersed with relatively asymptomatic periods. There is enormous variability on many dimensions of psychotic episodes, including frequency, duration, overall severity, quality of symptoms, type and degree of cognitive impairment during the episode, and the overall difference in functioning between acute psychosis and baseline. In some individuals, baseline functioning is so similar to acute psychosis that the episodic course of the illness is undetectable. Similarly, in some individuals the acute psychosis is so protracted that episodes cannot be observed. At the other extreme, some people experience a complete breakdown in personal and social functioning during acute psychosis but no significant difficulties between episodes.

It is clear that the dimensions of psychotic episodes are related to clinical outcome. The more severe and protracted the acute psychosis, and the more frequent the episodes, the more guarded the prognosis (see Cromwell, 1975). This interrelationship is not to be confused with the prognostic significance of untreated psychosis early in the course of illness, or the prognostic significance of various characteristics of early psychosis, both of which remain controversial (de Haan, van der Gaag, & Wolthaus, 2000; McGlashan, 1999). The classic finding that long-term outcome is related to the severity, duration, and frequency of psychotic episodes over the course of the illness is uncontroversial. For the affected individual, psychosis is an extremely distressing and undesirable state. It disrupts most aspects of routine daily functioning and often precludes benefiting from rehabilitation. For these reasons, and because episodic psychoses are ubiquitous in disabling mental illness, eliminating them or at least minimizing their effects is one of the most common rehabilitation and recovery goals.

Not all forms of psychosis are episodic. Many individuals with mental illness experience psychotic symptoms and related problems (e.g., neurocognitive impairments, discussed in Chapters 5–7) between psychotic episodes. The episodes may be marked only by an increase in the severity of symptoms that are present all the time. This omnipresence of symptoms indicates that the CNS dysregulation underlying psychosis has *tonic* as well as episodic aspects. In neo-Kraepelinian terms, this idea is most clearly represented in the concept of residual schizophrenia, although there is no reason to believe that residual psychosis is unique to schizophrenia. Psychopathology is paying increased attention to residual symptoms and residual cognitive impairments, partly in response to a recent accumulation of evidence that the severity of residual cognitive impairments is a strong predictor of personal and social functioning. Atypical antipsychotics appear to reduce the neurocognitive impairment associated with the residual phase of psychosis, relative to neuroleptics, suggesting that they more effectively address the tonic aspects of the dysregulation.

Even when there is no evident functional problem between episodes, a covert level of dysregulation might operate in the form of a vulnerability to more overt dysfunction. For example, in limbic–cortical dysregulation, a tonic state may lower the threshold for catastrophic limbic arousal under stress.

The CNS dysregulations associated with depression, dysthymia, explosiveness, and anxiety (to the degree that they are really neurophysiological at all) appear generally to produce tonic rather than episodic problems (episodic severe depression would be an exception). Depression, dysthymia, extreme irritability, explosiveness, and anxiety are all problems potentially relevant to rehabilitation and recovery.

## Identifying CNS Dysregulation

Although the accumulation of scientific evidence overwhelmingly supports the existence of neurophysiological dysregulations related to mental illness, there is no specific measurement paradigm or test that directly and conclusively indicates the presence of a dysregulation in a specific individual. It must be inferred from behavioral and phenomenological data—that is, from observation of behavior and the subjective report of the affected individual. Such inferences can be made more confidently in some cases than others. All the signs and symptoms of neurophysiological dysregulation can be produced by other etiologies.

Rehabilitation usually begins after an individual has been receiving conventional psychiatric treatment long enough to have produced some data on the individual's response to pharmacotherapy. Further drug trials are often helpful in supporting the existence, and articulating the nature, of a neurophysiological dysregulation. In some cases, a systematic process of elimination must be performed to rule out alternative explanations of psychosis or other behavioral or psychological problems. Ultimately, successful identification and treatment of a neurophysiological dysregulation requires careful and systematic hypothetico-deductive analysis throughout the assessment and rehabilitation process.

Assessment and rehabilitation of neurophysiological dysregulation requires two different sets of technology. The first set includes the biomedical technologies that make it possible to safely administer any drug (psychiatric and other), monitor the patient's biological response, and manage biomedical side effects. The second set includes the assessment technologies by which a drug's psychological and behavioral effects can be measured, and the hypothetico-deductive methods that shape the team's understanding of the dysregulation and its impact on personal and social functioning. The first set is traditionally the province of medical professionals. However, in the field of rehabilitation, resolving biomedical issues requires broader participation of the rehabilitation team because choices that have broader implications for personal and social functioning must be made. For example, sometimes difficult choices must be made between optimal control of psychosis, minimizing side effects, and managing residual symptoms and impairments. Biomedical technology illuminates the options, but determining the best option falls to the team members. The second set of technologies also requires the participation of the entire team, because the psychological and behavioral effects of psychiatric drugs may pervade all levels and domains of personal and social functioning.

## FORMULATING NEUROPHYSIOLOGICAL
## PROBLEMS IN THE INTEGRATED PARADIGM

### Rationale

The prototype problem set (Appendix 1) lists two types of CNS dysregulation, episodic and tonic. This formulation is a departure from the conventional PROMIS system, in that PROMIS problems are usually identified in terms of reports of delusions, hallucinations, and disorganized behavior, not hypothetical neurophysiological processes. However, defining a problem in purely behavioral terms neglects etiology and provides no logical link to treatment. Diagnosis offers nothing better in this regard. In the integrated paradigm, the neurophysiological problem titles specifically reflect a hypothesis that there is a neurophysiological problem, producing a significant barrier to optimal functioning, which is within the reach of current psychopharmacotherapeutic technology—that is, a problem that will respond to pharmacological intervention. If the problem proves to be beyond the reach of pharmacotherapy, it must be identified with a different problem title.

The existence of distinct drug families (antipsychotics, antidepressants, etc.) may seem to suggest that CNS dysregulations be subcategorized accordingly—for example, "CNS dysregulation of the psychotic type" or "CNS dysregulation of the depression type." However, drug families are derived in part from earlier and unsupported assumptions about the correspondence between drug action and diagnostic categories. "Antidepressants" are now the drug treatment of choice for "anxiety disorders." Optimal treatment of psychosis sometimes requires drugs from other than the antipsychotic family. Although the old drug families will probably be replaced by drug categories with names that reflect their molecular actions (as occurred with the appearance of the selective serotonin reuptake inhibitors [SSRIs]), it remains unclear whether these categories will correspond more closely to clinical effects. In many cases a neurophysiological problem is optimally resolved with a single drug. Nevertheless, the expression of the problem and its optimal psychopharmacotherapy are highly variable and idiosyncratic, especially in the case of severe and disabling mental illness. There is no particular value in categorizing neurophysiological problems according to behavioral expression or presumed treatment regimen, because each problem requires a unique problem description and unique intervention regimen.

In contrast, there are both conceptual and practical reasons to distinguish between tonic and episodic dysregulations. The latter typically generate intervention goals that are focused on resolving the episode and preventing its recurrence; the former typically generate intervention goals that are focused on continuous treatment, with the expectation of a gradual improvement in functioning. In addition, the day-to-day clinical management strategies tend to be different, and there is a fairly clear qualitative distinction, in that psychotic and depressive dysregulations are often episodic, while the other types seldom are.

At the start of rehabilitation there is often compelling evidence that an episodic CNS dysregulation is creating significant barriers to better functioning. In the least ambiguous case, the clinical history would report a distinct onset of psychotic symptoms in late adolescence, a premorbid history of normal personal and social functioning, absence of extraordinary stress or medical conditions that could account for the symptoms, a well-managed clinical trial of a psychiatric drug, resulting in elimination of the psychotic symptoms and a rapid return to baseline personal and social functioning, and a return of psychotic symptoms after discontinuation of the drug. The recovering person would recognize that the episode had recurred, would identify phenomenological and behavioral characteristics of it, and would perceive that the drug intervention had indeed affected the psychotic state. (It is important to note that if all, or even most, assessment issues held so little ambiguity, rehabilitation of severe mental illness would be a lot easier than it is.)

In the terminology of the integrated paradigm, the rehabilitation team would respond to this evidence by identifying an "episodic CNS dysregulation" as one problem. The problem description would detail the symptoms, related characteristics, frequency, and other relevant parameters of the acute psychosis. The long-term goal probably would be to prevent psychotic episodes. The short-term goals probably would be to increase the periods of time without acute psychosis and to foster specific knowledge and skills acquisition related to identifying early signs of an impending episode. The interventions would include a regimen of medication to prevent recurrence of the CNS dysregulation, plus psychoeducational procedures related to prevention and early warning. In addition, there probably would be a contingency plan describing what the various team members would do in the event of warning signs or recurrence of acute psychosis.

Even in an unambiguous case such as this, new data could undermine the team's confidence in their hypothesis of an episodic CNS dysregulation. Occasional recurrence of acute psychosis would not be disconfirmatory, as people do experience recurrences even when taking antipsychotic drugs. However, multiple recurrences or the appearance of psychotic symptoms without a clear recurrence of the episode would suggest that other problems might be present. Similarly, continuing difficulties in personal or social functioning, despite good response to medication, would suggest additional problems, whether or not they may be linked to the neurophysiological dysfunction. Interventions other than those originally planned may be necessary for optimal recovery.

## Case Application

The case of Joe, described in Chapter 2, presents a clinical picture more typical of rehabilitation. The neurophysiological dysregulation hypothesis is reasonably well supported by the data, but effective treatment of the episodic psychosis is insufficient, by itself, to bring about full recovery. In fact, there are factors that appear to interfere with direct treatment of the neurophysiological problem; for example, Joe appears to believe that he does not need medication. Such circumstances usually complicate the process of testing hypotheses about neurophysiological dysregulation. Later in rehabilitation, while Joe's refusal of treatment is temporarily overruled by his legal status, there is evidence, suggested by the presence of neuro-cognitive impairments that were not evident in Joe's premorbid history, that he may have a tonic CNS dysregulation in addition to the episodic one. Furthermore, there appears to be a period during Joe's recovery when his sense of hopelessness and failure are suggestive of depression, with its underlying independent neurophysiological component (reflected in choice of an antidepressant drug intervention).

Joe's nonadherence to drug treatment in the face of strong evidence of a serious but treatable problem may require extensive intervention at the cognitive level, by helping him develop more adaptive beliefs about, and understandings of, his illness. (Cognitive interventions are discussed further in Chapter 6.) Sometimes legal mechanisms present additional alternatives (as will be discussed in Chapter 10), and sometimes judicious manipulation of the pharmacotherapy regimen itself can resolve nonadherence problems. Nonadherence is often associated with drug side effects the recovering person finds significantly aversive. These side effects can be reduced sometimes by simply switching to a different antipsychotic drug (different people experience different side effects with a given drug), or using anticholinergic drugs or selective dopamine agonists to counteract the unwanted effects. Similarly, simplifying the dosage regimen is sometimes sufficient to achieve adherence without effecting extensive attitudinal changes. After resolution of the psychotic episode, it may be possible to reduce the dosage to a level more acceptable to the recovering person but still sufficient to reduce the risk of recurrence. In some cases (e.g., when side effects are severe or persistent), the most workable strategy may be to discontinue the drug after resolution of the episode, but with a "rapid response" plan in place, to be activated upon the first warning signs of recurrence. This last strategy is not usually advisable, as the evidence that "rapid response" effectively prevents recurrence of psychosis is weak (Herz & Melville, 1980). However, this might be the best option in some cases, and it is certainly better than nothing.

The appearance of a possible tonic CNS dysregulation presents the rehabilitation team with a number of options. One option is to hypothesize that the tonic dysregulation and its residual functional impairments represent an incomplete response to treatment of the episodic psychosis. The superiority of atypical antipsychotics over neuroleptics in producing fewer residual cognitive impairments may be attributable, in part, to a more complete resolution of the episodic dysregulation due to the atypicals. Switching to an atypical antipsychotic would thus be a logical intervention. If the residual impairments persist even with atypicals, additional alternative hypotheses must be considered.

Cognitive deficits are associated with depression-related dysregulation, which also fits Joe's clinical picture. A hypothesis based on this possibility is that there is a second CNS dysregulation problem, of the type associated with depression, requiring a different set of interventions. A trial of antidepressant drug treatment would be expected to provide the quickest test of this hypothesis. The comparable effectiveness of drug versus psychosocial treatment of depression (Schmidt et al., 2001) indicates that, over time, depression has significant neurophysiological *and* sociocognitive components. Drug treatment tends to produce faster symptom reduction, but psychotherapy produces a lower risk of relapse after discontinuation of treatment. For the purpose of testing hypotheses in a particular case, the rapidity of drug treatment is a salient factor. For the larger purposes of rehabilitation, the team also should consider treating the sociocognitive component of depression with appropriate psychotherapy. The success of reducing both the depressive symptoms and the cognitive impairments would constitute the strongest support for the hypothesis; reducing one but not the other would indicate partial support. This partial resolution would indicate the need to define a third problem in recognition of the functional independence of the cognitive impairments and the depression. None of these possibilities is unexpected in the rehabilitation of people with severe mental illness.

Complications multiply even more quickly when psychotic episodes are not clearly defined by the appearance of symptoms and their reduction in response to treatment. Many individuals experience only partial relief from psychotic symptoms in response to antipsychotic drugs. Others experience none at all. The difference between acute psychosis and residual psychotic symptoms is a relative one and qualitatively unique to individuals. Complicated pictures predominate in rehabilitation of severe mental illness. In most cases, the primary challenge to the rehabilitation team is to identify precisely what parts of the clinical picture are amenable to interventions based on a hypothesis of neurophysiological dysregulation—in other words, determining which parts are drug-responsive and which are not. However, the neurophysiological armamentarium is not completely limited to drugs. Electroconvulsive therapy, psychosurgery, and respite in a low-demand, low-stress environment are other options (not of comparable popularity) for treating proposed CNS dysregulations. (Cognitive and sociobehavioral technologies also can produce neurophysiological changes; however, such changes are presumably mediated by cognitive and/or sociobehavioral processes and therefore are discussed in subsequent chapters.) Over time, the response of specific aspects of the clinical picture to specific interventions refines and validates (or invalidates) the hypotheses reflected in the team's selection of problems.

Articulating the problem description is an important part of the team's work toward understanding interrelationships between neurophysiological dysregulation, symptoms, functional impairments, and clinical problems. The team might hypothesize that a number of elements in a particular clinical picture is part of a single cascade of neurophysiological events that culminate in psychotic episodes. In the rehabilitation plan this hypothesis would be represented by enumeration of a single problem, with all of its various consequences. For example:

PROBLEM 1

*Problem title*: Episodic CNS dysregulation

*Problem description*: Periods of acute distress accompanied by auditory hallucinations (voices making personal, disparaging remarks), confusion, extreme anxiety, neglect of self-care, intense feelings of guilt and hopelessness.

Alternatively, the team might hypothesize that the clinical picture reflects two functionally separate CNS dysregulations, producing different consequences and requiring different interventions. For example:

PROBLEM 1

*Problem title*: Episodic CNS dysregulation

*Problem description*: Periods of acute distress accompanied by auditory hallucinations (voices making personal, disparaging remarks), confusion, and extreme anxiety.

PROBLEM 2

*Problem title*: Tonic CNS dysregulation

*Problem Description*: Intense feelings of guilt and hopelessness, neglect of personal care, difficulty with routine problem solving.

Note that in adding the second problem, the team has separated elements in the single problem's description and added features to the second problem's description. Thus formulating some problems at any particular level of functioning can affect how other problems are formulated at different levels.

Goal setting is an important part of the team's deliberations about neurophysiological problems. Permanent elimination of psychotic episodes is a straightforward long-term goal with obvious implications for the recovering person's personal and social functioning. However, the high rate of relapse of even optimally medicated people makes it statistically unlikely that such a goal could be achieved. It is therefore always appropriate to include goals that address the probability of eventual relapse. A formal *relapse prevention plan* is often the best vehicle for this purpose (discussed further in Chapter 9). Relapse prevention plans are constructed by the rehabilitation team and based on information about the particular characteristics of the recovering person's psychotic episodes and personal circumstances. The plan identifies stressful conditions suspected of precipitating episodes, behavioral strategies for avoiding or managing those conditions, early warning signs of impending psychosis, and behavioral strategies for responding when those signs appear.

Residual symptoms and impairments present further challenges to goal setting. Not all psychotic symptoms can be eliminated, even temporarily. Perpetual pursuit of unresponsive symptoms with alternative drugs and higher doses can lead to overmedication, demoralization, and neglect of alternative strategies. At some point, the team must elect to limit the treatment goals or relegate the persisting symptoms or impairments to another problem formulation with a different intervention strategy. An example of the former would be to adjust the goal to one in which symptoms are stabilized at a level of severity that does not prohibit performance of routine daily activities. An example of the latter would be to select the problem of "disorder management deficit" and designate the goal as the acquisition and effective use of skills necessary to minimize the impact of the residual symptoms or impairment.

An important short-term goal of interventions based on psychopharmacotherapy is to determine the drug regimen that produces *optimal medication*. Achieving this optimal level is a highly individualized process because the complex interaction of symptom suppression, relapse prevention, degree of sedation (desirable and undesirable), and iatrogenic factors (side effects, including motor impairment, restlessness, cognitive impairment, and long-term health consequences of drug use) is different for everyone. Factors that render a regimen "optimal" include not only type of drug and dosage but the schedule of administration and involvement of others in ensuring adherence. All these variables must be determined through a comprehensive evaluation of the recovering person's functioning in response to systematic manipulation of the various dimensions of the regimen.

## ASSESSMENT AND PROGRESS EVALUATION TOOLS FOR NEUROPHYSIOLOGICAL DYSREGULATION

At the beginning of the rehabilitation process, the two most important sources of information about the possible presence of neurophysiological dysregulation are the recovering person and the case history. Hence, two key assessment technologies are anamnestic interviewing and case history interpretation. Other clinical assessment domains of special relevance include behavioral observation, neuropsychological assessment, and functional skills assessment. (For a general discussion of assessing the need for and response to interventions, with special consideration of the combined use of psychopharmacological and psychosocial modalities, see Meredith, Lambert, & Drozd, 2001; for sources on specific instruments, see Burns, 1995; Fischer & Corcoran, 1994.)

## Anamnestic Assessment

The basic skills for gathering information about a person's phenomenological experiences relevant to neurophysiological dysregulation are included in the general assessment repertoire of most mental health professionals. Evidence for the presence of a dysregulation includes subjective reports (of psychotic symptoms, depression, euphoria, etc.) and behavior (agitation, despondent mood, hostility, confusion, etc.) during the interview. Structured interview schedules for psychiatric diagnosis can be helpful to ensure complete coverage of potentially significant symptoms (see Ventura, Liberman, Green, Shaner, & Mintz, 1998). Quantitative rating scales (e.g., Andreasen, 1986) provide more precise indications of severity but address a limited range of symptoms and other behavioral characteristics. Generally, diagnostic schedules are more helpful at the outset, and quantitative rating scales are more helpful for assessing changes over time. It is always important to remember that CNS dysregulations can have unique and idiosyncratic expressions, and that a subjective report of an anomalous experience should not be dismissed because it does not correspond to any item on a schedule or rating scale.

Formal questionnaires can be used to augment anamnestic interview data. These questionnaires are typically in a problem checklist format, wherein the assessment subject indicates which items on a list of problems are applicable. Probably the most commonly used of these is the Symptom Checklist (SCL-90; Peveler & Fairburn, 1990), which lists 90 symptoms and other problems encountered in mental health settings. Self-report instruments such as the SCL-90 ensure comprehensive coverage of a person's clinically relevant experiences and may provide helpful clues about possible neurophysiological dysregulation. However, they have the same problems as other self-report measures: They depend on the subject's perceptions and recollections and therefore may convey deceptive information. In addition, although they may indicate what problems are present at one point in time, they are not reliable indicators of the severity, intensity, or frequency of the problems and hence have limited usefulness for evaluating progress, at least in the short term.

The subjective nature of anamnestic data puts it in the expansive domain of *social cognition*. In the integrated paradigm, the sociocognitive level of functioning includes beliefs, attitudes, and other complex cognitive processes. Sometimes the boundaries between symptoms and sociocognitive processes are unclear. For example, a delusion is a psychotic symptom, but it is also a belief. It may be a direct expression of neurophysiological dysregulation, or it may be a belief that is maintained by circumstances comparable to those that maintain "normal" beliefs, or some combination of the two (the latter is discussed further in Chapter 8). Similarly, the subjective distress associated with depression may be a direct expression of neurophysiological dysregulation of mood, or it may be a response to a plethora of environmental, behavioral, and cognitive factors (which is normally the case with subjective distress). In rehabilitation settings, we encounter a myriad of beliefs, values, attributions, and related phenomena whose relationship to neurophysiological functioning is a central issue. Assessment at the sociocognitive level requires careful analysis and sophisticated tools (these will be discussed in detail in Chapter 8). For present purposes, it suffices to say that people's beliefs about their illness, their symptoms and related problems, their subjective distress, the effectiveness of past and present interventions, and their own personal and social functioning are vastly more complex than can be assessed in an anamnestic interview. It is a serious but common error to mistake specific aspects of a person's social cognition as a symptom or other direct expression of neurophysiological dysregulation when it is a product of complex socioenvironmental factors. This error can be avoided by performing a complete assessment of social cognition, carefully identifying specific aspects hypothesized to be direct expressions of neurophysiological dysregulation, and recognizing that problems in social cognition that do not respond to neurophysiological intervention must be addressed in other ways.

## Case History

By the time a person comes to the attention of rehabilitation professionals, there is usually a considerable accumulation of historical data from health care providers and other sources. This data provide an important adjunct to the person's own recollections. Unfortunately, there is much variation in the completeness and focus of such histories. Details about the suddenness of symptom onset, the presence of extraordinary stress, reactions of family and friends, and the particular behavior expressed at particular times—important factors in ascertaining the nature of neurophysiological dysregulations—are often absent in historical documents. A key assessment resource for a rehabilitation program is a staff person who has the skill to identify signs of neurophysiological dysregulation in a historical narrative, and the time to construct a historical narrative when it is absent or incomplete. Historical data contribute heavily to the selection of initial hypotheses about the nature of a neurophysiological dysregulation and are instructive resources when choosing more precise and quantitative measures as key indicators for evaluating intervention effects.

## Behavioral Observation

Behavioral observation is the oldest and most commonly used approach to assessing people's neurophysiological status relevant to mental illness—although, of course, neurophysiological status can only be inferred from observable behavior. Neo-Kraepelinian diagnosis is based on observation of behavior during the interview and as recorded in case history. In that sense, structured diagnostic interviews combine anamnestic and behavioral observational methods. However, both methods have some serious limitations. First, the usefulness of interviews is contingent on the person's memory, and when severe mental illness is present, memory is often impaired. Second, a person's behavior during an interview is not necessarily consistent with his or her behavior in other settings. As a result, it is often necessary to collect data from other sources, even for the purpose of neo-Kraepelinian diagnosis. This need for multiple sources introduces uncertainty and imprecision. The reliability of interview-based assessment and diagnosis can be increased through use of structured interview protocols and behavioral rating scales. Since 1980, diagnostic interview protocols have been published along with each new version of the DSM. However, interview-based assessments must be complemented by systematic behavioral observation in more natural settings.

*Interview-based measures not closely linked to diagnostic categorization* include the Brief Psychiatric Rating Scale (BPRS; Ventura, Green, Shaner, & Liberman, 1993) and the Positive and Negative Symptom Scale (PANSS; Kay, Fizbein, & Opler, 1987). The BPRS evolved from predecessors developed in the 1960s to assess antipsychotic drug effects. It is one of the most commonly used rating scales in mental health, especially for the purpose of monitoring psychotic symptoms and episodes. In its most modern version, it includes 24 items describing behaviors ranging from subjective reports of hallucinations to mood to motor behavior. Most, but not all, of the BPRS items rate behaviors associated with psychosis. The items are rated for severity, intensity, or frequency on a seven-point scale, according to scoring criteria specific to each item. The items can be interpreted individually, on an a priori basis (e.g., an increase on the "confusion" item means the subject is more confused). Factor analyses of the BPRS group the items into five independent dimensions, which also aids interpretation (e.g., an increase in the suspiciousness, hostility, and persecutory delusion items means an increase in the paranoia factor). The PANSS was developed to augment diagnosis with more precise and differentiated assessment of specific symptoms. It also yields ratings for individual items (e.g., hallucinations, blunted affect) and item categories (e.g., positive vs. negative symptoms). BPRS and PANSS items and derived scores often provide informative key indicators for evaluating interventions on the neurophysiological level, especially drug interventions.

*Milieu-based observational instruments* can provide valuable information without the limitations of an interview-based format. Some lack the specificity of interview-based measures, but they are more reliable indicators of what the subject is actually doing in less contrived situations. One of the first such instruments, developed for assessing antipsychotic drug effects, was the Nurses Observational Scale for Inpatient Evaluation (NOSIE; Honigfeld, Gillis, & Klett, 1966). In its most recent form, it includes 30 items that describe behavioral assets (e.g., ability to perform a daily schedule, interact socially) and deficits (e.g., bizarre motor behavior, irritability, social withdrawal). Ratings are made by care staff who have had opportunities to observe the person in the inpatient milieu over a period of at least 72 hours. The NOSIE yields six subscale scores and an overall score. The subscales include three that reflect behavioral assets and three that reflect abnormal or impaired behavior. Individual NOSIE items are not generally reliable or stable enough to serve as key indicators, but the subscales and overall score are sensitive indicators of acute psychosis and drug effects. Furthermore, the NOSIE's different subscales yield qualitative assessment of behavioral change. This is helpful in discriminating true antipsychotic drug effects from sedation or other effects that may reduce psychotic behavior but with undesirable reduction of positive behavior as well. The NOSIE is also useful for assessing behavioral risks (Swett & Mills, 1997), effects of the atypical antipsychotics (Dennis, McBride, Peterson, & Corley-Wheeler, 1996), and trajectories of progress in rehabilitation (Hoffman & Kupper, 1996).

*Time-sampled observational instruments* provide more reliable, sensitive, and valid milieu-based measures of behavior in the ambient environment, but they are considerably more expensive in terms of staff time and training. Consequently, they are seldom used outside a clinical research context, although arguably they are worth the investment in any intensive rehabilitation setting. The "gold standards" are the Time-Sampled Behavior Checklist (TSBC) and the Staff–Resident Interaction Chronograph (S-RIC), both developed for Paul and Lentz's (1977) outcome study (discussed in Chapter 1). The former focuses on the personal and social functioning of the recovering person, and the latter focuses on interactions between the recovering person and rehabilitation staff. Both are extremely useful for general assessment, progress evaluation, as well as specific assessment of drug effects. (For detailed descriptions, discussion, and implementation guidelines, see Paul, 1986a, 1986b, 1988a, 1988b, 1988c).

*Event logs* are recording systems by which significant behavioral events are recorded as they occur. The observational recording systems used in contingency management programs (discussed further in Chapter 10) are essentially event logs. They require a set of operationally defined events (behaviors) and a staff trained to identify and record those events. The set of events may be generally defined for an entire milieu or program, or specifically tailored to an individual. When expected drug effects include a change in the frequency or intensity of specific behaviors (e.g., a reduction of bizarre verbalizations or delusional statements), event logs are a very useful tool for progress evaluation.

## Neuropsychological Assessment

Neuropsychology is a discipline that focuses primarily on the neurocognitive level of functioning but also seeks to establish relationships between neurocognitive functioning, neurophysiological functioning, and more molar behavior. A dramatic expansion in the neuropsychological level of analysis occurred during the 1990s and continues today. There are a number of technological applications in rehabilitation, including tracking the effects of treating neurophysiological dysregulation (discussed in detail in the next chapter). Understanding the role of neurophysiological dysregulation in a person's overall functioning and evaluating the effects of interventions directed at the neurophysiological level are both augmented valuably by neuropsychological assessment.

## Functional Skills Assessment

It is increasingly clear that the detrimental effects of neurophysiological dysregulation extend far beyond those directly associated with psychotic symptoms and related behavioral expressions. Neurocognitive consequences such as impairments in memory, attention, and behavioral organization can have pervasive effects on personal and social functioning. In some individuals, there is a psychopathological cascade so linear and so direct that resolution of the neurophysiological dysregulation brings about normalization of molar behavioral functioning. Unfortunately, this is the exception rather than the rule in rehabilitation settings. In most cases, treatment at the neurophysiological level produces some degree of improvement at other levels of functioning, but significant impairments remain. Therefore, *nothing* can be taken for granted. In each individual case it is necessary to determine, precisely and quantitatively, the effects of neurophysiological intervention at other levels of functioning. Functional skills assessment provides a systematic approach to measuring relatively molar behavior in ways relevant to rehabilitation. (The extensive skills assessment armamentarium available for this purpose is discussed in detail in subsequent chapters.) As with neuropsychological assessment, functional skills assessment complements behavioral observation in evaluating the effects of neurophysiological interventions.

## INTERVENTIONS FOR NEUROPHYSIOLOGICAL DYSREGULATION

Intervention options for neurophysiological dysregulation include psychiatric drugs, psychoeducational and psychosocial interventions, electroconvulsive therapy, and psychosurgery.

### Psychiatric Drugs

Drugs are by far the most widespread and accepted approach to resolving neurophysiological dysregulation in people with severe mental illness. The scientific and technical literature on this application is voluminous. There are several comprehensive sources that describe the theoretical foundations of neurophysiological models as well as guidelines for the clinical use of drugs (e.g., Meltzer & Fatemi, 1998; Spaulding, Johnson, & Coursey, 2001). This literature is mostly organized according to neo-Kraepelinian categories, but the diligent student can derive from it a sufficient account of the effects of specific drugs on specific behavioral problems. For complete familiarity with the biomedical considerations of psychopharmacotherapy, consider the following sources.

Several sets of practice guidelines have been formulated and published by various entities within the biological psychiatry community (see Smith & Docherty, 1998). *Guidelines for Treatment of Schizophrenia,* by the American Psychiatric Association (1997), provides practical advice for the prescribing pharmacotherapist, including dosing strategies, management of comorbid conditions, and side effects. These guidelines also list the panoply of psychosocial approaches of known effectiveness but do not describe or provide further information. The *Expert Consensus Guideline Series Treatment of Schizophrenia* (McEvoy et al., 1999) includes detailed protocols for selecting pharmacological treatments and related services. Spaulding, Johnson, and Coursey (2001) provide a comprehensive review of pharmacological and psychosocial treatment options for schizophrenia and related conditions, plus a logical algorithm that codifies the specific judgments and decisions required for administering drug treatment in the context of comprehensive rehabilitation. This algorithm is reproduced in Appendix 3 of this book.

## Psychoeducational and Psychosocial Treatment

Although standards of practice generally identify pharmacotherapy as a sine qua non in treating severe mental illness, especially schizophrenia, there is considerable evidence that, at least for some individuals, CNS dysregulation of the type associated with episodic psychosis can be managed with combinations of psychosocial and psychoeducational interventions. This evidence comes from studies of drug-free treatment programs, and from studies of drug reduction during psychosocial treatment. The most complete example of the drug-free treatment program is a 12-year study of drug-free treatment, the Soteria Project (reviewed by Mosher, 1999), in which a series of controlled studies revealed that the drug-free condition was comparable to conventional hospital and medication treatment for a large majority of recipients *and* was considerably less expensive. The most complete example of drug reduction during psychosocial treatment is the research of Paul and Lentz (1977), in which a large percentage of patients was able to reduce or discontinue antipsychotic medication. Interestingly, one of the comparison conditions in this study was a therapeutic community program similar to the Soteria model. Paul and Lentz's social-learning condition produced the best outcome, and the therapeutic community condition was superior to conventional medical model treatment; both social-learning and therapeutic community treatments produced dramatic reductions in use of antipsychotic drugs. Strauss and Carpenter (1977) also report a successful drug-free treatment approach that focused on shorter-term treatment of the acute episode.

Psychoeducational interventions are increasingly a standard part of psychopharmacotherapy, but they are intended to improve adherence rather than reduce the need for medication (Beckman, Liberman, Phi, & Blair, 1990). There have been no systematic studies to determine whether such interventions reduce the need for antipsychotic drugs. The interventions generally include a substantial relapse prevention component, emphasizing self-monitoring for early warning signs and preventive intervention. This component might be expected to reduce the need for maintenance medication. However, studies of drug intervention based on early warning signs have been disappointing (Herz, 1986; Herz et al., 2000): By the time a psychotic episode is detectable, findings indicate that it may be too late to abort it. These studies emphasized detection by professionals in an interview situation, however; it remains unknown whether more extensive relapse prevention training, in which the individual acquires a very high level of self-monitoring skills and the ability to respond rapidly to warning signs, would be more effective. Medication-related psychoeducation, best conceptualized as a skills training intervention, is discussed further as a sociobehavioral intervention in Chapter 9.

Despite the success of programs using a drug-free treatment protocol for schizophrenia, they remain outside the generally accepted standards of practice, especially in the acute phase. There are too many risks and liabilities to attempt routine drug-free treatment of episodic psychosis. On the other hand, it is reasonable to expect that some individuals may be able to function safely without maintenance medication, if provided sufficient education and training in self-monitoring and a reliable early intervention plan. This possibility can be evaluated through careful and gradual titration of medication and ongoing assessment of the recovering person's relevant skills in the later stages of rehabilitation.

Another implication of the findings on drug-free treatment is that certain psychosocial and environmental conditions facilitate recovery from acute neurophysiological dysregulation. There is no reason to expect that conditions beneficial in drug-free treatment would not be beneficial when drugs are used. There is evidence that antipsychotic drugs interfere with skills acquisition in ways relevant to rehabilitation (Corrigan & Penn, 1995; Paul, Tobias, & Holly, 1972). However, this evidence dates from an earlier era of psychopharmacotherapy and pertains to treatment in the residual phase of the disorder, not the acute phase. The optimal treatment of acute psychosis should be expected to combine pharmacotherapy with maintenance of therapeutic environmental conditions.

Systematic attention to the therapeutic milieu is a familiar principle in psychiatry and psychiatric nursing. The data on drug-free treatment suggest that the key features of a therapeutic milieu, optimized to treat acute psychosis, include:

1. Twenty-four-hour supervision of the psychotic person to ensure safety and provide social and emotional support
2. Clear expectations of behavior (e.g., to not be aggressive, attend to basic personal care and hygiene, maintain a daily schedule of activity, etc.)
3. An empathetic, nonjudgmental attitude on the part of caregivers toward the psychotic person's ongoing experience
4. A matter-of-fact psychoeducational approach to symptoms and other features of psychosis, highly tailored to the psychotic person's individual experience and presentation
5. Systematic management (not necessarily avoidance) of significant stresses (e.g., assistance with personal finances, resolution of interpersonal conflicts, respite from a stressful environment, etc.)
6. Systematic engagement of the psychotic person in problem-solving activities related to the person's situation and status (e.g., managing symptoms, resolving legal problems, planning for a return to normal functioning)

It has been argued that inpatient psychiatric units—the milieu in which acute psychosis is most commonly treated—are not particularly conducive to these conditions. Alternative settings are sometimes available, but current trends in health care do not suggest that such alternatives will become common in the forseeable future. Ultimately, maintenance of an optimal therapeutic milieu of any kind is a management task, not a psychopharmacological one. Success depends on exploiting the opportunities and neutralizing the liabilities that any particular setting might present to the milieu manager. Various aspects of creating and maintaining a therapeutic milieu are discussed in Chapters 10–12.

Finally, the need for psychosocial treatment of tonic neurophysiological dysregulation should always be considered. Depression is known to respond well to specific types of interpersonal psychotherapy and cognitive-behavioral therapy. Explosive behavior may be responsive to relaxation training, stress management, and social skills training. Reciprocal relationships between neurophysiological functioning, cognition, and behavior appear to pervade these conditions. Interventions at the cognitive and behavioral levels may be as efficacious in producing neurophysiological benefits as neurophysiological interventions are at producing cognitive and behavioral benefits.

## Electroconvulsive Therapy (ECT)

ECT is a controversial treatment due to a history of indiscriminate use and abusive application. Nevertheless, there is ample evidence that it sometimes successfully resolves psychotic states when all other alternatives fail. A clinical picture of severe depression or mania appears to be the strongest indication of potential benefit, and it is possible to construct a theoretical model in which ECT emulates the neurophysiological mechanisms of antidepressant drug effects. Contemporary anesthesiologist techniques make ECT a painless and humane procedure. It should be available as a last recourse to rehabilitation teams. At the same time, it is unlikely that ECT alone can permanently resolve neurophysiological dysregulation, so additional interventions (pharmacological, psychosocial, or both) to sustain its effects are also required.

## Psychosurgery

Psychosurgery also has a bad reputation from years of institutional abuse (for a historical perspective, see Pressman, 1998). Frontal lobotomy is no longer an acceptable practice, but in rare situations, psychosurgery may be justifiable as a last-recourse treatment for severely disabling or life-threatening symptoms (Baker et al., 1995; Mindus, Edman, & Andreewitch, 1999; Morgan & Crisp, 2000; Price et al., 2001).

## FORMULATING NEUROPHYSIOLOGICAL PROBLEMS
## OVER THE COURSE OF REHABILITATION

Effective progress evaluation requires a carefully articulated description of the elements hypothesized to be expressions of a CNS dysregulation. As data accumulate, the description should be amplified by formal measures and the revealed parameters of the clinical picture. For example, a problem description that includes only sketchy details of the symptoms and other parameters of a person's psychotic episodes at the beginning of rehabilitation would include much more information after several months of assessment, intervention, and progress evaluation. For example:

PROBLEM 1 (at initial assessment)

*Problem title*: Episodic CNS dysregulation

*Problem description*: Periods of acute distress accompanied by auditory hallucinations (voices making personal, disparaging remarks), confusion, extreme anxiety, and inability to perform routine activities of daily living.

PROBLEM 1 (after 6 months of rehabilitation)

*Problem title*: Episodic CNS dysregulation

*Problem description*: Periods of acute distress accompanied by auditory hallucinations (voices making personal, disparaging remarks), confusion, extreme anxiety, and inability to perform routine activities of daily living. Episode has not been observed to remit spontaneously, but fairly complete remission is achieved within 6 weeks of treatment with 20 mg/day of olanzapine. Early warning signs include anxiety, self-disparaging thoughts, and inattention to daily schedule. Episode resolution is effectively tracked by reductions on the BPRS's Disorganization and Hallucination factors and increases on the NOSIE-30 Total Assets scale.

The rehabilitation process incorporates a process of increasingly precise and quantitative characterizations of identified problems. This is especially important in the case of neurophysiological problems for four reasons: (1) There are no direct neurophysiological measures of episodic or tonic dysregulation; (2) the expressions of neurophysiology dysregulation are so idiosyncratic; (3) a full characterization of the dysregulation's expressions and dimensions is prerequisite to effective prevention of psychotic episodes; and (4) there are so many other possible etiologies for the behaviors produced by dysregulation. This is one reason why a continuing process of formulation, testing, and reformulation is so crucial in the rehabilitation enterprise.

# Chapter 5

# The Neurocognitive Level
# of Functioning

The term *cognition* can be used to refer to any of the brain's information-processing activity, from the most elemental sensory processes to the most complex levels of thought. Cognition thus spans a broad continuum of organizational levels. If it were possible to divide this continuum in half, with the more molecular levels of cognition in one half and the more molar levels in another, the more molecular category would be *neuro*cognition. The prefix *neuro-* indicates a closer, more isomorphic relationship between specific neurological structures and processes and the specific types of cognitive activity they support. For example, the cognitive process of *visual feature detection*, which allows us to perceive the boundaries of objects in our visual field, is a relatively molecular process closely associated with specific neurons in the retina, optic tract, and various brain structures. *Manipulation of spatial relations* is a more molar cognitive process, by which we use visual feature information to track and manipulate objects in space. This activity involves a greater number of neurons distributed more widely across the brain, but it still falls along the neurocognitive continuum. Other processes generally included in the neurocognitive continuum include simple problem solving, memory storage and retrieval, concept formation, organization and execution of behavioral responses, and elemental language processes. These all involve widely distributed, but still identifiable, neurological structures and processes. Complex language and problem solving, abstract reasoning, formation of beliefs, attitudes, and complex habits generally fall outside the neurocognitive continuum, and for our purposes are categorized as *social cognition.*

The distinction between neurocognition and social cognition is imprecise, somewhat arbitrary, and may even reflect the limits of our scientific understanding of cognition and the brain as much as a real difference between types of cognition. For example, the assumption that social cognition always occurs at a molar level of organization is questionable. The human brain may have evolved particular molecular mechanisms that are highly specialized for processing social information (Penn, 1991; Penn et al., 1997). Perhaps the feature detection mechanisms for processing human faces are different from the ones that process the boundaries of inanimate objects of comparable size. These specialized processes would be more molecular than more complex processes not specialized for social information. Future advances in cognitive science and neuroscience may provide a better way of organizing discussions of different cognitive levels. For the time being, for the purpose of organizing what we know about cognition and mental illness, the social–neurocognitive distinction is as good as any.

*Neuropsychology* is a scientific and professional discipline whose primary concern is the neurocognitive level of functioning. Neuropsychology evolved out of the application of experimental psychological analysis to relationships between brain structure and behavior. As an academic discipline its roots extend to the very origins of modern psychology in the late 19th century. However, neuropsychology did not become a professional clinical discipline until the 1960s, when its assessment technology proved useful for assessing brain injury and disease. Throughout the late 20th century, neuropsychology developed an increasingly complete theoretical and empirical foundation and increasingly useful clinical technologies. For practical purposes, the neurocognitive level of functioning can be operationally defined as the level whose processes are measured by neuropsychological assessment technology.[1]

Although early neuropsychological research addressed severe mental illness, it fell into a Kraepelinian conundrum. At that time, schizophrenia and related conditions were classified as "functional" disorders, whereas brain injury and known neuropathy were classified as "organic brain syndrome." Neuropsychological studies inspired little confidence that chronic schizophrenia could be reliably discriminated from organic brain syndrome (Goldstein, 1978; Shelly & Goldstein, 1983). Ironically, this ambiguity was interpreted by some as a technological limitation of neuropsychological assessment—an inability to distinguish between functional and organic disorders. By the end of the 1980s the view had evolved that schizophrenia *is* an "organic brain syndrome" in some sense (David & Cutting, 1994; Goldstein, 1986, 1991; Levin, Yurgelun-Todd, & Craft, 1989; Randolph, Goldberg, & Weinberger, 1993); for a comprehensive survey of neuropsychological and related research on schizophrenia at the end of the 1980s,

---

[1] For the purposes of science, the neurocognitive level of functioning is addressed by a number of disciplines within the broader cognitive neuroscience community. In this context, the boundaries between neuropsychology and other disciplines are indistinct.

see Steinhauer, Gruzelier, & Zubin, 1991). Intensive research on the neuro-psychology of schizophrenia occurred during the 1990s. The assessment technology expanded from its original base (i.e., use of behavioral tests to assess brain injury) to include the laboratory paradigms of experimental psychopathology. In this way, a broad and integrated understanding of neurocognition in mental illness began to evolve (Green, 2001).

By the end of the 20th century, schizophrenia was being conceptualized as "a neurocognitive disorder" (Green, 1998; Green & Neuchterlein, 1999), based on both scientific findings and clinical outcome. In basic science, neuropsychological principles played a central role in *neuro-developmental* theories of schizophrenia, which in turn made sense of much of the genetic, developmental, pharmacological, and clinical data on severe mental illness (McClure & Weinberger, 2001; Meinecke, 2001; Walker, 1994; Weinberger, 1996). In neurodevelopmental models, the various neurophysiological, cognitive, and behavioral characteristics of mental illness are understood as the consequences of relatively subtle disruptions of brain development stemming from injury, infection, extreme stress, or genetically related abnormalities occurring as early as the second trimester of gestation. These consequences manifest in changing ways over the course of a person's development, demonstrated most dramatically by the events of adolescence and early adulthood that we recognize as "the onset of schizophrenia." Neuropsychological research identified many of the earlier and later sequelae of neurodevelopmental abnormalities.

Some find validation of Kraepelin's view of a specific, progressive neurological disease in the neuropsychological research on schizophrenia (e.g., Randolph et al., 1993). However, the larger picture of neuropsychological impairment in severe mental illness does not support such a view. There is considerable overlap in the neuropsychological functioning of people diagnosed with schizophrenia and those with other known neuropathology (Goldstein, 1978; Shelly & Goldstein, 1983). Neurocognitive functioning in schizophrenia varies along the same major dimensions as it varies in other brain impairments and in people in general (the major dimensions are attention/distractibility, memory, and abstract reasoning; Allen et al., 1998). People who are diagnosed with schizophrenia comprise a heterogeneous group with respect to neuropsychological impairments (Goldstein, 1990; Goldstein & Shemansky, 1995). Diagnostic subtypes of schizophrenia do not reflect corresponding differences in severity or type of neuropsychological impairment (Goldstein & Halperin, 1977; Kremen, Seidman, Goldstein, Faraone, & Tsuang, 1994). On the other hand, in people with severe and disabling mental illness, including people diagnosed with schizophrenia, neuropsychological factors are strongly linked to personal and social functioning and to rehabilitation outcome (reviewed by Green, 1998).

Without accepting neo-Kraepelinian assumptions about diagnostic categories, it is reasonable to conclude from several decades of research that neurocognitive problems, as articulated by neuropsychological assessment technology, are often key factors in disabling mental illness. There are often statistical differences on neuropsychological measures between groups based on psychiatric diagnosis, but no diagnosis is associated with a unique or distinctive pattern of neurocognitive impairments. Individual people have unique constellations of impairments and problems, and each individual may require a unique treatment and rehabilitation approach.

## DIMENSIONS OF NEUROCOGNITIVE IMPAIRMENT IN SEVERE MENTAL ILLNESS

Despite the heterogeneity of neurocognitive impairment in mental illness, it is possible to utilize superordinate dimensions to organize our understanding:

- Episodic
- Quality and localization
- Lateral and fronto–occipital
- Explicit–implicit

### Episodic Dimension

As discussed in the previous chapter, severe mental illness has an episodic dimension. The course of illness includes periods of relatively stable functioning interspersed with periods of pronounced debilitation. The latter are generally recognized as psychotic episodes. Although there is great individual variation in the frequency, severity, duration, and quality of psychotic episodes, some sort of distinct episode plays an important role in the functioning of a substantial majority of people with disabling mental illness. Interventions directed at hypothetical dysregulation of the CNS are often helpful in reducing or eliminating psychotic episodes.

Neurocognitive functioning often fluctuates with the occurrence of psychotic episodes (Neuchterlein & Dawson, 1984; Spaulding, Fleming, Sullivan, Storzbach, & Lam, 1999; Spohn & Strauss, 1989). During acute psychosis new neurocognitive impairments may appear, and preexisting ones may worsen. In some instances, certain aspects of neurocognitive functioning may paradoxically appear to improve during acute psychosis. For example, people who experience paranoia perform better than people without any mental illness on laboratory tasks requiring sensitivity to subtle social cues. Generally, however, neurocognitive functioning is more severely impaired during acute psychosis.

Some areas of neurocognitive functioning appear to be more prone to disruption by acute psychosis than others. Despite considerable individual variation, research shows a general tendency for relatively molar processes to be more prone to disruption than relatively molecular processes (Neuchterlein et al., 1992; Spaulding et al., 1994). For example, visual feature processing and simple reaction time are relatively unaffected by acute psychosis, whereas higher-level problem solving and concept manipulation are affected. Some of the processes unaffected by acute psychosis are also thought to reflect *vulnerability* to mental illness, because they are impaired in individuals at risk (usually because of family history), before the onset of the illness. If such preexisting impairments are severe, the distinction between them and the impairments made worse by acute psychosis may be obscured.

Psychotic episodes are followed by a post-acute period characterized by a gradual dissipation of psychotic symptoms and related expressions and a return to baseline functioning. This period may be brief or protracted. Accordingly, neurocognitive impairments that accompany acute psychosis may dissipate quickly or slowly over time. As the psychotic episode continues to resolve during the residual phase, some of its expressions may persist, including positive or negative symptoms, impairments in personal and social functioning, and neurocognitive impairments. The residual phase of mental illness is not well understood; it is probably the product of a multiplicity of etiological factors. It may be that, for some individuals, resolution of the acute episode is so protracted that it is undetectable. It may be that, for others, the CNS dysregulation associated with the acute phase produces permanent structural changes in the brain, resulting in new impairments. It is possible to construct neurophysiological models for how this might happen (Arango, Kirkpatrick, & Koenig, 2001; Ashe, Berry, & Boulton, 2001; Benes, 1997), but whether it *does* happen in one way or another remains controversial (reviewed by Arango et al., 2001). Whatever the etiology, it is clear that residual neurocognitive impairments sometimes accumulate over the course of severe mental illness. In fact, this cumulative aspect may have led Kraepelin to conclude that schizophrenia (actually, he used the predecessor term, "dementia praecox") is a progressive dementia whose lifelong course is toward an eventual vegetative state. Today it is clear that only some individuals with disabling mental illness (including some of those who meet diagnostic criteria for schizophrenia) experience a lifelong progressive loss of neurocognitive functioning. However, a large proportion do experience significant neurocognitive impairment in the residual phase of their illness.

## Quality and Localization Dimensions

The success of neuropsychology is based, in large part, on the fact that laboratory tests can detect discrete impairments in neurocognitive functioning.

"Discrete impairments" show qualitatively distinct characteristics relative to other impairments. For example, loss of tactile perception in one hand but not the other reflects a discrete impairment in left-hand tactile perception. Loss of memory for recent events but not older events reflects a discrete impairment in short-term memory. Discrete neurocognitive impairments are often traceable to damage in discrete areas of the brain. For over two decades, before the advent of computerized brain imaging techniques such as CAT, PET, and MRI, this detection ability made neuropsychological testing the most reliable and accurate method for determining the presence and location of discrete brain lesions. Today, localization is a less central concern in neuropsychology, but the relationship between neurocognitive functions and discrete brain areas or subsystems remains an important area of psychopathological investigation.

It is surprisingly difficult to demonstrate scientifically that people with mental illness have discrete neurocognitive impairments. There are several reasons for this difficulty. First, research efforts have been overly influenced by psychiatric diagnostic categories. Diagnostic groups associated with severe mental illness, including schizophrenia, bipolar disorder, and depression, are quite heterogeneous with respect to neurocognitive functioning. Trying to find the one true "neuropsychological profile" of particular diagnostic groups has not been particularly fruitful. Second, whether mental illness is associated with discrete impairments or not, it is clearly associated with overall or *global* impairment (Chapman & Chapman, 1978). This globality makes it difficult methodologically to prove that impaired performance on a laboratory test reflects a truly discrete deficit. It may simply mean that that particular task is more sensitive than others to the global impairment in functioning usually observed in people with severe mental illness. Third, mental illness has a significant episodic dimension, whereas both discrete and global impairments fluctuate over time. Until recently, neuropsychological research on severe mental illness tended to ignore the longitudinal dimension, rendering most conclusions limited (the work of Neuchterlein & Dawson, 1984, cited above in reference to episodic fluctuations, is a significant exception).

Present-day research is gradually overcoming the historical barriers to understanding the discrete nature of neurocognitive impairments in mental illness, but the picture is far from complete. The next few years will probably bring substantial progress, perhaps even a revision of current organizational schemes. For the time being, however, there is reasonable consensus in the neuropsychological and psychopathological communities about four relevant principles:

1. Global neurocognitive impairment, though ubiquitous in mental illness, covers the complete range of severity across individuals.

2. Impairments in executive functioning (concept manipulation, response planning and organization, and working memory) are ubiquitous and somewhat independent of global impairments.
3. Impairments in verbal and nonverbal memory are common and somewhat independent of global impairment.
4. Many people with disabling mental illness have individually unique constellations of neurocognitive abnormalities in executive, memory, sensorimotor, perceptual, and other functions.

## Fronto-Occipital and Lateral Dimensions

Beyond localization of specific neurocognitive functions to specific brain areas, neuropsychological analysis uses overall anatomical dimensions to characterize patterns of neurocognitive impairment. Neurodevelopmental models of severe mental illness emphasize malformation and/or neurophysiological dysfunction of neural pathways that project forward from the limbic system and subcortical structures to the frontal cortex (see Meinecke, 2001). This malformation and/or dysfunction is consistent with neuropsychological data indicating impairment in executive functioning, which is primarily associated with frontal cortex. (Executive functioning is probably supported by a number of brain structures and areas other than the frontal cortex, but the latter area appears to support a number of specific functions, including motor response planning and working memory, that are central to executive operations [Lezak, 1982, 1994]). Theories based on psychiatric diagnosis interpret these relationships to mean that schizophrenia is a "frontal dementia," that is, a specific loss of the neurocognitive abilities associated with the frontal lobe (Weinberger, 1994). However, such theories neglect the variable severity of frontal impairment within and across diagnostic groups. Without necessarily accepting neo-Kraepelinian assumptions, neurodevelopmental theories suggest that individuals suffer brain malformation to varying degrees, reflecting the severity of the vulnerabilities and stresses that produce the malformation. Thus the severity of *hypofrontality* (i.e., impairment of neurocognitive functions associated with the frontal lobe) is an important source of individual variance among people with severe mental illness.

Neuropsychological investigation of the frontal lobes has revealed at least two relatively distinct syndromes, behavioral disinhibition and attentional neglect, reflecting the failure of two relatively distinct frontal lobe functions (Vellig .n et al., 2000). *Behavioral disinhibition* is a failure to inhibit inappropriate responses to immediate situations, whereas *attentional neglect* is a failure to activate appropriate responses. Behavioral disinhibition may be expressed as impulsive, socially inappropriate, or situationally inappropriate behavior. Obvious examples include talking to oneself, verbalizing thoughts about other people that are best kept private, or impulsively engaging in dangerous behavior. Less obvious would be bizarre behavior such as wearing inappropriate clothing, which may occur because the person puts on whatever clothes he or she encounters in the wardrobe (i.e., failure to inhibit dressing behavior). Attentional neglect may be expressed as dishevelment (failure to activate appropriate self-care behavior), social withdrawal (failure to activate appropriate social behavior), or anhedonia and apathy (failure to activate appropriate emotional responses). Either disinhibition or neglect, or both, may appear when the frontal lobe is damaged. Appearance of such behaviors in severe mental illness may indicate frontal neurocognitive impairment.

The lateral dimension of impairment reflects a predominance of neurocognitive impairments associated with one or the other brain hemisphere. The left hemisphere is associated with sensory and motor processing for the right side of the body, plus language and related abilities. The right hemisphere is associated with sensory and motor processing for the left side of the body, plus nonverbal and emotional functioning. Severe mental illness often appears to be associated with neuropsychological lateralization, both anatomical and functional (Gruzelier, 1991; Gruzelier, Wilson, & Richardson, 1999; Gur & Chin, 1999; Gur & Gur, 1991; Petty, 1999; Sommer, Aleman, Ramsey, Bouma, & Kahn, 2001; Spaulding, Fleming, et al., 1999), but this finding is difficult to interpret in a neo-Kraepelinian context. There is unresolved debate, for example, about whether schizophrenia involves lateralized deficits or absence of normal asymmetry. The latter may reflect slower rates of development rather than actual injury or compromise of brain functioning (Saugstad, 1999). In part, lateralization may be secondary to fronto–cortical compromise (Bradshaw & Sheppard, 2000). What is clear is that individuals with severe mental illness often experience lateralized impairments. There is some evidence that lateralization to the left may represent a more serious barrier to recovery than lateralization to the right. The neurophysiological basis for lateralization in severe mental illness is poorly understood and its implications are controversial, but it clearly occurs, and in both directions and to varying degrees.

## The Explicit–Implicit Dimension

There appear to be two relatively distinct subsystems involved in activities generally subsumed under the rubrics of *learning* (which, in contemporary neuropsychological terms, incorporates a number of executive processes) and *memory*. Processes associated with one or the other of these subsystems are termed *explicit* or *implicit* (Nelson, Schreiber, & McEvoy, 1992). In the context of rehabilitation, acquisition of skills is enhanced by both types of learning and memory. Explicit learning involves verbal representation of acquired information, making it possible for the individual to understand tasks and situations in verbal terms and to communicate with others about them. Implicit learning, also termed *procedural* learning, does not include such representation, and therefore the individual is unaware that skill acquisition has taken place. Procedural learning underlies complex perceptual and motor abilities associated with performing complex tasks, as in athletic performance. Acquisition of any complex skill normally involves both explicit and implicit components.

There is some evidence that explicit and implicit processes can be impaired differentially (Abrams & Reber, 1988). For example, people with neuropathological conditions (e.g., Alzheimer's disease) sometimes can improve their performance on a task through repeated practice, even though they demonstrate no recognition or memory of the task. Studies of implicit learning in people diagnosed with schizophrenia yield contradictory results (Bressi et al., 1998; Danion, Meulemans, Kauffmann-Muller, & Vermaat, 2001), suggesting, once again, heterogeneous impairments within that group. Finer distinctions may be necessary within the categories of implicit and explicit learning (Bressi et al., 1998; Green, Kern, Williams, McGurk, & Kee, 1997). In any case, implicit learning is a potentially important factor in neurocognitive recovery (Wexler et al., 1997). The next few years will probably bring important developments in our understanding of the role of implicit versus explicit learning in rehabilitation.

## A Three-Factor Model

The qualitative and episodic dimensions of neurocognitive impairment can be integrated into a three-factor model that is heuristically useful for clinical assessment and rehabilitation planning (Spaulding et al., 1994): baseline functioning, episode-linked impairment, and post-acute recovery. It is important to remember that these factors are *sources of variance* and not types or categories. In the present context, a three-factor model describes ways that individuals *within* the population of people with severe mental illness are different from each other. An individual may occupy any point along the quantitative continuums that the factors define.

### Baseline Functioning

The first factor in this model, *baseline functioning*, reflects the severity of global neurocognitive impairment at times of optimal neurophysiological stability (i.e., not during psychotic episodes). Statistically, people with disabling mental illness show more impairment in baseline functioning than populations without mental illness. In subgroups with the most severe disabilities, the subgroup mean on this factor is near the 95th percentile of the total population (Spaulding, 1992). However, even at that extreme level there is substantial overlap between the two distributions; this overlap reflects two seemingly incompatible realities about severe mental illness. On the one hand, global neurocognitive impairment is ubiquitous in severe mental illness and probably reflects key etiological processes. On the other hand, many people with severe mental illness show a normal range of neurocognitive functioning, at least during periods of optimal stability.

Impaired baseline neurocognitive functioning is *pervasive*, meaning that a broad range of specific processes, spanning the molar–molecular continuum, is affected. In this sense, the baseline functioning factor is somewhat like the concept of intelligence, in that it reflects a person's overall adaptability and behavioral functioning. Unlike intelligence, however, baseline impairment is not equally distributed across all neurocognitive processes. Some processes appear to be more affected than others. Although research does not yet allow confident conclusions about which areas are most affected by baseline impairment, executive processes appear to be especially vulnerable, and impairments in concept formation, planning, complex problem solving, and working memory appear to be common. This impairment on the executive level is consistent with neurodevelopmental models of etiology that emphasize malformation of limbic–frontal activation pathways; executive processes involve many brain areas and mechanisms, but limbic and frontal cortex are especially heavily involved.

If this baseline impairment is a product of neurodevelopmental processes, then it reflects not only structural and neurophysiological abnormalities but also their consequences, operating over a lifetime. In adulthood, baseline impairment may therefore include a deficient repertoire of acquired abilities. These deficiencies affect not only areas we normally think of as involving "skills" (e.g., personal care skills, interpersonal relationship skills, athletic skills) but also the cognitive *microskills* (e.g., apprehending one's own and others' emotional states, understanding various social roles, analyzing the trajectory of a fly ball) that are a prerequisite to developing important adult abilities. The possibility that baseline impairment is a product of neurodevelopmental processes has recently inspired interest among psychopathologists in the cognitive developmental processes of adolescence, frequently the time of onset for disabling mental illness (e.g., Benes, 1989; Karp et al., 2001). It is increasingly clear that some areas of the frontal cortex do not begin to function until adolescence, probably making it possible for the person to acquire the more subtle and sophisticated cognitive abilities of adulthood. Failure to acquire these abilities, as a consequence of severe mental illness in adolescence, would leave the person with serious impairments. It is possible that, just as language acquisition occurs most effectively during certain periods of development, acquisition of these abilities can only occur during specific developmental windows. A more complete understanding of adolescent cognitive development is expected to inform our understanding of adult psychopathology in important ways.

The severity of baseline neurocognitive impairment is probably determined by a multiplicity of factors, including genetic vulnerability, the severity of prenatal stress or injury, and the supportiveness of the person's environment during development. Obviously, the severity of various factors affecting various parts of the brain, and various domains of learning and development, at different times, can produce impairments of different severity in different neurocognitive processes. This means that despite the pervasive, global tendency of baseline impairment, individuals have unique constellations of impairments. It is common for a single disease process to produce individually unique constellations of impairments. Even identical lesions can produce different neurocognitive consequences in different individuals, because the functional organization of the brain is highly individualized.

The baseline factor is a treatment refractory factor, since science and technology currently do not provide the means to correct structural problems in brain development. Even deficits in acquired abilities may not be treatable if acquisition is restricted to developmental windows. If an impairment diminishes, then it is not a baseline impairment. However, baseline impairment can certainly worsen over time, as in the Kraepelinian view of schizophrenia. Whether by accumulation of impairments associated with acute psychosis or another progressive neurophysiological factor, some individuals' baseline impairment may worsen over time, despite all efforts to prevent it.

The baseline factor thus includes two subtypes of neurocognitive impairment: *vulnerability-linked* impairments, which were present before the onset of illness, and *residual* impairments, which are acquired over the course of the illness.

## Episode-Linked Impairment

The second factor in the three-factor model, *episode-linked impairment*, presumably reflects a cascade of events originating with neurophysiological dysregulation. During acute psychosis, baseline neurocognitive impairment worsens, and new impairments appear. There is considerable individual variation in how neurocognition changes over the course of an episode. High levels of baseline impairment may obscure the episode-linked factor, because detection of the second factor requires relatively good test performance at some point in time. There is some evidence that the executive domain is affected differentially by episode-linked impairment, at least in individuals with little baseline impairment. As previously discussed, some processes at the molecular end of the neurocognitive spectrum appear to be distinctly invulnerable to acute psychosis.

### Post-Acute Recovery

The third factor in this model is a *post-acute recovery* factor, whose existence is supported by the clinical observation that some individuals require more time than others to regain baseline functioning in the wake of a psychotic episode. It is further evidenced in the finding that people sometimes experience slow but significant improvement in personal and social functioning over protracted periods of neurophysiological stability, suggesting that this improvement is made possible (at least, in part) by improved neurocognitive functioning. The most important evidence for a post-acute recovery factor in neurocognition comes from studies in which neurocognitive impairment was treated directly, using environmental or psychological interventions (discussed in detail in Chapter 7). A number of interventions, from residing in a highly structured therapeutic milieu to receiving training and practice on laboratory tasks, appears to bring about improvements in neurocognitive functioning, especially in the executive domain. Improvement on laboratory tasks can be explained as the result of ordinary learning, but more generalized changes, or changes in response to a therapeutic milieu, are more feasibly explained as acceleration of a natural recovery process that, for some individuals, is so slow as to be indiscernible.

At least three mechanisms have been proposed to explain how post-acute recovery could be influenced by environmental manipulations or psychological interventions: (1) learning compensatory microskills, (2) providing supportive therapeutic and environmental conditions that facilitate rebalancing of the dopaminergic neuronal subsystems, and (3) rebalancing of cortisol functioning. The first mechanism is a conventional learning process, wherein the affected individual learns microskills that help compensate for deficits in other areas. For example, to compensate for deficits in sustained attention and vigilance, a person might learn to take frequent breaks, use self-talk as a cue to pay attention, and avoid situations where attentional deficits are especially detrimental. (This is not really a model of post-acute recovery, as one could learn compensatory skills any time, not just in the post-acute phase. However, baseline deficits tend to appear in the wake of acute episodes, so the post-acute phase would be the period in which the preponderance of such learning would take place.)

The second mechanism involves a behavioral response organization process thought to be supported by dopaminergic neuronal subsystems in the limbic system, basal ganglia, and primitive frontal cortex. This mechanism monitors the environment and organizes the person's behavioral repertoire to meet environmental demands in the most efficient manner; in the dopaminergic firestorm of an acute psychotic episode, it is temporarily disabled. After the episode is resolved on the neurophysiological level, experience with the environment, over time, is required to reorganize the behavioral repertoire. The structure of a therapeutic milieu or a psychological intervention condenses the environmental factors that must be reorganized, thereby facilitating more rapid improvement in behavioral functioning.

The third explanatory mechanism is the neuroendocrine system. A loss of the activating effects of the stress hormone cortisol appears to be associated with chronic mental illness. Cortisol acts directly upon cortical neurons to mediate cognitive activity. The predictable routines of a therapeutic milieu may help reestablish cortisol rhythms and enhance cortical activation.

The mechanisms of third factor impairment during post-acute recovery and their implications for rehabilitation are discussed in more detail in the next chapter.

Applying the three-factor model elucidates important questions about neurocognition processes in the rehabilitation context:

1. Is the person's current functioning and recovery potential limited by baseline neurocognitive impairment that will not respond to any available treatment, and if so, what could be done to minimize the impact of the impairment?
2. Is the person's current functioning and recovery potential limited by neurocognitive impairment that would be reduced or eliminated by resolution of a psychotic episode?
3. Is the person's current functioning and recovery potential limited by neurocognitive impairment residual to psychosis that would be reduced or eliminated by a structured milieu and/or psychological interventions?

Assessment and intervention at the neurocognitive level are organized by these questions.

## FORMULATING NEUROCOGNITIVE PROBLEMS IN THE INTEGRATED PARADIGM

In the integrated paradigm problem set (Appendix 1) there are two titles for neurocognitive problems, *post-acute neurocognitive impairment* and *baseline neurocognitive impairment*. These correspond to third-factor and first-factor impairments, respectively, as discussed above. Second factor or episode-linked impairment is not defined as a neurocognitive problem because it is consequent to episodic psychosis associated with CNS dysregulation. A description of the neurocognitive level of impairment can be included as part of the problem description for a CNS dysregulation problem, in which the impairment is expected to diminish or even disappear as the acute episode is resolved. Neurocognitive impairment that remains after resolution of acute psychosis must be reformulated under a new problem, as either post-acute or baseline impairment. Whether acute, post-acute, or residual, the particular nature of the impairment is described under the problem description. When sufficient data are available, this description includes specification of whether the impairment is pervasive or discrete, and if the latter, the particular qualities of the neurocognitive impairment and the behavioral consequences.

Evidence for neurocognitive impairment includes behavior suggestive of failures at that level of functioning, including memory difficulty, concrete thinking or language, confusion, and difficulty with attention or concentration. Of course, these may also be indications of acute psychosis. Longitudinal assessment of neurocognitive impairments during resolution of acute psychosis is key to determining whether the impairments are baseline, acute, or post-acute. Although no particular pattern of neuropsychological test performance can be confidently identified as characteristically baseline, acute, or post-acute, repeated testing may reveal an individual's pattern of longitudinal change. For example, in individuals with low baseline impairment, discrete abnormalities in working memory and concept manipulation may come and go with psychotic episodes. In some individuals, this relationship may even be reliable enough to use (along with others) as an indicator of an impending episode or its resolution. Discriminating post-acute from baseline impairments may require extensive longitudinal assessment. There is no accepted time frame for the post-acute period. Ultimately, a neurocognitive impairment is indisputably baseline in nature only if it persists after a protracted period free of acute psychosis and exhaustive but unsuccessful attempts to treat it as a post-acute impairment. Historical data may increase confidence that the impairment is baseline. For example, a person with neurocognitive impairment associated with a known head injury or present prior to the onset of mental illness would be expected to show that pattern in the post-acute and residual phase of the illness.

The rehabilitation team's hypotheses about the baseline, acute, or post-acute status of a recovering person's neurocognitive impairments have straightforward implications for intervention. Baseline impairments, being refractory to all known technologies for improvement, require compensatory strategies and environmental prosthetics. The permanence of baseline impairments gives special importance to the particular pattern of the person's neurocognitive strengths and weaknesses, and so they must be articulated in detail. Acute and post-acute impairments demand trials of corrective interventions. Treatment of acute neurocognitive impairment is essentially treatment of acute psychosis. Post-acute impairments can be addressed with environmental and specialized interventions, such as a therapeutic milieu and individual and group therapies, respectively. Intervention principles, strategies, and techniques for residual and post-acute neurocognitive impairments are discussed in Chapters 6 and 7.

## ASSESSMENT AND PROGRESS EVALUATION TOOLS FOR NEUROCOGNITIVE IMPAIRMENT

Neuropsychological assessment methods provide the technology for directly assessing neurocognitive impairment. However, as a result of neuropsychology's origins in neuropathology and neurosurgery, the traditional technology is well suited only to assessing baseline impairments in the residual phase of the disorder. Tests and related procedures were originally developed to detect and localize lesions in the context of a one-time assessment, so there was no investment in developing instruments for repeated or longitudinal assessment. Traditional neuropsychological testing is a powerful and accurate method for characterizing brain impairments and their behavioral consequences, but only if the person being assessed is in a stable state. In severe mental illness, interpretation of neuropsychological test results is contingent on whether the person is in an acute, post-acute, or residual phase, which cannot be determined by test data alone.

### Assessment of Baseline Impairment

The purpose of neuropsychological assessment in the residual phase is primarily to identify neurocognitive impairments that are barriers to rehabilitation. These impairments are expected to be distributed pervasively and to cover a wide range of severity. Considering the ubiquity of baseline neurocognitive impairment in people with severe mental illness, and the strength of the evidence that it is a significant limiting factor in rehabilitation, quantitative assessment of its nature and severity should be a sine qua non.

Instruments for comprehensive assessment of intellectual functioning (e.g., the WAIS-III) are useful for assessing the severity of baseline impairment. Overall summative test scores such as a WAIS IQ provide information about the rate at which a person can acquire new skills, a central concern in rehabilitation. Similarly, a WAIS IQ score guides formulation of general expectations about the nature of a person's functioning after maximal recovery. The pattern of WAIS subtest scores also provide a picture of the individual's relative strengths and weaknesses. In this particular sense, pervasive baseline neurocognitive impairment, as measured by IQ tests, is comparable to the concept of intelligence. However, IQ and subtest patterns do not provide sufficient measurement of executive dysfunction and related impairments associated with hypofrontality (insufficient functioning of the frontal lobe). Therefore, assessment of baseline impairment should routinely include additional instruments to measure fronto–cortical functioning. There is no generally accepted battery for this purpose, especially for assessment of people with severe mental illness. New instruments are currently being developed at a rapid pace, so practically any recommendation in this regard may be quickly dated. Generally speaking, however, a reasonably complete battery for assessment of frontal functioning should include measures of concept formation and manipulation, working memory, inhibitory functioning, and simple problem solving. Neuropsychological instruments often used to assess hypofrontality in people with mental illness include the Wisconsin Card Sorting Task (WCST), verbal fluency tasks (thought to measure inhibitory functions), Trailmaking, Halstead Categories, and backward digit span (thought to measure working memory) (see Goldstein, 1991; Erickson, 1994). Instruments and batteries specialized for measuring baseline hypofrontality in severe mental illness hopefully will emerge in the next few years.

Indications of additional discrete neurocognitive impairments in the residual phase may necessitate further assessment. Such indications may include a history of head trauma, significant variability across WAIS subtests and/or measures of hypofrontality, behavior indicative of memory failure, or difficulties in behavioral performance that are not accounted for by low IQ or executive dysfunction. At this point, assessment in the integrated paradigm becomes indistinguishable from traditional neuropsychological assessment, in which the primary purpose is to develop a complete profile of the recovering person's neurocognitive strengths and weaknesses. Because assessing individual constellations of impairments and their functional implications requires skills different from those usually required of rehabilitation professionals, the consulting services of a traditional neuropsychologist should be available to the rehabilitation team.

Theoretically, baseline cognitive impairment is not subject to change, so its assessment is not directly relevant to evaluating rehabilitation progress. Nevertheless, progress must be interpreted in light of what is known about baseline impairment. A rate of progress slower than that predicted by baseline impairment may indicate that undetected factors are creating barriers. A rate of progress faster than that predicted by baseline impairment may indicate that the impairment is not really baseline, which suggests that the recovering person was not in a fully stable residual state when assessed. In turn, this may mean that the person is experiencing undetected fluctuations, possibly undetected psychotic episodes. Such a fluctuation would be corroborated by changes in test performance during ostensibly stable periods. Little is known about the prospects for long-term improvement in the cognitive functioning of people who have disabling mental illness, so nothing can be taken for granted in this regard. Periodic reassessment of baseline neurocognitive functioning is necessary to ensure against mistaking slowly improving impairments for permanent ones.

## ASSESSMENT OF EPISODE-LINKED IMPAIRMENT

The purpose of assessing second-factor neurocognitive impairment is twofold: (1) to assist in determining the presence of an acute psychotic state, and (2) to determine how neurocognitive impairments associated with acute psychosis may disrupt or compromise rehabilitation efforts. For both purposes, the key element is *repeated assessment over time*—a weak point in traditional neuropsychology. Little is known about the effects of repeated assessment on test performance. Under some circumstances, learning and practice effects could be so strong as to disallow confident interpretation. Much effort is currently being invested in developing instruments with known longitudinal properties, but for now cautious use of familiar instruments is the only alternative.

Neuropsychological assessment may be useful for detecting acute psychosis under conditions of (1) limited baseline impairment, permitting substantial performance change between acute and residual phases, and (2) a relatively slow, insidious onset of acute psychosis. Some individuals experience or exhibit warning signs of impending psychosis for days or even weeks before the episode becomes clearly discernible, and neurocognitive impairment may appear relatively early in this process. Detection may alert the treatment team to an impending episode, so that preventive action can be taken. To take advantage of a known episode-linked neurocognitive warning sign, it is generally necessary to formalize a plan for performing a laboratory assessment upon the appearance of earlier warning signs. This plan could be part of a comprehensive relapse prevention plan, as discussed in the previous chapter.

Identifying a neurocognitive warning sign as a marker of an impending psychotic episode usually depends on fortuitous observation of a change in test performance associated with the onset of a psychotic episode. A prerequisite to such an observation would be the enforcement of a routine assessment program whenever acute psychosis is a recurring part of the clinical picture. Since rehabilitation often begins as a person is recovering from an acute psychotic episode, tracking the resolution of the episode usually provides the first indications of a potentially useful neurocognitive marker. Measures that show significant change as the recovery proceeds point to initial candidates. A number of measures may have to be administered several times, across a number of episodes, before reliable markers can be identified. Even though practice effects may obscure the recovery process, a sudden unexplained deterioration of performance would be a strong indicator of an episode-linked impairment.

As discussed earlier, episode-linked impairments are thought to occur primarily in the domain of memory and executive functioning. Instruments that measure these types of neurocognition are the most likely to prove useful as episode markers. The frontal–executive measures that augment the WAIS (or similar instrument) in assessment of baseline impairment may be the best candidates for routine use. However, because individuals appear to show unique constellations of episode-linked impairments, all available measures should be examined for episode-marker properties in cases where early detection of acute psychosis is especially important. The particular instruments known to be useful for episode detection must be clearly identified for the purposes of a relapse prevention plan.

The second purpose of conducting assessments of episode-linked impairment—determining the consequences of this type of impairment for other aspects of rehabilitation—is essential to maintaining program efficiency and facilitating timely progress in the patient. Episode-linked impairment may severely compromise response to an array of rehabilitation modalities, especially those involving acquisition of new skills. (Many individuals, however, do not experience severe changes in neurocognition during acute psychosis.) It might be a waste of time and resources, not to mention a needless source of stress for the recovering person, to attempt certain types of rehabilitation activities while episode-linked impairments are still active. Some rehabilitation activities are amenable to modification to compensate for neurocognitive impairments, and these modification activities may be a better option than postponement for some individuals. The severity and nature of episode-linked impairment must be assessed individually to determine their immediate implications for rehabilitation.

The episode-linked neurocognitive impairments most likely to interfere with rehabilitation interventions are gross disruption of sustained attention and vigilance. The behavioral consequences are readily observable when the impairments are especially severe; people are unable to attend to even simple tasks or function in a skills training group. As the episode resolves, it may be more difficult to determine to what degree behavioral performance is being compromised by these impairments. Abatement of extreme agitation and anxiety may create an impression that the person is better able to focus his or her attention when, in fact, attentional impairment continues to be severe. Simple laboratory measures, such as the Continuous Performance Task (CPT; Neuchterlein, 1991; Rosvold, Mirsky, Sarason, Bransome, & Beck, 1956) provide quantitative measurement of sustained attention and vigilance and are probably not affected significantly by practice. Repeated use of such measures is thus a useful adjunct to the traditional means of evaluating resolution of psychosis, such as behavioral observation and structured interviews.

As resolution proceeds, gross disruption of attention and vigilance may subside but nevertheless leave significant impairment in learning processes and working memory, as measured by various learning and memory tasks. These impairments greatly compromise a person's ability to benefit from skills training and related rehabilitation interventions. Clinical decisions can be usefully informed by repeated assessment in these domains. Still later, more complex tasks involving executive functioning, such as the WCST, can be useful for tracking the last stages of cognitive recovery from acute psychosis. However, the more complex tasks are also more prone to practice and learning effects and therefore must be interpreted with caution.

## Assessment of the Post-Acute Recovery Factor

There is no distinct point at which episode-linked impairment becomes post-acute impairment. For practical purposes, the best criterion is the point at which the recovering person has attained maximum benefit from the interventions intended to resolve the acute psychosis. Usually, but not always, this time period would correspond to the point at which psychotic symptoms and other expressions of acute psychosis, including neurocognitive impairments, have decreased to a plateau. At that point, the rehabilitation team's hypotheses about post-acute neurocognitive impairments become operative, and the target of treatment shifts from the neurophysiological dysregulation underlying acute psychosis to the neurocognitive impairments themselves.

Little is known about the nature of post-acute neurocognitive impairment. Findings indicate that it is qualitatively similar to episode-linked impairment and may be produced by the same etiological processes. Treatments directed at neurocognitive impairment appear to exert their most definitive effects in the executive domain. Therefore, the transition from post-acute to residual is generally expected to be characterized by a differential improvement in executive cognition, relative to other domains. The WCST, Halstead Categories, and tests of verbal learning have proven sensitive indicators of post-acute neurocognitive recovery.

In a sense, assessment of post-acute impairment is actually the beginning of assessment of baseline or residual impairment: The latter is what is left after all approaches to treating the former have been exhausted.

# Chapter 6

# Mechanisms of
# Neurocognitive Recovery

There is little doubt that neurocognitive recovery occurs in people with severe mental illness. At least since the 1970s, interventions ranging from practice on laboratory tasks to comprehensive rehabilitation approaches have shown that specific aspects of performance can improve (Corrigan & Storzbach, 1993; Spaulding, Storms, Goodrich, & Sullivan, 1986; Storzbach & Corrigan, 1996). Because much of this improvement may be attributable to recovery from acute psychosis, this part of the recovery process has been increasingly studied (Olbrich, Kirsch, Pfeiffer, & Mussgay, 2001; Spaulding, Fleming, et al., 1999). However, in many individuals, significant cognitive impairment persists after other indications of acute psychosis have resolved. Some of these post-acute impairments respond to psychosocial interventions directed at the neurocognitive level of functioning. As of this writing, researchers conducting three large-scale controlled clinical trails (Bell, Bryson, Greig, Corcoran, & Wexler, 2001; Hogarty & Flesher, 1999b; Spaulding, Reed, Sullivan, Richardson, & Weiler, 1999) have reported that interventions explicitly targeting neurocognitive functioning contribute uniquely and importantly to rehabilitation progress. An additional six studies report successful interventions but with smaller subject samples, incomplete control conditions, and limited generalization of improvement or dependent measures that fall short of a priori clinical importance (Benedict et al., 1996; Brown, Harwood, Hays, Heckman, & Short, 2000; Corrigan, Hirschbeck, & Wolfe, 1995; Hermanutz & Gestrich, 1991; Medalia, Aluma, Tyron, & Merriam, 1998; Wykes, Reeder, Corner, Williams, & Everitt, 1999). Many others, too numerous to list, report improved performance on neurocognitive measures under laboratory conditions, induced by learning, practice, or related procedures. The research literature has moved beyond exploring the simple question of whether neurocognitive recovery can be enhanced by such interventions, to questions about the extent of the effects, the conditions under which they occur, and the neurophysiological and neurocognitive mechanisms by which recovery occurs. The pressing research question is no longer "whether" but "when" and "for whom."

Extensive further research is now required to determine empirically the optimal conditions for treatment and the ways in which interventions should be tailored to individual needs. Meanwhile, the current state of scientific understanding allows formulation of principles and models to guide rehabilitation. The neuropsychological analysis in the previous chapter provides a conceptual foundation for this formulation by articulating the nature of impairments over the course of the disorder and identifying an assessment approach. This chapter discusses possible mechanisms by which neurocognitive recovery occurs and concludes with a formulation of principles and guidelines for addressing neurocognitive impairments in rehabilitation. The following chapter discusses specific neurocognitive interventions.

## LEVELS AND MECHANISMS OF RECOVERY

### Structural versus Functional Levels of Recovery

The psychopathology of severe mental illness generally suggests that neurocognitive impairments have four partially discrete origins: (1) structural brain lesions or anomalies caused by genetic flaws, infectious disease, and/or injury early in life (probably pre- and perinatal); (2) ongoing deterioration of the brain's structural integrity, whose causes, though not well understood, probably involve subtle neurophysiological processes[1]; (3) neurophysiological consequences of general health factors associated with severe mental illness, from malnutrition to side effects of psychiatric medication; (4) functional consequences of episodic neurophysiological dysregulation. Recovery of neurocognitive functioning presumably involves one or more of those originating sources.

A conventional understanding of brain biology allows a strong pre-

---

[1]As discussed in Chapter 4, it remains controversial whether this type of deterioration actually occurs, much less whether it is inevitable. Clinical studies and experience indicate that at least some individuals suffer a progressive deterioration clinically similar to that observed in progressive dementias that have known neuropathological causes. However, it is difficult to rule out the effects of extraneous variables, such as generally poor health, vulnerability to head injury, long-term effects of psychiatric drugs, accelerated aging, or deprivation associated with institutionalization. Whatever the etiology, however, a progressive dementia-like deterioration in neurocognitive functioning may be part of the clinical picture for some individuals.

sumption that adaptive changes of any kind, including neurocognitive changes, do not result from the correction of structural abnormalities, whether congenital (e.g., from prenatal viral infection) or acquired (e.g., head injury). The cellular architecture of the brain, once developed, does not change. Physical injury is permanent; dead neurons are not replaced. It is highly unlikely that any intervention, psychological or biological, operates by healing anatomical lesions or reshaping malformations. (However, therapeutic intervention could indirectly prevent or reduce accumulation of acquired neurophysiological impairment and deterioration by preventing acute psychosis and by helping patients maintain a healthy diet and avoid harmful substances.) This baseline reality leaves a limited number of possibilities:

1. Neurocognitive functioning does not really change, beyond resolution of acute psychosis; it may appear to change because people with residual impairments can still learn new skills, including skills to compensate behaviorally for neurocognitive impairments.
2. Neurocognitive impairments that respond to treatment do not have a structural substrate but result from a lingering functional abnormality, and this abnormality changes in response to environmental events and the person's own behavior.
3. The structural substrate of some impairments is at a subcellular level (e.g., the distribution of synaptic sites and related structures, neurotransmitter metabolism, gene activation, and neuroendocrine factors), and some of these microstructural "lesions" are amenable to change through person–environment interactions.

At this point in time, these are all viable hypotheses and not necessarily mutually exclusive. All three of the hypotheses have a common element: the implication that *patterns of interaction between people and their environments can bring about changes in brain functioning at the neurocognitive level.* Time (and research) will tell whether these interactions involve a unique type of skills acquisition, or whether they have a "structural" substrate. For a complete understanding, some of our customary ways of thinking about the brain may need to change. For example, ultimately it may not prove useful to distinguish "functional changes" from "structural changes," or "skills acquisition" from other "functional changes" at the neurocognitive level. At the level of neurophysiological organization, it is customary (and heuristically expedient) to distinguish between neural "structures"—configurations of cells and their physical components (axons, dendrites, terminal boutons, synapses, etc.)—and the biochemical activity that interacts with those configurations (metabolic processes, synaptic transmission, deployment of receptor sites, gene activation and deactivation, etc.). However, the distinction between *structural* and *functional* is inherently problematic. Neural structures involve an assemblage of interacting chemicals. Ultimately, the *behavior* of these chemicals contribute as much to neural "structure" as the chemicals' physical characteristics. As the science and technology relevant to neurophysiological functioning advance, it may eventually be necessary to abandon this distinction.

As with the structural–functional distinction, the distinction between *neurophysiological* and *neurocognitive* breaks down in, for example, neurophysiological explanations of learning. "Skills" are customarily conceptualized as "functional" products of learning because they can be acquired and lost. Ultimately, however, we must expect that learned skills have a "structural" basis as particular distributions of neural dendrites, synapses, receptor sites, enzymes, or gene activation factors. The conceptual issue is less about structure versus function than about what level of structure in the CNS is amenable to modification through interaction with the environment. It is also important to note that the "environment" can range from the social environment to the biochemical one (it is the latter we manipulate through pharmacotherapy). Interestingly, the success of antipsychotic drugs has not created a debate about whether the mechanisms of action could possibly be structural or functional—the distinction is tacitly recognized as unimportant—yet much of the skepticism in the scientific community about psychosocial neurocognitive treatment stems from a presumption that the mechanism could not possibly be structural.

## Specific and Nonspecific Treatment Effects

The research on neurocognitive-level interventions has generated two phenomena in need of explanation: specific and nonspecific treatment effects. A *specific* treatment effect is one that operates on a particular process, with particular results, preferably according to predictions generated by the theory behind the treatment. For example, penicillin exerts a specific treatment effect, killing specific bacteria that cause specific diseases. A *nonspecific* effect is one that operates on a diversity of processes, producing more diverse (but usually smaller) therapeutic benefits, not necessarily in ways addressed by the theory behind the treatment. For example, aspirin exerts a nonspecific treatment effect, blocking the physiological mechanisms that produce pain and inflammation, regardless of the specific cause of the pain and inflammation. Researchers became familiar with specific and nonspecific treatment effects in the psychotherapy research of the 1950s and 1960s, when they found that although patients tend to benefit from psychotherapy, it is not necessarily in the ways or for the reasons described by theories of psychotherapy. Ultimately, treatment is best understood when both its specific and nonspecific effects are understood.

In one large-scale controlled trial of neurocognitive intervention (Spaulding, Reed, et al., 1999), it was clear that the intervention produced better progress in social functioning, compared to comprehensive rehabilitation without the neurocognitive intervention. However, *all* the participants in the study showed substantial improvement in their neurocognitive functioning, whether they received the explicitly neurocognitive treatment or not. In fact, the degree of improvement was substantially greater than the additional improvement added by the neurocognitive intervention. This was unexpected, as previous studies in the same laboratory had shown little or no neurocognitive improvement associated with conventional treatment or rehabilitation. The only feasible explanation for the finding was that the intensive rehabilitation program produced nonspecific neurocognitive benefits that less intensive programs do not produce. A complete model of neurocognitive treatment effects thus needs to explain the nonspecific benefits of comprehensive rehabilitation in addition to the specific benefits of explicit treatment of neurocognitive deficits.

Our current understanding of neurophysiology and neuropsychology permits two plausible mechanisms of functional neurocognitive impairment and recovery in the post-acute phase of severe mental illness: One is a neuroendocrine mechanism, and the other is a neuropsychological mechanism.

## A Neuroendocrine Model

The hormone cortisol is one component of a neuroendocrine regulatory system whose structural components include the hypothalamus, pituitary, and adrenal glands, collectively termed the *hypothalamic–pituitary–adrenal* (HPA) *axis*. Cortisol is secreted by the adrenal gland in response to the secretion of adrenocorticotrophic hormone (ACH) by the pituitary. In turn, ACH is secreted in response to neurophysiological signals from the hypothalamus. It is well known that cortisol is secreted in response to stressful environmental events. Cortisol is usually present in the blood at abnormally high levels in people with acute psychosis. This heightened secretion could indicate that high cortisol levels are directly implicated in neurophysiological dysregulation, or that acute psychosis is extremely stressful. *Hypercortisolemia* (i.e., accelerated secretion of cortisol) generally abates as acute psychosis remits. In the residual phase, cortisol levels may recede to abnormally low levels. The implications of low cortisol levels have been fully appreciated only relatively recently, in part because of the traditional (and limiting) view of cortisol as a "stress hormone."

Cortisol secretion is indeed activated by stressful events, but its role in the stress response is only part of the picture. Healthy individuals show a diurnal cycle of cortisol secretion, with a peak in the early morning hours (before rising) and a trough in the evening. This cycle is generally interpreted as part of a mechanism for regulating an overall level of biological activation, corresponding to fluctuating diurnal demands. Furthermore, stress-related cortisol responses show considerable plasticity over time. When the stressful event is unfamiliar and the individual lacks an effective behavioral repertoire for coping with it, the cortisol response proceeds relatively slowly, resulting in slower increases and decreases in blood levels. This gradual dissipation of cortisol is probably responsible for the biological damage that results from protracted stress. However, as stressful situations become more familiar and the individual acquires a repertoire of effective coping behaviors, the cortisol response becomes more discrete. It may reach a higher peak level than occurs in response to unfamiliar stress, but it dissipates quickly. Phenomenologically, this pattern of fluctuating cortisol levels is reflected by the tranformation of an initially aversive experience of stress into a desirable experience of mastery and exhilaration.

The role of cortisol in diurnal regulation and its changing levels during acquisition of coping skills have led to a reformulation of its role as an "activating" hormone (Dienstbier, 1991). Accordingly, the HPA axis is increasingly seen as playing an important role in regulating broad patterns of activation as well as patterns of responding to stressful events. Cortisol secretion is linked to the metabolism of brain catecholamines (Silbergeld & Noble, 1973), indicating a role in the activity of this family of neurotransmitters. Recently the discovery of cortisol receptors in the frontal cortex has implicated HPA functioning more directly in neurocognitive activation (Kellendonk et al., 2002).

Hypocortisolemia (i.e., low levels of cortisol) is often observed in neuropathological conditions, especially those associated with aging (Basavaraju & Phillips, 1989), and in chronic disabling mental illness (Spaulding, Fleming et al., 1999). In mental illness, hypocortisolemia may be largely iatrogenic, given that antipsychotic drugs generally suppress cortisol secretion. The environmental homogenization of institutions and the inactive, featureless lifestyle to which mentally ill individuals are often consigned may also contribute. The diurnal cortisol cycle may disappear entirely in some individuals, resulting in a blunted response to specific stressful events. Recently it has been demonstrated that among individuals with severe mental illness, those with the lowest cortisol levels have the most severe cognitive impairments. There appears to be a three-way relationship between hypocortisolemia, cognitive impairment, and preference for a passive–avoidant style of coping (Jansen et al., 1998).

The link between cognitive impairment and hypocortisolemia suggests a problem in neurophysiological functioning. In the integrated paradigm, cognitive impairments and other consequences of hypocortisolemia that could be treated effectively at the neurophysiological level would justify identifying the underlying problem as a CNS dysregulation. However, there are no reports, as yet, in the scientific literature of successfully targeting hypocortisolemia for treatment in severe mental illness. It is possible to manipulate cortisol levels using current pharmacological technology, but the effectiveness or advisability of doing so to correct hypocortisolemia in people with mental illness has not been evaluated systematically.

The plasticity of the cortisol response indicates that environmental events have significant influence over the neurophysiological level at which both stress and coping patterns of response are mediated. There is some evidence that cortisol levels change toward more normal diurnal patterns in people with disabling mental illness who are undergoing rehabilitation (Spaulding, Wyss, & Littrell, 1990). Many characteristics of rehabilitation could be responsible, at least in part, for improved HPA functioning, ranging from following daily routines (perhaps reestablishing a diurnal activation cycle) to skills training in stress management.

It remains to be seen whether treatments directed at hypocortisolemia (be they pharmacological or psychosocial) might produce improvement in neurocognitive functioning. This is an important topic for systematic clinical research. Future research will determine whether HPA dysregulation should be formulated best as a neurophysiological problem or as a psychophysiological problem involving socioenvironmental, psychological, and neurophysiological components. For the time being, the neuroendocrine model suggests one way in which improvements may occur in nonspecific cognitive impairment in the postacute recovery phase. The orderliness and predictability of an intensive rehabilitation environment, with its focus on performance of daily routines and activities, together with a skills training emphasis on coping and stress management help normalize diurnal HPA regulation. In turn, HPA regulation enhances the activating role of cortisol, which produces more efficient and timely activation of the frontal cortex, resulting in overall improvements in neurocognition, especially in the executive domain. These are nonspecific effects of intensive rehabilitation. It remains unclear how this neuroendocrine mechanism could explain the *specific* effects of explicitly neurocognitive interventions.

## A Neuropsychological Model

The second model explaining treatment effects on post-acute recovery neurocognitive impairments is a neuropsychological one, in that it combines principles of neurophysiological and neurocognitive functioning with concepts associated with more molar levels of cognitive and behavioral functioning, including the processes of learning, conditioning, and skills acquisition. At the center of this model is a hypothetical neurocognitive mechanism whose function is to match the availability of specific cognitive operations with the demand for those operations in the current environment. Evidence for the existence of such a mechanism, which has been identified in lower mammals, may help explain the advances in behavioral complexity that mammals gained over reptiles and dinosaurs. (For a general discussion of these mechanisms, see Bradshaw & Sheppard, 2000; Gabrielli, 1995; Houk, 1995; Houk & Wise, 1993; Ito, 1990). In the human brain, a comparable mechanism almost certainly exists, located in phylogenetically primitive parts of the frontal cortex and frontal subcortical structures, especially the basal ganglia. Failure of this mechanism during acute psychosis could explain post-acute recovery neurocognitive impairment, and its repair could explain the effects of treatment directed at the neurocognitive level of functioning.

Evolution of a mechanism for continuously adjusting the availability of elements constituting a complex response repertoire would have had to occur to support the behavioral complexity of primates. As the mammalian brain became larger and more complex, it became capable of acquiring and storing an increasingly extensive repertoire of responses. This repertoire included not only molar skills, such as cooperative hunting and foraging, but also the more molecular-level perceptual and analytical abilities needed to support the molar skills. Uniquely human activities, such as tool making, engaging in tactical combat, and conducting business require special *acquired* abilities across the range of cognitive levels of functioning, from visual feature analysis to analytical problem solving. In the previous chapter the term *microskills* was introduced to characterize the molecular abilities required to support more complex skills. The "most molecular" microskills lie within the neurocognitive level of functioning.

Specific microskills are often components of a variety of more molar skills. For example, some of the microskills involved in reading are used to support many other skills, from story telling to bridge building. At the same time, different tasks require different combinations of microskills. For example, the perceptual, attentional, and memory operations that best support writing a book are very different from the ones that best support playing baseball. Thus, in the course of human evolution, the ability to select and activate specific skills and microskills from a very large repertoire became a crucial attribute of responding to environmental demands.

The modern human brain has a seemingly limitless capacity for storing information and acquiring complex skills that have both molar and molecular components. However, a large storage capacity creates a problem of *access*. If our protohuman ancestors had to sort through their entire response repertoire to select the specific neurocognitive operations they needed for particular situations, they would have been eaten by lions before they could select the appropriate response. The evolutionary solution was

to organize the availability of complex responses according to how frequently they are needed.

## Activation Thresholds

The brain accomplishes this fluctuation in availability by adjusting the *activation thresholds* of information stored in memory. Generally, contemporary models of skills performance contend that the information that guides
performance is stored in the form of potential patterns of neurophysiological activity across populations of memory-related neurons. The potential is maintained by configurations of synaptic interconnections (the
*junctional microstructure*), patterns of neurotransmitter activity, and patterns of gene activation (Davis, 2001). (Gene activation is a process
whereby specific areas on nuclear DNA are made available for protein synthesis. Studies of the molecular neurophysiology of learning and memory
implicate gene activation patterns as a possible locus for the storage of
memory information, perhaps through its effects on local neural activity.) A
memory is accessed when its particular pattern is activated physiologically,
which makes the information it contains available to other brain processes.
Frequently used information is given a low activation threshold, so that it is
more quickly activated when circumstances demand it. Thus the *hierarchical ordering of activation thresholds* is a basic principle in the organization
of cognitive activity and the basis of a person's ability to activate crucial
abilities when they are needed. Timely selection and execution of responses
to environmental circumstances are the essence of executive functioning,
and the ongoing process of adjusting activation thresholds represents a molecular level of executive cognition. In the modern human brain, executive
cognition involves a much more complex array of processes than those
characterizing our protohuman forebears, but the threshold activation
mechanism continues to play a crucial role in behavioral organization.

   We experience the operation of the response organization mechanism
whenever we encounter environmental changes that significantly shift the
demand for previously learned skills. For example, after living in a foreign
country for a long period of time, people experience a lack of fluency when
shifting back to their native language. It takes some time for the environmental demand to use the native language to effect the readjustment of the
activation thresholds for relevant vocabulary and grammar memory stores.
We also learn to manage environmental demands to perform special skills
not ordinarily demanded by a natural environment. For example, athletes
and musicians practice every day to maintain their "performance edge."
Practicing creates an artificial environmental demand, keeping the activation thresholds of the relevant skills low enough for the rapid access required for athletic competition or musical performance. (However, this

mechanism is quite distinct from the anatomical, metabolic, and cardiovascular conditions we associate with "physical fitness." Through inappropriate "practice," an athlete or musician could maintain the muscle strength and stamina to perform optimally without maintaining sufficient cognitive and psychomotor ability.)

In ordinary daily life we maintain low activation thresholds for complex skill repertoires that we take for granted. For example, routine social interaction requires a number of acquired microskills, such as the ability to rapidly scan the visual features of a person's facial expression and interpret them in terms of the person's emotional state. Humans are rarely removed from environments wherein these skills are in high continuous demand, so we seldom experience loss of access to them. Theoretically, long periods of social isolation (e.g., being marooned on an uninhabited island) would elevate activation thresholds in favor of the skills needed for solitary survival. People who experience such deprivation might be expected to undergo a period of difficulty, after their return to a social environment, in conducting ordinary social interaction. Perhaps this difficult reentry period approximates the experience of a person recovering from an acute psychotic episode.

## Response Hierarchy

The concept of an activation threshold hierarchy is comparable to the concept of a *response hierarchy* in learning theory (see Broen & Storms, 1966; Storms & Broen, 1969). A response hierarchy is composed of a group of possible behavioral responses, organized with respect to the relative probability that any particular response in the group will be performed in a given situation. *Reinforcement* is crucial to the original construction and maintenance of response hierarchies. Reinforcement is the process of increasing the probability of specific behaviors when environmental events associated with those behaviors result in reduction of some appetitive drive. For example, a hungry rat learns to press a lever when that behavior consistently results in delivery of a food pellet. The lever-pressing response is acquired because of the reinforcement value of its consequences. As long as lever pressing is reinforced, it will remain dominant in the hierarchy of possible behaviors. Another way to say this is to say that its activation threshold will remain low. If more complex responses are required for reinforcement (e.g., pressing the lever only when a green light is turned on, or performing a series of lever presses), those responses collectively gain dominance in the hierarchy.

As acquired or learned responses become very complex, they become more recognizable as "skills" and their cognitive and neurocognitive underpinnings become increasingly significant. In humans, social events acquire reinforcing properties (e.g., the approval of valued others), vastly extending the scope and increasing the speed with which learning can occur. Reinforcement alone does not account for the full complexity of acquired behavior in humans (or even lower animals), but it clearly exerts a significant influence beyond the original acquisition of skills. In natural environments, the activation thresholds of acquired behaviors and their associated microskills are influenced by the interplay of environmental demand for those behaviors and the rate at which they are reinforced. (Ultimately, the distinction between *demand* and *rate of reinforcement* may be tautological. In a sense, there is no demand for behavior that is never reinforced. The semantic distinction in the context of the integrated paradigm serves to direct our attention to two separable characteristics of the environment: the general circumstances that create demand, and the specific events that reinforce specific responses.)

## The Immediacy Hypothesis

The plausibility of the response hierarchy model as a mechanism to account for the complexity of neurocognitive recovery suggests another heuristically useful principle, the *immediacy hypothesis* (Salzinger, 1973, 1984). Originally formulated in the 1970s, the immediacy hypothesis provides an account of the overall impact of neurocognitive impairment on functional behavior. The key idea is that neurocognitive impairment generally reduces an individual's ability to respond to environmental circumstances (*stimuli*, in behaviorist terminology) that are physically, temporally, or conceptually distant. Responding to increasingly distant events is central in human development. As children, our behavior is influenced primarily by events that occur in the proximal environment. As we become adults we comport our behavior in relation to increasingly distant events—a monthly paycheck, college graduation, success in a career. Failures in this developmental process create distinct behavioral problems, including impulsiveness and inadequate socialization, in older children and adolescents; in adults, behavior that is overly controlled by immediate circumstances can be disastrous. The immediacy hypothesis not only provides a plausible, unifying concept for understanding some of the behavioral characteristics of adults with severe mental illness, but also accounts for an impressive array of findings from experimental psychopathology laboratories.

The immediacy hypothesis was formulated before there was widespread appreciation of the episodic nature of mental illness and hence does not distinguish between acute, post-acute, and residual neurocognitive impairments as contributors to stimulus–response immediacy. It is equally applicable to all three types and has comparable implications. Part of the therapeutic benefits of an intensive rehabilitation milieu, especially that part associated with token economy or other forms of formal contingency management, accrues from making stimulus–response contingencies very concrete and very immediate. A person with neurocognitive impairment can function and be successful in such an environment, when a more natural environment with more abstract and more distant contingencies would produce functional failure. This environmental effect further reinforces the importance of predictability and consistency in a therapeutic milieu, and the importance of concrete and immediate consequences for key behaviors. An updated version of the immediacy hypothesis would suggest that with recovery from acute and post-acute neurocognitive impairment, the proximity of stimulus–response relationships could be gradually relaxed. In fact, the "fading" of contingency management interventions (discussed in Chapter 10) may turn out to be an important indicator of neurocognitive recovery, at least for some individuals. The relationship between neurocognitive impairment, immediacy, and environmental conditions also sheds light on the phenomenon of institutionalization. People with severe mental illness are notoriously vulnerable to the effects of institutionalization; behavior that is adaptive within an institution is inadequate in a more normal environment. Although institutional environments can be described as "predictable," they are not usually predictable in a therapeutic way. Daily routines and demands in an institutional environment may be consistent, but they tend to be the routines and demands of the institutional staff, not normal life. The most immediately available reinforcers (e.g., staff attention) tend to be contingent on inappropriate behavior. That is, the most predictable way to get the attention of a staff person is to engage in disruptive behavior. Consequences that would normally guide behavior (e.g., release from the institution) are too temporally distant and abstract to be apprehended by people with severe cognitive impairment. As a result, institutional environments tend to selectively reinforce inappropriate behavior. Therapeutic uses of environmental contingencies to promote adaptive behavior and prevent institutionalization are further discussed in Chapter 10.

## The Role of Dopamine

Dopamine appears to be an important neurotransmitter in the neural structures associated with the response organization mechanism. Dopamine is heavily implicated in the CNS dysregulation associated with episodic psychosis. The dopamine dysregulation that accompanies acute psychosis would produce a temporary malfunction of the response organization mechanism. For a time, the hierarchical organization of activation thresholds would be compromised (Figure 6.1).

Depending on the severity and duration of the dopamine dysregulation, access to the highly rehearsed microskills required for routine social functioning could be reduced. The activation thresholds themselves could

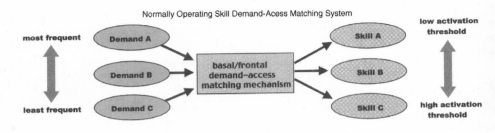

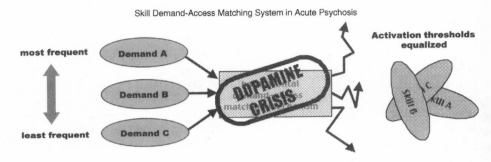

**FIGURE 6.1.** The consequences of disrupting a dopamine-regulated mechanism for matching response hierarchies to changing environmental demands are collapse of the response hierarchy and randomization of access to needed skills.

be equalized, meaning that no skill is any more accessible than any other. The operations needed for routine social interaction would be no more accessible than arcane, rarely used microskills. Most importantly, the optimal hierarchical organization would not be expected to return spontaneously upon resolution of the dopamine dysregulation. Organization of the hierarchy requires not just a properly working mechanism but also *experience with the environment.* It is the frequency of environmental demand, translated into activation thresholds by the response organization mechanism, that establishes the optimal organizational hierarchy. The homogeneous, low-demand environments in most institutions and the reinforcement-depleted lifestyle of the chronic mental patient would sustain a state of suboptimal response organization.

In this neuropsychological model, recovery from the acute-phase neurocognitive impairment occurs as environmental conditions interact with a restabilized response organization mechanism to reestablish a functional hierarchy of relevant neurocognitive microskills. This mechanism provides an explanation of the specific and nonspecific treatment effects found in the Spaulding, Reed, and colleagues (1999) study. The nonspecific effects accrue from the rehabilitation milieu's orderly and predictable routines and contingencies, which create a demand for apprehending contingencies, conceptualizing circumstances, and solving problems. Furthermore, appropriate exercise of the relevant microskills usually produces behavior that is immediately and specifically reinforced, thereby lowering the activation thresholds of those skills. The cognitive operations for apprehending the demands of a task and activating the needed microskills become more accessible; in turn, this enhanced accessibility is reflected in better performance on laboratory tasks, especially tasks that demand executive cognition. Rehabilitation emphasis on social skills lowers the activation thresholds for the microskills most important for interpersonal functioning, resulting in better social skills acquisition and higher levels of social competence. The additional benefit (i.e., the specific treatment effect) of neurocognitive intervention accrues from an even more intensive focus on activating the microskills most pertinent to particular tasks, especially tasks involving social interaction. This narrowed focus results in even greater gains in social competence.

## Specificity of Neurocognitive Changes

In keeping with the three-factor model, executive- and memory-related functions are the most prone to change in the post-acute phase. At this time, there is insufficient data to determine whether these are the same or different functions that most respond to the treatment of acute psychosis. There is probably considerable individual variability in the specific constellations of impairments that fluctuate with a person's acute and post-acute status, even within the domains we now identify as executive and memory. These domains are vast and still relatively unexplored. Nevertheless, there is much clinical relevance in the general findings that (1) tasks that measure executive and memory abilities tend to be the first to show post-acute improvement, and (2) baseline executive and memory functioning is predictive of success in rehabilitative skill acquisition.

The executive domain of cognition, which is primarily concerned with the selection and execution of skills, incorporates a complex repertoire of microskills specific to situational demands. Closely related to situation-identification is the function of allocating cognitive resources, also referred to as information-processing capacity, to handle the information necessary to further analyze the situation and support a response. Short-term memory tasks, which directly and specifically demand allocation of the immediate storage space, are particularly vulnerable to failures in the allocation function. This vulnerability makes sense of the parallel failure and recovery of conceptual, executive, and memory functions in mental illness.

For practical purposes, situation-identification and capacity allocation functions represent functionally distinct types of microskills, by their nature prerequisite to the proper functioning of other microskills. For present purposes they are termed *executive microskills* to distinguish them from *performance microskills*, which are the ones activated during performance of the behavioral skill itself. In the performance of complex tasks, sequences of microskills become *automated*, meaning they activate each other in proper sequence without ongoing involvement of executive microskills. Experimental findings suggest that severe mental illness is associated with insufficient automatization of cognitive processes, which may result from impairments in the executive processes that facilitate automatization (Gray, Buhusi, & Schmajuk, 1997). Insufficient automatization of performance microskills would decrease efficiency beyond that produced by impaired executive microskills. Executive microskills are expected to be the first to reappear during post-acute recovery simply because others cannot function without them. They are analogous to the operating system of a computer—those components that monitor input devices, allocate central memory to run programs, activate output devices, and so on. When a computer crashes, the operating system must be restarted before the computer can do anything else. Indeed, stabilization of the power supply is usually not sufficient to restore all functioning post-crash. The operating system must be "re-bootstrapped," meaning that a set sequence of operations must be systematically initialized by loading software programs into the computer's core memory and executing them. Similarly, the nonspecific treatment effects on executive functioning suggest that parts of the human "operating system" crash in the wake of acute psychosis and reorganize themselves in response to the environmental characteristics of intensive rehabilitation.

Short of a total "crash," the human operating system shows great variability in the efficiency with which microskills are activated in response to changing environmental demands. Detection of situational demands can be a complex task, especially in the domain of interpersonal functioning, so failure can occur at many points. Complex task performance requires ongoing detection of changing demands and ongoing revisions of resource allocation and microskill activation. Gradual recovery from post-acute neurocognitive impairment reflects the gradual readjustment of the activation thresholds for all these microskills, one microskill at a time.

The acquisition of complex skills does not proceed in a linear sequence from acquisition of executive microskills to that of performance microskills. Rather, the process is a cyclic one, alternating between acquisition of executive and performance skills of increasing complexity. Post-acute reorganization of microskill hierarchies would presumably undergo a similar

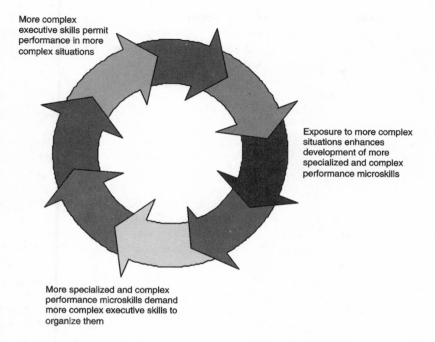

More complex
executive skills permit
performance in more
complex situations

Exposure to more complex
situations enhances
development of more
specialized and complex
performance microskills

More specialized and complex
performance microskills demand
more complex executive skills to
organize them

**FIGURE 6.2.** Acquisition and reorganization of performance abilities are cyclic processes involving the development and specialization of increasingly complex microskills, along with increasingly complex executive skills to organize them.

process. Proper functioning of some executive microskills will require proper functioning of some performance microskills. Therefore, recovery of neurocognitive functioning in the post-acute phase is not expected to proceed in a linear sequence, from executive to performance microskills, but as a cyclic interplay between executive and performance microskills (Figure 6.2). This nonlinear view is a departure from earlier constructions of mental illness that presumed a linear, hierarchical relationship between levels of functioning (Cromwell & Spaulding, 1978) and prescribed a corresponding linear sequence of treatment (Brenner, 1987; Spaulding et al., 1986). Ironically, this view inspired the original version of integrated psychological therapy (IPT), which produced the data (Spaulding, Reed, et al., 1999) that requires a nonlinear model of cognitive change.

Explicitly neurocognitive interventions include specific procedures for activating and exercising the executive microskills associated with those performance microskills relevant to rehabilitation. The nonspecific treatment effects of the intensive rehabilitation milieu accrue from its demand for and reinforcement of the executive microskills associated with performing activities of routine daily functioning (e.g., self-care, being at the right place at the right time, responding to other people).

## IMPLICATIONS FOR TREATMENT

The models of neurocognitive failure and recovery in mental illness described above generates five principles for constructing a treatment strategy:

1. Recovery of executive and memory functions, which mediates subsequent recovery of personal and social functioning, is enhanced by an environment rich in salient reinforcing events, with clear and consistent relationships between individual behaviors and their environmental antecedents and consequences, and where behavior associated with appropriate attention to routine environmental demands is heavily and differentially reinforced.

2. Recovery of the neurocognitive abilities that support basic social and interpersonal functioning is enhanced by an environment that provides frequent opportunities and support for appropriate social behavior, with consistent and perceptible reinforcement of effective and/or appropriate behavior and minimal inadvertent reinforcement of ineffective or inappropriate behavior.

3. The relatively nonspecific effects of an orderly, consistent, prosocial, and contingency-rich environment are further enhanced by specific interventions that explicitly invoke the neurocognitive microskills that underlie performance of social and interpersonal skills.

4. For both specific and nonspecific interventions, the ability to identify specific situations requiring specific microskills, and to allocate resources to perform those microskills, are as important as performance of the microskills themselves. Exercising the ability to recognize various task demands and to modify one's cognition (i.e., activate microskills) in response to changing demands is as important as exercising the ability to perform a particular skill.

5. Although restoring functioning on the executive and memory levels mediates subsequent recovery, it is not a strict prerequisite. Identifying situational demands, allocating capacity, and activating the appropriate microskills are complex cognitive activities, some of which are highly specific to particular situations and skills. As recovery progresses, restoration of advanced executive functions may require intact performance functions. Achieving this level of recov-

ery requires a cyclic rather than linear approach to neurocognitive intervention. Exercise of fundamental microskills should be preceded by exercise in detecting relevant situational demands, but treatment should then address detection of more complex situations and demands, followed by exercise of more complex skill performance, and so on.

In the next chapter, these general guidelines are discussed in relation to specific intervention technologies.

# Chapter 7

# Neurocognitive Interventions

Neurocognitive interventions address (1) post-acute and (2) residual impairments. Interventions for post-acute impairments are designed to facilitate recovery from the neurocognitive disorganization that accompanies acute psychosis. In the sense that residual impairments are not amenable to change, interventions for these impairments are generally *prosthetic* in nature. That is, they are designed to compensate for the functional disabilities that the neurocognitive impairment produces, rather than change the neurocognitive impairment itself.

Interventions for post-acute neurocognitive impairment can be subdivided into those that operate in the early stages of recovery from acute psychosis (Drury, Birchwood, Cochrane, & MacMillan, 1996a, 1996b), and those that operate in later stages (Bell et al., 2001; Hogarty & Flesher, 1999a; Medalia, Aluma, Tyron, & Merriam, 1998; Silverstein, Menditto, & Stuve, 2000; Spaulding, Reed, et al., 1999; Wykes, Reeder, Corner, Williams, & Everitt, 1999). In the former case, clinical circumstances overlap with those of treating the acute phase itself. There is no universally endorsed criterion for marking the resolution of an acute episode, and there is significant individual variation on any objective measure. Recovery of neurocognitive functioning is only weakly correlated with other indications (e.g., positive symptom suppression). In the case of later-stage interventions, clinical circumstances may overlap with those of treating the residual state of the illness, with the attendant residual neurocognitive impairment, except that intervention produces improvement. Outcome data suggest that interventions for post-acute neurocognitive impairment are most usefully conducted from the earliest to the latest periods of the post-acute phase. The amenability to neurocognitive recovery long after resolution of the acute phase suggests that, in some circumstances, the post-acute recovery phase is a highly stable one. As discussed in Chapter 6, homogenous institutional environments with no demand for scheduled activity or appropriate interpersonal interaction are expected to help perpetuate response hierarchy disorganization. Even outside an institutional environment, an impoverished lifestyle with low demand for appropriate functioning could perpetuate post-acute phase impairment. In contemporary mental health services, it is not uncommon for people to begin rehabilitation after an extended period in such environments. It should therefore be no surprise that individuals show significant neurocognitive recovery in an intensive rehabilitation milieu, even after a protracted period of neurophysiological stability.

Although there is strong evidence that neurocognitive functioning can improve in response to intervention, the mechanisms by which this improvement occurs are not fully understood. It is possible that all such mechanisms involve acquisition of particular skills or microskills that compensate for, but do not eliminate, the impairments. Such a situation would blur the distinction between prosthesis and recovery. Research will undoubtedly clarify this point over the next few years. For the time being, it is reasonable and heuristically convenient to classify interventions designed to improve functioning separately from those designed to minimize the impact of apparently permanent impairments. Ultimately, it will be important to determine which interventions are prosthetic and which foster recovery. A prosthetic intervention is needed to maintain functioning in the foreseeable future. Recovery means functioning without prostheses; that is, a greater degree of independence and autonomy.

## EARLY-STAGE NEUROCOGNITIVE INTERVENTIONS

The presence of acute psychosis is the first evidence of post-acute neurocognitive impairment. As the psychotic episode dissipates, remaining neurocognitive impairments are decreasingly likely indicators of ongoing acute neurophysiological dysregulation. Current neuropsychological technology provides a means of quantitatively tracking the changes in neurocognition as an episode subsides, but it does not provide a simple criterion for determining if the impairments constitute independent problems. Choosing to activate "post-acute neurocognitive impairment" as a problem on a rehabilitation plan reflects the rehabilitation team's collective judgment that there are neurocognitive impairments that are not being addressed through interventions directed at neurophysiological dysregulation. When the problem is entered on the rehabilitation plan, it represents the team's hypothesis that neurocognitive, as opposed to neurophysiological, interventions are required for further progress.

Theoretically, intervention for post-acute neurocognitive impairment would be demarcated by a shift in the therapeutic milieu, away from conditions optimized for resolving acute neurophysiological dysregulation and toward conditions optimized for reorganizing microskill hierarchies. However, this shift is a subtle one, as can be seen by comparing the two sets of conditions (Table 7.1). In practice, it is often imperceptible, as ongoing adjustments to individualized environmental demands create a continuous segue. As a result, the task of initiating treatment of neurocognitive deficits early in the post-acute phase is, in large part, one of effecting a gradual and systematic transition from milieu-based treatment of acute neurophysiological dysregulation.

TABLE 7.1. Milieu Characteristics for Optimizing Recovery in the Acute and Post-Acute Stages (bold type indicates changes; for details, see discussion in Chapters 4 and 6)

| *Acute Stage* | *Post-Acute Stage* |
|---|---|
| Supervision and restriction necessary for safety in acute psychotic state | Supervision and restriction necessary for safety, **adjusted as recovery progresses** |
| Highly consistent schedule of daily routines | Highly consistent schedule of daily routines |
| Empathetic, nonjudgmental, matter-of-fact staff attitudes and behaviors | Empathetic, nonjudgmental, matter-of-fact staff attitudes and behaviors |
| Clear expectations for behavioral comportment (e.g., no aggression, attendance to basic personal care and hygiene and daily schedule) | Clear expectations for behavioral comportment (e.g., no aggression, attendance to basic personal care and hygiene and daily schedule) |
| Social support and encouragement to adhere to behavioral expectations | **Systematic contingency management as necessary to maintain** adherence to behavioral expectations |
| Minimal ambient stress, demands for interpersonal functioning adjusted to individual characteristics of acute psychotic state | **Systematically graduated demands for normal** interpersonal functioning, **adjusted as recovery progresses** |
| Psychoeducation and counseling focused on acute aspects of disorder (e.g., recognizing the illness state, significance of symptoms, and role of medication and related treatment for acute psychosis) | Psychoeducation and counseling focused on **post**-acute aspects of disorder (e.g., **neurocognitive recovery, self-monitoring of mental status and symptoms, participating in team processes**) |
| Systematic engagement in problem solving related to immediate situation (e.g., managing symptoms, resolving legal problems, planning return of normal functioning) | Systematic engagement in problem solving related to **post-acute recovery** (e.g., **interpersonal interactions, regaining independence, planning for long-term rehabilitation**) |

The transition from a neurophysiological to a neurocognitive focus involves shifts in the focus and emphasis of specific rehabilitation interventions as well as the therapeutic milieu. In the acute phase, the most useful foci of rehabilitation counseling, psychoeducation, and skills training are expected to help the recovering person recognize the presence of the illness and the need for intervention, whereas in the post-acute phase, attention gradually turns to the person's ability to participate in clinical assessment and planning, monitor recovery processes, and otherwise actively engage in the rehabilitation enterprise.

Initiating post-acute neurocognitive interventions is thus a task of gradually modifying the rehabilitation plan in response to ongoing clinical assessment of neurophysiological and neurocognitive functioning. The rehabilitation team must be able to (1) provide a therapeutic milieu and specific treatment modalities that are optimized for the resolution of acute psychosis, and (2) gradually modify the milieu and the specific modalities over the course of recovery. These rehabilitative requirements are essentially management tasks and are discussed in more detail in Chapters 11 and 12. The component unique to addressing neurocognitive functioning is that of utilizing neuropsychological assessment data as a guide for making gradual adjustments in the rehabilitation regimen as recovery proceeds.

## LATER-STAGE NEUROCOGNITIVE INTERVENTIONS

### Preliminary Considerations

The nonspecific effects of intensive rehabilitation on neurocognitive functioning observed by Spaulding, Reed, and colleagues (1999) occurred over a 6-month time period in individuals who were well beyond stabilization of an acute episode and who, on average, had been ill for over 10 years. Although the nonspecific benefits of neurocognitive treatment have yet to be verified by independent researchers, there is reason to believe that the milieu and other nonspecific rehabilitation factors most conducive to neurocognitive recovery can exert beneficial effects at any time in the course of the illness. However, a person's functioning in the later post-acute phase is expected to differ substantially from earlier phases. The demands of the milieu must be gradually increased as the person's capabilities return, so that demand for, and reinforcement of, essential microskills continue. The complexity and requirements of counseling, psychoeducation, and skills training must be increased gradually, so that the recovering person is challenged to use recovered cognitive capacities without becoming overwhelmed.

As in the earlier phase of post-acute recovery, repeated neuropsychological assessment is a key guide for this process, and the person's ability to adhere to a daily routine, measured by observable behavior, reflects a key parameter of this later post-acute phase. Until the person is able to consistently adhere to a daily routine, including attendance and participation in counseling, psychoeducation, and skills training activities, the impact of more specific neurocognitive interventions will be compromised. Careful, systematic use of contingency management interventions and/or behavioral contracting is often necessary to achieve this degree of behavioral stability (these techniques are discussed in more detail in Chapter 10). The person's stability provides the optimal condition for specific neurocognitive interventions.

At some point *prior to* behavioral stabilization (i.e., consistent adherence to a routine daily schedule), however, the character of the clinical decision to intervene at the neurocognitive level begins to change. In the acute and early post-acute phases of illness, clinical decisions are strongly influenced by the urgency and risk associated with the circumstances of treatment. The short-term goals of treatment often involve the immediate physical safety of the recovering person, and there is often little choice about whether to provide treatment. In some cases, the recovering person may lose legal competence to make key decisions. As these circumstances change and treatment for the acute psychosis segues into rehabilitation in the post-acute phase, alternatives may multiply and decisions may become more complex and difficult. Now there is a greater degree of separation between the decisions and prerogatives of the recovering person (and others legally responsible to make decisions on behalf of the recovering person) and the mental health service system. Progress in rehabilitation counseling may be necessary before the recovering person agrees to invest in neurocognitive interventions.

Even if the recovering person desires services, the system may not provide them. In some venues, the prevailing mental health service model may not even recognize the need for, or value of, any treatment or rehabilitation beyond that associated with resolving the acute episode.[1] In venues where rehabilitation is routinely available, it may not be intensive enough to generate nonspecific neurocognitive benefits. The clinical decision as to whether to provide explicit post-acute intervention for neurocognitive impairment can thus be preempted by the desires of the recovering person or the limitations of the mental health system. As the early post-acute phase

[1]It is noteworthy that Assertive Community Treatment and related forms of aftercare case management, probably the services most commonly available in the United States to people with severe and disabling mental illness, have produced no evidence of rehabilitative benefits. Their value is in providing compensatory and support services to prevent relapse and/or rehospitalization, not in improving peoples' personal and social functioning.

becomes the later post-acute phase, the decision to address neurocognitive impairments, with either specific or nonspecific interventions, requires an increasingly distinct commitment on the part of both service recipients and service providers.

Some individuals experience such a rapid and complete return of their baseline neurocognitive functioning that provisions for post-acute neurocognitive recovery are a minor factor in their continuing progress. Other individuals—disproportionately those with the most disabling conditions—experience such protracted and severe post-acute neurocognitive impairment that success in addressing it may determine the overall success of rehabilitation. Continuous assessment of their neurophysiological and neurocognitive status is necessary to determine which circumstance is applicable, for it obviously will influence the setting of priorities for neurocognitive intervention. In most mental health systems, a key decision point arrives when the recovering person is ready to leave the environment in which the acute psychosis has been treated—generally an acute inpatient psychiatric unit, less often an alternative setting such as a respite program or crisis shelter. Sometimes the acute phase can be managed while the recovering person maintains his or her usual place of residence. When it is time for the post-acute treatment environment to change, specific consideration should be given to the therapeutic value of the destination milieu (see Table 7.1). If the environment does not change, consideration should be given to enhancing its therapeutic characteristics pertinent to the later post-acute phase of treatment.

Theoretically, a key factor in assessing the degree of need for neurocognitive intervention in the later post-acute phase is the degree to which the person's neurocognitive functioning has returned to a reliably established baseline when other indicators (disappearance or diminishment of psychotic symptoms, behavioral stabilization, etc.) suggest resolution of the acute episode. However, it may be impossible to establish a reliable estimate of baseline neurocognitive functioning in people with severe and disabling mental illness. Furthermore, it is questionable whether there are individual differences in the benefits of post-acute neurocognitive interventions. The large-scale outcome studies investigating this area have included people who were at different points along the severity continuum. Those in the Spaulding, Reed, and colleagues (1999) study were extremely disabled, unable to function outside an institutional setting, whereas those in the Hogarty and colleagues (1999b) study were living in the community with relatively mild functional deficits. Those of the Bell and colleagues (2001) study were in between, living outside an institution but with severe functional impairments. There is insufficient data to identify any particular subgroup or characteristic as indicative of beneficial response to neurocognitive intervention. From a scientific standpoint, the most defensible clinical decision is to provide both specific and nonspecific interventions, whenever possible, to *everyone* in the later post-acute phase of a severe mental illness.

For individuals at the most extreme end of the severity continuum, an operant theory-based approach may be the best intervention choice (Silverstein et al., 2000). In this approach, the motor behavior associated with attending is selectively reinforced with tokens during group skills training. This approach is potentially applicable to most any skills training intervention, from basic conversation to work skills. Early outcome studies are promising, although large-scale studies sufficient to identify the characteristics of individuals who benefit the most have yet to be performed.

Nonspecific intervention for neurocognitive impairment in the later post-acute phase is basically an extension of intervention in the earlier phase. Maximum neurocognitive benefit is expected from comprehensive rehabilitation at the highest intensity the recovering person can comfortably tolerate. Specific interventions enhance the nonspecific benefits of intensive rehabilitation and should be provided whenever possible. Specific neurocognitive interventions can be categorized as dyadic or group in format. The optimal format, or combination of formats, is jointly determined by the needs and preferences of the individual recipient, and the resources and capabilities of the mental health service system.

All specific interventions for neurocognitive impairment have in common some procedure(s) for isolating hypothetical neurocognitive abilities (*microskills* in the terms of this discussion) and exercising those abilities by engaging the recovering person in activities designed to invoke their use.

## Dyadic Therapy Techniques

The literature provides procedural descriptions of specific techniques easily adapted to a dyadic psychotherapy-like format (e.g., Corrigan & Storzbach, 1993; Medalia et al., 1998; Reed, Sullivan, Penn, Stuve, & Spaulding, 1992; Spaulding et al., 1986; vanderGaag, 1992; vanderGaag et al., 1994; Wykes et al., 1999). In this approach, exercises are constructed in an ad hoc manner, derived from the results of laboratory testing, direct observation, and functional assessment. Progress toward short-term treatment goals is typically assessed by using laboratory tasks adapted to measure the specific impairments targeted for treatment, such as attention deficits. Generalization of treatment effects and progress toward longer-term goals are assessed by measuring changes in performance of ecologically significant abilities (e.g., daily hygiene activities) hypothesized to be affected by the targeted cognitive impairments. For example, when performance in a work setting is hypothesized to be compromised by distractibility and deficits in continuous attention, improvement on laboratory measures of attention and vigilance is expected following neurocognitive treatment, followed, in turn, by improvement on in vivo measures of work performance. In a clinical (as opposed to research) context, multiple-baseline quasi-experimental designs capable of detecting the distinct effects of medication, neurocognitive treatment, and other interventions are generally well suited to this purpose.

Individualized neurocognitive treatment is usually provided by including the specific techniques in a broader, dyadic rehabilitation counseling and psychotherapy context. These techniques are accompanied by (1) the team's collaborative formulation of relevant treatment and rehabilitation goals, (2) discussion of the abilities addressed by the exercises and their role in naturalistic settings, (3) assignment and review of "homework" (*in vivo* applications of the exercises), and (4) review and evaluation of overall rehabilitation progress. For example, "better interactions with people" may be identified as a treatment goal. Functional and laboratory assessment may indicate that the problem derives from a social skills deficit, to which distractibility, poor interpersonal problem solving, and a rigid, stereotypic way of analyzing complex social situations all contribute (the assessment would also indicate that these do not derive from a transient, acute psychotic state). Exercises demanding focused attention, resistance to distraction, and conceptual flexibility would be included in dyadic sessions, accompanied by interpersonal problem solving and social skills training in group formats. In addition to the neurocognitive exercises, the dyadic sessions include (1) reviewing performance data in therapy and in vivo situations, (2) discussing the role of neurocognitive factors in ongoing experiences relevant to social competence and comfort, (3) reviewing objective measures of social performance, and (4) appraising overall progress toward the goal.

In addition to a dyadic psychotherapy-like setting, individualized neurocognitive exercises can be integrated into occupational and recreational therapy, work, and other rehabilitative activities. For example, continuous attention exercises are easily integrated with simple workshop tasks. The optimal setting varies with individual needs and rehabilitation goals.

## Group Format Modalities

At least two comprehensive, systematic approaches to treatment of neurocognitive impairments in people with schizophrenia have evolved over the past two decades: integrated psychological therapy (IPT; Brenner et al., 1994) and cognitive enhancement therapy (CET; Hogarty & Flesher, 1999a, 1999b). They share the strategy of identifying, isolating, and exercising specific cognitive abilities typically impaired in people with chronic schizophrenia. They also use somewhat similar procedures, including a diversity of specific exercises, formatted as group activities, targeting specific abilities. Both combine a primary focus on cognitive *processes* (i.e., emphasis on strengthening information processing) with didactic provision of factual information (i.e., the *content* of cognition) pertinent to personal and social functioning. Both are highly manualized, and the IPT manual is commercially available (Brenner et al., 1994). There have been no studies of therapist skills or qualifications required for effectively administering these modalities. However, considerable clinical judgment is required to determine when to persist with a particular exercise, when to provide special assistance to group members, and when to move on. Considerable experience with neuropsychological assessment, functional assessment, and group skills training are also probably necessary.

There is a noteworthy theoretical difference between the two approaches. IPT was developed from classical ideas in experimental psychopathology that predated contemporary interest in distinctively social cognition. CET also draws heavily from experimental psychopathology and neuropsychology but, in addition, is heavily influenced by developmental theories of social cognition. This theoretical difference implies two different types of treatment mechanisms. In IPT, treatment effects are thought to accrue in a stepwise fashion. Molecular cognitive processes are exercised first so that, later, those strengthened molecular processes can enhance acquisition of more molar abilities. The rehabilitation process progresses from process-focused therapy to more conventional social skills and interpersonal problem-solving training.

CET is less linear and stepwise. It draws heavily on the theory that a crucial problem in schizophrenia is deficient apprehension of the "gist" of social problems and situations. "Gistful" social cognition does not involve a gradual compilation of information from more molecular processes (i.e., the gradual synthesis of the "Big Picture" from informational elements) but a rapid and conceptual apprehension, inferred from a relatively small amount of information about a situation, when that information correlates with specific social schemata (declarative relationships, social roles, procedural scripts, etc.) stored in memory and acquired in the course of development. The CET approach is guided by the hypothesis (among others) that impairment of processes that identify and respond to the "gist" of social situations and interactions is a key limiting factor in the social performance of people with schizophrenia.

Controlled outcome studies have shown both IPT and CET to be effective in enhancing social competence and performance (Hogarty & Flesher, 1999b; Spaulding, Reed, et al., 1999). So far, however, there is insufficient data to conclude whether the mechanisms of their respective treatment effects are as different as their respective theoretical premises. Indeed, the actual procedural differences between the two approaches have yet to be assessed systematically. (Given that research on IPT militates for revision of its assumptions about the linear, hierarchical nature of its treatment effects, there may be even less difference between the CET theoretical model and an updated version of the IPT model.) The subject samples in the two studies were quite different (the IPT participants were severely disabled and involuntarily institutionalized, whereas the CET participants were less severely disabled voluntary outpatients), and any differences in outcome or treatment effect mechanisms are potentially attributable to that. In addition to sheer severity of impairment, participants in the two samples likely differed in their position on the continuum from acute to post-acute to residual phase. Systematic comparative studies of the two approaches, across a range of subpopulations, will be necessary to draw any valid conclusions.

The original developers of IPT recommend providing this modality separately to recipients with higher and lower overall cognitive functioning. The therapy procedures do not differ, but the rate of progress through the modality is expected to be slower with lower-functioning participants. Comprehensive neuropsychological assessment is not required for group assignment, but a reliable overall evaluation of baseline cognitive and neurocognitive functioning, taking into account episodic psychosis, is necessary. Such assessment capability should be in the repertoire of any program or agency that serves people with severe and disabling psychiatric disorders.

The IPT subprograms proceed as a sequence of structured group activities, each demanding various combinations of cognitive abilities and operations. The therapist introduces each activity, guides the participation of the members, and evaluates their responses. The therapist is given some flexibility to repeat specific activities when patients have difficulties that might be overcome with further practice. All the activities are designed to include social interaction between patients, which the therapist selectively facilitates. The cognitive differentiation subprogram includes activities designed to exercise concept manipulation and related operations. A representative activity is a sorting task that engages the group in alternative strategies for sorting objects of different color, size, and shape. The social perception subprogram includes activities designed to exercise the processing of social information. A representative activity involves systematic examination and description of pictures of individuals involved in social situations. The group members are guided through a discussion of their differing perceptions of the ambiguous situations and encouraged to find areas of agreement and disagreement. The verbal communication subprogram is designed to exercise the cognitive substrates, including attention and short-term memory, of verbal interaction. A representative activity engages patients in carefully listening to each others' verbal statements, then repeating them verbatim, then paraphrasing them. Across all the subprograms, the activities are graduated in complexity and amount of required social interaction.

To manage group dynamics, the therapist follows a set of interaction rules. These include (1) maintaining a friendly but matter-of-fact social atmosphere, (2) eliciting group feedback and discussion rather than telling patients they are wrong or factually incorrect, (3) empathetically reflecting emotional expressions when they occur, (4) clarifying patients' verbalizations, and (5) encouraging participation by all group members. Bizarre behavior can be met with a brief reflection of its affective component (e.g., "Mr. Smith, it appears you find this topic distressing") but is otherwise ignored. Disruptive behavior is met with a request to desist, and if it continues the patient is excused from the session. When participant populations include individuals who are involuntary recipients of treatment or who otherwise have difficulty engaging in treatment, a contingency management system may be a necessary adjunct to IPT (Spaulding et al., 2001).

The cognitive intervention modalities developed by Wykes and colleagues (1999) and Bell and colleagues (2001) combine individual, dyadic, and group activities with special attention to work functioning. Bell and colleagues' intervention produced more robust results, probably because it includes more systematic integration of neurocognitive and behavioral objectives.

## Monitoring Progress of Post-Acute Interventions

With currently available technology, the benefits of specific and nonspecific neurocognitive interventions may not be directly measurable in individual cases. Some dramatic individual responses have been reported (e.g., Reed et al., 1992; Spaulding et al., 1986), no doubt familiar to most clinicians who use neurocognitive interventions, but these are clearly exceptions. The research that supports the effectiveness of neurocognitive interventions (Drury et al., 1996a, 1996b; Bell et al., 2001; Hogarty & Flesher, 1999a; Medalia et al., 1998; Silverstein et al., 2000; Spaulding, Reed, et al., 1999; Wykes et al., 1999) relies on statistical differences between people in different treatment conditions. There is no guarantee that measures that reveal group-wide effects also will be optimal for tracking individual progress. Nor has there been sufficient research on the mechanisms and moderators of treatment effects to allow conclusions about which laboratory or clinical measures represent good tools for assessing them clinically. It is even unclear whether gaining facility with the exercises in specific interventions is necessary for, or predictive of, overall benefits. Simple exposure and engagement may be sufficient. This (hypothetical) finding would be consistent with the response organization model of the treatment effect, in which the limiting factor is not faulty performance of particular microskills but, rather, failure to activate them in a timely manner. Activation, rather than mastery, of the microskills may therefore be the key factor in the treatment effect. So far, the domains that show the most robust effects are at the behavioral level (e.g., progress in acquisition of social skills), which reflects a more overall level of rehabilitation progress.

Some neuropsychological measures (e.g., WCST; Heaton, 1981) have been found to be sensitive to specific neurocognitive intervention, but they also are quite sensitive to nonspecific rehabilitation effects (Spaulding, Reed, et al., 1999). These measures would not necessarily be expected to show the differential effects of a specific intervention in an individual case. As a result, the role of neuropsychological assessment diminishes as the acute psychosis is resolved and attention shifts to post-acute interventions. Neuropsychological assessment becomes central again after specific and nonspecific neurocognitive intervention options have been exhausted, and it is time to assess the quality and severity of truly residual impairment.

Thus the justification for neurocognitive intervention in the later post-acute phase comes primarily from research on its efficacy in enhancing rehabilitation progress. Treatment responses in individual recipients typically do not confirm a rehabilitation team's hypothesis of post-acute neurocognitive impairment. Nevertheless, the research evidence is arguably strong enough to justify making specific interventions available to all individuals who may benefit, including all individuals with a disabling mental illness that has an episodic course (however cryptic the episodes may be). With respect to nonspecific neurocognitive intervention, there is reason enough to make intensive rehabilitation available to those who need it, independent of its neurocognitive benefits. In the terminology of the integrated paradigm, post-acute neurocognitive impairment should be considered as a problem on the rehabilitation plan of any individual with a history of psychosis who is undergoing intensive rehabilitation. Evidence of neurocognitive impairment, from the laboratory or from observations in the natural environment, compel its inclusion as a problem.

In lieu of reliable tracking measures, neurocognitive intervention must be conducted in terms of the dosages and time frames reported in outcome research. The Spaulding, Reed, and colleagues (1999) study provided 6 months of the cognitive subprograms of IPT at 3 hours per week. For a severely disabled recipient population, this dosage and time frame could be considered the minimum required for a fair trial. Hogarty and Flesher (1999b) reported using a comparable time and dose with a less severely impaired population, and their treatment effects appear to be substantially larger than those found in the Spaulding, Reed, and colleagues study. Therefore, a shorter or less intensive trial period may be justifiable for less severely impaired recipients. The Bell and colleagues (2001) intervention spanned 5 months, and the intensity (hours per week) was generally comparable to the other two trials. However, the differences between inpatient, day treatment, and therapeutic work settings make precise comparisons problematic. Regardless of the time and dose of specific interventions, neurocognitive impairment should be considered truly residual only after sufficient exposure to intensive rehabilitation. As with the specific interventions, 6 months is a minimal trial period.

## PROSTHETIC NEUROCOGNITIVE INTERVENTIONS

When all options for improving post-acute neurocognitive impairment have been exhausted, the next step is to evaluate the remaining impairment as truly residual. At this point, qualitative distinctions between different impairments again become important. Unlike intervention for post-acute impairment, prosthesis for residual impairment often must be highly tailored to the particular impaired ability. Neuropsychological assessment performs a key role in articulating the quality as well as the severity of any residual impairment. However, neuropsychological assessment alone is insufficient to design a prosthetic intervention. Ultimately, the target of the intervention is a functional behavior that is (hypothetically) compromised by neurocognitive impairment(s). Although neuropsychological tests can provide important clues as to the underlying causes of behavioral failures, they cannot *predict* behavioral failures. Similarly, providing a prosthetic intervention that enables a person to perform a neuropsychological task in a therapeutic setting does not guarantee that the prosthetic will be beneficial in a naturalistic environment. Designing effective prosthetic interventions requires joint application of functional behavioral and neuropsychological assessments. The functional assessment identifies the behavioral failures and the circumstances in which they occur, and the neuropsychological assessment provides guidance as to what types of prosthesis may most effectively compensate for the behavioral failure.

### Cognitively Sensitive Skills Training

In the 1980s, as the neurocognitive level of severe mental illness was brought to light, there was increasing concern about the implications of this level for psychosocial interventions (Liberman, Nuechterlein, & Wallace, 1982). For example, social skills training—by then one of the most ubiquitous rehabilitation modalities—made no assumptions about the neurocognitive underpinnings of skill acquisition or performance. Research was already beginning to show that neurocognitive impairment is a limiting factor in response to social skills training. In response, developers of social skills training and related modalities began enhancing the therapeutic procedures to make them "more sensitive" to the possible neurocognitive limitations of the participants (Wallace, 1982; Wallace & Boone, 1984). These "cognitively sensitive" training techniques were not intended to enhance neurocognitive recovery. At that time, there was little evidence that such recovery could take place. They were designed to enhance skill acquisition *despite* neurocognitive impairment—which is why they are classified as prosthetic.

No treatment trials pitting "cognitively sensitive" skills training against "cognitively insensitive" skills training were conducted, however. The premise that the former would produce better skill acquisition in people with severe mental illness was generally accepted without argument. In retrospect, it seems likely that the cognitive sensitivity of skills training probably enhances not only skills training, as initially expected, but also contributes significantly to the nonspecific neurocognitive benefits of intensive rehabilitation. Nevertheless, since these techniques are presumably also useful for helping people with truly residual impairments enhance their social competence, they are best discussed under the rubric of prosthetic interventions.

Over the years, the principles of cognitively sensitive skills training have evolved and sorted themselves into discrete categories of *attention, learning,* and *memory.* Even though the concept of inattention is problematic in experimental psychology and neuropsychology, it remains a useful descriptor of a particular difficulty a person with mental illness may have in a skills training group. Learning and memory are more closely related to formal concepts in psychology and neuropsychology. All the principles of cognitively sensitive skills training have applications that go beyond the original one of enhancing skill acquisition. They can be used in a diversity of settings and circumstances (e.g., occupational therapy, vocational skills development, therapeutic community activities, and rehabilitation counseling) to help the recovering person derive maximum benefit. The principles are summarized in Tables 7.2 and 7.3.

## Contingency Management

Another traditional modality for severe mental illness, contingency management, also can serve as a prosthetic, as well as therapeutic, intervention. As the immediacy hypothesis (discussed in Chapter 6) indicates, people who have neurocognitive impairments that prevent normal functioning in a natural environment may be able to function in a therapeutic milieu where stimulus–response relationships are made more proximal, immediate, and concrete. To the degree that the neurocognitive impairments are truly residual, a contingency management intervention may serve to sustain more normal functioning. Although contingency management is usually associated with rehabilitation in relatively restrictive settings, especially institu-

**TABLE 7.2. Techniques to Facilitate Attention in Group Skills Training**

1. *Introduce topics.* Explain what you intend to do before beginning discussion or initiating activity. Introducing the topic orients group members and focuses attention: "Now we will talk about it . . . "

2. *Advise the group when changing topics.* Prepare group members to refocus attention: "We've been talking about. . . . Now we will change topics. The new topic of discussion is . . . "

3. *Call members by name and make eye contact.* Saying a person's name and making eye contact before giving information or asking a question alerts the person to attend and increases the probability that what you say will be heard: "Mr. Smith, please bring your workbook to class on Wednesday."

4. *Decrease competing stimuli.* To reduce distractions, remove or cover competing visual stimuli (e.g., wall pictures, bulletin boards, signs). Erect room partitions and close the room door to decrease noise from the hallway.

5. *Use cues or prompts liberally.* Direct attention by using verbal or visual prompts. Be specific: "Mr. Smith, look at the bottom of your worksheet. . . . Ms. Jones, look at the first line of this poster . . . "

6. *Give advance notice of expectations.* Telling group members ahead of time what you will be expecting them to do assists them in focusing their attention: "We will watch the videotape for a few minutes. Then I will stop the tape and ask you whether you saw a problem situation in the video."

7. *Ask group members for help.* When working with one individual in a group situation, ask the other group members to help. This request keeps other group members involved and increases their self-esteem by being able to assist: "Mr. Smith, can you help Ms. Jones out? What is the fourth problem-solving step? . . . Ms. Jones, would you help by watching the role-play to see if Mr. Smith uses good eye contact and clear voice tone?"

tions, newer approaches are adaptable to more naturalistic settings and circumstances (discussed in detail in Chapter 10). Under these circumstances, formalized contingencies can be part of a "cognitive exoskeleton" that compensates for an individual's inability to respond to the more distant or abstract circumstances that normally motivate functional behavior (Heinssen, 1996).

## Environmental Prosthesis

The literature on traumatic brain injury and other neuropathological conditions is rich in strategies for compensating for the neurocognitive consequences of those conditions (Ben-Yishay et al., 1985; Sohlberg & Mateer,

1989). Living environments can be designed to compensate for memory impairments by locating key prompts (e.g., written signs) at central locations to support particular activities. Individuals can be trained to make special use of personal calendars and date books. All such interventions are potentially useful for people with disabling mental illness, whose residual neurocognitive impairments are primarily in the memory domain.

Specialized neuropsychological interventions have been developed for people with specific impairments in the executive domain. Such impairments are ubiquitous in people with frontal head injury, as is caused by hitting the dashboard in a car accident. Because of the predominance of executive impairment in severe mental illness, there has been special interest in

**TABLE 7.3. Techniques to Facilitate Learning and Memory in Group Skills Training**

1. *Simplify complex tasks.* Reduce complexity of verbal information and physical tasks by building, step by step, from the simple to the more complex: "There are six steps to remember when self-administering medications. We will practice each step separately. Later, when each step is familiar, we will put them all together."

2. *Use short, clear sentences.* Be literal and explicit and use concrete examples to illustrate what you mean. Avoid the use of double negatives and complex grammar: "First we will review the problem-solving steps. Next we will practice with role-plays."

3. *Use visual aids.* Posters, demonstrations, training videos, and other visual displays help reinforce auditory information and promote understanding. Some people learn better visually, some aurally.

4. *Use active learning techniques.* Role-plays, homework assignments, discussion, and taking notes are all active learning techniques that increase the probability that group members will remember the information.

5. *Emphasize through repetition.* Reiterate information as often as necessary to ensure learning.

6. *Confirm reception.* Monitor how well group members are attending and remembering by asking them to repeat back what you have just told them. Make sure they remember and understand the information before going to the next step or point: "Ms. Jones, can you tell us the first step in identifying resources for leisure activities?"

7. *Liberally apply positive reinforcement.* Use praise and social reinforcement for any and all successful endeavors. When success is partial, reinforce the successful part; systematically reinforce approximations to correct or adequate responses. When there is no success, reinforce attempts. Break down tasks into smaller steps that can be reinforced: "Good, you remembered one of the three steps. Now let's go over them again and learn the other ones too."

these techniques in rehabilitation. An approach to compensating for severe frontal/executive impairment, specialized for people with disabling mental illness, has been developed by Velligan and her colleagues (Velligan et al., 2000). The approach uses the distinction between disinhibitory impairment and attentional impairment (discussed in Chapter 5) to design individualized compensatory strategies. For example, severe disinhibitory problems are hypothesized to be instrumental in the wearing of inappropriate clothing, which is often observed in people with severe mental illness. The underlying mechanism is hypothesized to be a failure to inhibit dressing behaviors when a varied wardrobe is the stimulus. A person who cannot inhibit dressing behavior puts on whatever clothing he or she encounters, regardless of what he or she has already donned. The solution is to package each day's clothing in a separate unit, so that the person only has to open the package and put on whatever it contains.

So far, research (Velligan et al., 2000) has suggested that this approach can be useful for behavioral problems ranging from inappropriate dressing to nonadherence to medication regimens. However, this research has not systematically distinguished between post-acute and residual neurocognitive impairments or compared the results with interventions intended to resolve post-acute impairments. Further research will doubtless clarify the relationship between post-acute and truly residual impairments as they respond to this approach. For the time being, great caution is indicated so that prosthetic solutions such as these are not used when a rehabilitative approach to post-acute impairment would reestablish more normal behavioral functioning. Fortunately, therapeutic and prosthetic interventions are not inherently incompatible and can be applied in complementary ways (Goldberg, 1994), as long as the individual's functioning is continually reassessed and adjustments are made in response to functional recovery.

# Chapter 8

# Social-Cognitive Processes in Research and Treatment

Social cognition is a heuristic term that conveniently distinguishes higher-level cognitive functions from the more basic neurocognitive functions. The theoretical relationship between social cognition and neurocognition is not yet clear, however. It appears likely that some neurocognitive functions are exclusively "social" in character; that is, information related to social processes (e.g., perception of facial cues, voice tone, etc.) may be identified and processed at very early or basic levels of cognition. Other social processes (those by which we understand what people are doing and why) are higher-level "consumers" of nonsocial neurocognitive operations. Much of the current discussion in evolutionary psychology and medicine centers on the evolution of distinctly social–cognitive abilities in humans (Barkow et al., 1992; Penn et al., 1997). Understanding these abilities is crucial to utilizing the next wave of developments in the field of cognitive psychopathology and treatment. Meanwhile, theoretical models and clinical technologies are available to address particular problems conventionally understood to be in the domain of social cognition (Higgins & Bargh, 1987; Newman, 2001). For now, social cognition is most usefully defined as cognition that is primarily involved with understanding people, interpersonal events, and social relationships.

It is important to understand that, generally, theories and models of cognition tend to have fewer direct links to neurophysiology and neuroanatomy than neurocognitive models. There is less isomorphism between social–cognitive constructs and their neural underpinnings, compared to neurocognitive (or neuropsychological) constructs and their neural underpinnings. This is not a scientific weakness, although it is often mistaken for one by those who indulge in a naive reductionistic understanding of behavior. One of the ascendant ideas in the cognitive revolution during the mid-20th century was that *information* has an objective scientific reality

157

independent of its medium, and that *information processing* can be scientifically studied and manipulated (as it is in computer programming). Contemporary cognitive psychology is based on experimental methods and quantitative analysis and provides empirically-based and lawful principles of cognitive functioning, including social cognition. However, one way in which cognitive models cannot be aligned with specific neural underpinnings is that many lawful and measurable cognitive processes could be accomplished by a variety of neural architectures and processes. Progress in science may articulate, in some cases, which of a variety of possibilities is the one that actually applies. However, in other cases this determination may not be possible because molar cognitive abilities are exercised in a variety of ways, across individuals and across situations. Similarly, the complexity of organism–environmental interactions at the level of social cognition may prohibit a direct account of this level of functioning solely in terms of neural underpinnings. The information processing that occurs in the brain at the level of social cognition is complex, but it is nevertheless information processing. A scientific understanding of social cognition informs rehabilitation technology, despite unknown links to biological neuroscience.

There is also more ambiguity, at the level of social cognition, about what is "normal." Neuropsychology focuses on processes thought to be common and relatively invariant across normal populations. Clinical neuropsychological assessment takes normal individual variation into account, but this is not the subject of its analysis. In social cognition, individual differences are vast even within the normal range. Many characteristics of social cognition are implicated within the concept of personality—that is, they are stable, trait-like characteristics that give people their psychological and behavioral uniqueness. It is therefore less clear that rehabilitation interventions, directed at the social–cognitive level, work by "correcting" an "impairment." It is more parsimonious to say that they work by changing a person's social cognition in a way that enhances progress toward rehabilitation goals.

## RELATIONSHIPS AMONG NEUROPHYSIOLOGICAL, NEUROCOGNITIVE, AND SOCIOCOGNITIVE PROBLEMS IN MENTAL ILLNESS

There are clinical problems expressed at the sociocognitive level of functioning that are functionally independent of neurophysiological dysregulation and neurocognitive impairment. (For a comprehensive account of social cognition pertinent to severe mental illness, see Corrigan & Penn, 2001.) For the purposes of rehabilitation, this means that no amount of treatment directed at those more molecular levels can be expected to resolve the problem. In the integrated paradigm, this nonresponsiveness is what justifies identifying them as sociocognitive, as opposed to neurophysiological or neurocognitive, problems. However, problems that are a fairly proximal consequence of neurophysiological dysregulation and/or neurocognitive impairment are often difficult to distinguish from true sociocognitive problems. Making this distinction is often a key step in assessment and rehabilitation planning. Rehabilitation can easily be stalled or derailed by persistently treating sociocognitive problems as neurophysiological or neurocognitive ones, and vice versa. The first prerequisite to avoiding this is to understand the potential causal complexity of the various problems that express themselves at the sociocognitive level.

## Problem Solving: An Interplay of Behavioral and Cognitive Processes

There is a gray area, a transitional zone, on the continuum that ranges from neurocognitive to sociocognitive processes. This is a zone of cognition customarily understood as "problem solving" (D'Zurilla & Nezu, 1982). Since its inception, experimental psychology has investigated problem solving in humans and other animals. Even through the era of behaviorist domination, problem-solving behavior provided a compelling demonstration of the need for cognitive constructs (see D'Zurrila & Goldfried, 1971). As neuropsychology emerged in the mid-20th century, investigators focused efforts on determining the neurological and neurocognitive underpinnings of problem solving. Similarly, as social learning theory and cognitive psychology overtook radical behaviorism in clinical applications, problem solving became a focus of interest for clinicians.

By the 1980s a fairly extensive assessment and intervention technology had evolved, mostly associated with the clinical and scientific approach known as *cognitive-behavioral therapy* (CBT), to enhance peoples' problem-solving ability (D'Zurilla, 1986, 1988). The CBT approach to problem solving had broad appeal for a number of reasons. First, problem solving applies to a range of human functioning. In contrast to the highly specific behavioral changes that were the goals of earlier behavior therapists, improving problem-solving abilities was expected to improve functioning across a range of situations. Second, assessment research indicated poor problem-solving ability in many individuals in need of mental health services, suggesting it is a common factor in many psychological and behavioral problems. Third, clinical outcome trials indicated that interventions intended to improve problem solving did produce benefits, across a range of clientele, from delinquent adolescents to people with depression and disabling mental illness. As psychiatric rehabilitation emerged in the 1980s as a comprehensive, social learning-based approach for treating people with disabling mental illness, problem-solving assessment and intervention technology became an important item in its service array (this will be discussed in more detail later in this chapter). Today, problem-solving training is widely used in applications to disabling mental illness (as well as other conditions), both as a specific, focused intervention and as a component in other skills training interventions (skills deficits and skills training involve more molar levels of behavioral organization than social cognition; they are discussed in the next chapter).

The notion of formulating a unified concept of problem solving did not fair so well under the scrutiny of experimental psychology and neuropsychology. The specific cognitive and neurocognitive processes that underlie problem-solving behavior are many and complex. Although they are generally associated with the frontal lobe in humans, neuronal underpinnings of problem-solving behavior are widely distributed across the brain. The components of the CBT model of problem solving do not correspond well to the specific cognitive processes identified in the psychology laboratory. The CBT model was derived from a purely functional analysis of behavior in problem situations, rather than from an experimental analysis of cognition. The differences between CBT problem solving and laboratory problem solving suggest distinct levels of cognitive activity. It is not at all clear that problem-solving impairments at the neurocognitive level are directly associated with impairments in behavioral problem solving. It is not even clear that people engage in cognitive problem solving under normal circumstances the way they do when undergoing CBT (Bellak, Morrison, & Mueser, 1989). This ambiguity creates a conceptual pitfall for rehabilitation. Unfounded presumptions of isomorphism between neurocognitive, sociocognitive, and social–behavioral levels of problem solving could seriously mislead formulation of problems. Nevertheless, the *behavior* involved—in CBT, in the laboratory, or in the natural environment—is still recognizably problem-solving behavior. At the behavioral level, the problem-solving model provides assessment and treatment technology of demonstrated usefulness to people who have severe mental illness (Bowen et al., 1994; Donahoe et al., 1990; Penn et al., 1993; Schotte & Clum, 1987; Toomey, Schuldberg, Green, & Corrigan, 1993).

In recent years, as sociocognitive models in psychopathology have become increasingly sophisticated, other aspects of social cognition have joined problem-solving skills as key processes in support of interpersonal functioning. For example, *social perception* (Leonhard & Corrigan, 2001) refers to a range of specific functions, from apprehension of facial expressions and social cues to the more molar processes by which people identify and recognize personality characteristics. Corcoran's (2001) *theory of mind* refers to the particular ability to anticipate and infer the intentions and other psychological states of other people. Like that of problem solving, these constructs lie in the gray zone between neurocognitive and sociocognitive levels. In addition to illuminating specific domains in which mental illness may produce impairment or disability, these constructs potentially inform development of advanced forms of sociobehavioral interventions, especially social skills training (discussed in the next chapter). (See also Penn, Combs, & Mohamed, 2001, for a general discussion of social cognition and interpersonal functioning.)

## Social Cognition and Neo-Kraepelinian Symptoms

In the psychopathology of severe mental illness, there is a related ambiguity concerning the relationship between neurocognitive impairments and neo-Kreapelinian symptoms that manifest primarily in the sociocognitive level. The most important example of the latter is *delusions*. Delusions are colloquially understood to be kinds of beliefs—and "everyone knows what beliefs are." (For an analysis of colloquial beliefs pertinent to social cognition, see Malle, 2001.) Beliefs are delusions when they are bizarre or otherwise patently false. The philosophical problems associated with distinguishing delusions from bizarre beliefs that are not symptoms are among the most persistent in psychopathology. The neo-Kraepelinian nosology attempts to inject social context into the criteria; for example, beliefs are not symptoms, no matter how bizarre, if they are shared in some social context. This formulation presumes that social mechanisms of belief formation are "normal," and neglects the inverse possibility, that people with similar abnormal beliefs tend to affiliate *because* of those beliefs and their social consequences. Psychological analysis of such phenomena as "group-think" show that false and even bizarre beliefs can be established and maintained by social processes. This social context does not make them any less false or bizarre.

As with problem-solving processes, experimental analysis of the cognitive components and processes underlying beliefs does not support the simple, unified concept derived from superficial observations of behavior. Experimental and social psychology have revealed that beliefs are more than simply items of declarative information that we categorize as "true" versus "untrue" (Bisiach, Meregalli, & Berti, 1985; Cheng & Novick, 1992; Jones et al., 1971; Leven, 1992; Lipe, 1991). The information contained in any single belief is pervasively associated with other information we use in our routine personal and social functioning. The "truth value" we attach to any particular belief reflects not only the specific information we hold that is pertinent to that belief, but also how the belief complements other information in our long-term memory. *Cognitive dissonance theory*, a framework for understanding how we construct and maintain our beliefs, evolved along with social learning theory and cognitive psychology in the 1970s. (For a historical account, critical review, and update of cognitive dissonance theory, see Harmon-Jones & Mills, 1999.) This theory describes how we shape our various beliefs so as to minimize incongruity. Incongruity within our self-perceptions is a frequent source of dissonance, and so we tend to shape our beliefs to be maximally congruent with what we believe about ourselves. For example, if we see ourselves as basically ethical, we will tend to interpret our own unethical behavior as coerced or as an exceptional response to extraordinary circumstances. When necessary, we ignore factual information that contradicts a belief in order to maintain its consistency with our other beliefs about ourselves and the world in general. For example, instead of rationalizing our unethical behavior, we might simply ignore or "forget" it.

*Attribution theory* is a similar psychological framework for understanding beliefs. It generally addresses the ways in which we understand or interpret new information, such as the arrival of a new coworker, in the context of our preexisting beliefs and other cognitive characteristics. (For a historical account, critical review, and update of attribution theory and related concepts, especially as applied to mental health, see Kowalski & Leary, 1999). The "attribution" in attribution theory refers specifically to how people attribute "causes" to events and states of affairs. For example, do we attribute our new coworker's quick promotion to her abilities (an internal, stable trait) or to her arrival at an opportune time (an external, unstable variable)? The former attribution gives her the credit, the latter denies her the credit.

Cognitive dissonance theory, attribution theory, and related cognitive–psychological frameworks revolutionized our understanding of how beliefs operate to support personal and social functioning. As is the case with psychoanalytic interpretations, these cognitive–psychological frameworks explain odd and counterintuitive behavior often observed in "normal" individuals—for example, persistent investment in a once-profitable business venture that has gone bad. However, whereas psychoanalysis relies on hypothetical psychic mechanisms such as repression and denial, the psychological theories of belief were derived from quantitative behavioral data considered in a rigorous experimental paradigm. Whereas psychoanalysis is largely limited to post-hoc interpretations, cognitive dissonance and attribution theories provide quantitatively precise predictions of how we form beliefs in particular circumstances. Psychoanalysis relegates these processes to "the unconscious." In contrast, cognitive–psychological theories do not require such a concept, although it is true that under normal circumstances, we are often unaware of cognitive dissonance and other factors that shape our beliefs. This unawareness requires no further explanation; we are unaware (until made aware) of many of the forces that shape our behavior.

Applying cognitive–psychological frameworks such as cognitive dissonance theory and attribution theory to clinical contexts provides a perspective entirely different from the neo-Kraepelinian notion that "abnormal" beliefs are "symptoms" of mental illness. The social and intrapersonal factors that cause "normal" individuals to adopt false or distorted beliefs presumably operate in people with mental illness as well. In some cases, delusions are the product of entirely "normal" cognition, perhaps responding to extraordinary circumstances, but nevertheless forming beliefs in ways no different from normal belief formation (Bentall, 2001; Bentall & Kinderman, 1998; Himadi & Kaiser, 1992; Oltmanns & Maher, 1988).

## Somatic Delusions

An uncomplicated illustration of this process is provided by *somatic delusions*, which are delusions concerning one's own bodily integrity or functions. For example, the delusion that one is dead or rotting may represent an attempt to give a "reasonable" attribution to the olfactory hallucinations of foul odors that are not uncommon in acute psychosis. Supporting this interpretation is the finding that somatic delusions are often accompanied by real somatic abnormalities; for example, individuals who express the belief that a snake is living in their stomach turn out to have gastric ulcers (Oltmanns & Maher, 1988). In some cases, the "real" origin of the belief lies so far outside normal experience (e.g., hallucinations) that no other mechanism seems required to account for the bizarre quality of the belief. In other cases, the ordinariness of the sensory–perceptual experience (e.g., stomach pains) demands an additional explanation of why a more ordinary belief about its source is not adopted. Neurocognitive compromise may provide such an explanation, although psychological and social processes also may be at work.

Another good example of this process is the *Capgras delusion*, a belief that familiar people or places have been replaced by robots, impersonators, or artificial substitutes (Ellis & dePauw, 1994). This delusion traditionally has been labeled paranoid rather than somatic, but in all probability it results from neurophysiological compromise of a specific brain mechanism that associates an affective "familiarity" signal with familiar people and places. Loss of this signal leaves intact the sensory–perceptual image of the familiar object but without its affective component—rendering the experience artificial to the perceiver.

## Paranoid Delusions

Paranoid delusions—that is, bizarre or otherwise patently false beliefs of persecution—are also amenable to analysis in terms of specific parameters of normal social cognition (Bentall, 2001), as delineated by attribution theory. A paranoid view of the world results from the convergence of several circumstantial and attributional characteristics, including (1) personal failure in some salient pursuit, (2) a strong tendency to attribute the causes of events to external (i.e., in the environment) rather than internal (i.e., one's own characteristics or agency) sources, and (3) a tendency to see the causes of events as stable and consistent (i.e., unchangeable), as opposed to unstable and variable (i.e., changeable). These parameters of cognition cover a wide range in normal populations, so it is not surprising that a large number of people in the extraordinary circumstances that mental illness creates develop paranoid attributions.

The concept of paranoia causes much confusion and miscommunication in mental health circles, partly because there are a number of distinct characteristics, all within the sociocognitive level, associated with both the colloquial and neo-Kraepelinian notions of paranoia. One of these characteristics is a tendency to attribute events to the persecutory intent of others, which, when bizarre or patently false, is labeled a paranoid delusion. However, suspiciousness and hostility are two other characteristics, which, although associated with paranoid delusions, vary independently. Individuals who express bizarre paranoid delusions do not necessarily behave in a hostile or suspicious manner, and extremely hostile individuals may be neither suspicious nor delusional. In clinical practice all possible combinations of delusional paranoia, hostility and suspiciousness are encountered. Hostility is primarily associated with the affective state of anger and with a cognitive and emotional intolerance of interpersonal differences. Suspiciousness is primarily associated with the affective state of fear and often with compromised neurocognitive functioning. Suspiciousness, sometimes misinterpreted as paranoia, is often associated with sensory–perceptual difficulties, such as deafness and memory failure, as occurs in Korsakoff's disease, a progressive dementia associated with alcoholism. Unreflective use of neo-Kraepelinian concepts such as paranoia can mislead clinicians, encouraging a monolithic interpretation of behavior that, in fact, represents a number of relatively independent components.

## Social Role Performance

Another major source of confusion in sociocognitive assessment is determining the function of beliefs in social role performance. For example, would a person profess a belief without really believing it? A moment's reflection reveals that there are many circumstances, usually that we take for granted, where the expression of a particular belief or set of beliefs is more associated with performance of a particular social role than with the truth or even relevance of the belief. When salespeople offer us a bargain, we do not think of them as liars, or delusional, if we subsequently find a better price. When a politician espouses a particular economic theory, we generally assume that it has more to do with the characteristics of the politician's voting constituency than the empirical support for the theory. This is not to say that the person does not have a phenomenological experience of "believing." In fact, cognitive dissonance theory stipulates that there would be a strong sense of believing what was professed if doing so were consistent with the believer's self-perception of being a good salesperson or the champion of a political cause. In the myriad of social roles that are routinely performed in our culture, many involve the adoption of some set of beliefs. This is no less true for people with mental illness. If espousing bizarre beliefs is perceived to be an expected and accepted part of the social role of a "mental patient," then the person in that role is subject to espousing and believing those beliefs, no less than politicians are subject to believing and espousing the beliefs their constituencies expect.

## Strategic Delusions

Espousing beliefs in the context of social role performance can have a definitive impact on the outcome of interpersonal interactions. We take for granted that, under normal circumstances, the first step in any problem-solving process that involves more than one person is to reach some kind of consensus about the particular problem and its solution. However, under some circumstances, it is the consensus or the lack of consensus, rather than the specifics of what the consensus might be about, that determines the context of interpersonal interaction. There are situations in politics, diplomacy, labor–management mediation, and interpersonal relations where agreeing or disagreeing about *anything* has implications more crucial than the content of the agreement or disagreement. When two parties are confronted with the need to negotiate, "strategic disagreement" can play a significant role in determining the balance of power and the options available to each party.

This type of dynamic occurs frequently between people with mental illness and their families, friends, and service providers. Typically, the person with mental illness is in a disadvantaged position, confronted by demands and pressures to subscribe to the agenda of others. In this situation, professing a belief that neutralizes or vitiates the agenda can be a powerful strategy. It is often most effective when the belief is not subject to rational dispute or falsification, and especially if it is a belief that nobody else could possibly endorse. For example, when the "patient" holds that the service providers are spies and medication is poison, rationality and social pressure to take the medications are effectively neutralized. (For an insightful discussion of this phenomenon applied to severe mental illness, see the title essay in Haley, 1986, pp. 19–54.) Of course, endorsing delusional beliefs in the context of interpersonal negotiation is risky. Being labeled "crazy" undermines one's credibility and overall interpersonal influence. It is a strategy born of desperation, but people with disabling mental illness often find themselves in desperate circumstances. When one has little else to lose, espousing bizarre, delusional beliefs may immobilize all the parties in a negotiating process where power and influence are otherwise disproportionately distributed. This is not to say that people with delusions cynically plot to disrupt or immobilize the interpersonal processes in which they engage, any more than sincere politicians or diplomats behave cynically when they make a strategic decision to agree and when to disagree. The short-term impact of delusional behavior simply creates an overwhelming incentive, phenomenologically experienced as an imperative, to believe and espouse the delusional ideas. Cognitive dissonance and attribution theories have clearly shown that incentives exert a powerful effect on what we decide to believe.

A simplistic view of delusions as symptoms of mental illness can seriously misguide the rehabilitation process. Like other beliefs, delusions are subject to the effects of interpersonal processes and circumstances. People with mental illness often confront extraordinary circumstances and difficult interpersonal situations. When constrained by neo-Kraepelinian presumptions, it is easy to forget that many people who are not labeled "mentally ill" harbor or even espouse quite bizarre beliefs. One has only to peruse a grocery store tabloid ("I had Elvis's love child aboard a UFO piloted by Jackie O") to become convinced of this basic reality. Although delusions in people with mental illness often originate in neurophysiological and neurocognitive abnormalities, the delusions are also the most notoriously persistent of psychotic symptoms, often remaining long after all other indicators of acute psychosis have abated. The success of psychosocial interventions in resolving delusions that exert a negative impact on personal and social functioning (Bentall, 2001) is strong evidence that in the residual phase of the disorder, propitious circumstantial, interpersonal, and psychological factors are important mediators of recovery.

## Insight into Illness

Closely related to the problem of sociocognitive symptoms is the concept of insight, which originated in the psychoanalytic tradition as one of the key avenues to "cure." Insight is traditionally thought to involve "making the unconscious conscious," which in turn enhances the control of higher, mature psychic processes (ego functions) over instinctive drives. The concept was rejected by radical behaviorism but revived in a scientifically credible form with the emergence of social learning theory. Today there is general agreement that insight, conceptualized as an articulated understanding of one's thoughts, emotions, motivations, habits, and skills, fosters effective and phenomenologically fulfilling personal and social functioning.

The concept of an *absence* of insight has a history in Kraepelinian psychiatry. For example, brain injury sometimes produces the condition of *anosognosia*, a dramatic unawareness of severe impairment, such as paralysis. Anosognosia seems comparable to the denial expressed by some people with mental illness—denial that they have an illness, that their psychotic symptoms are abnormal, or that anything is wrong at all. However, the *absence* of awareness was difficult to fit into Kraepelinian diagnostic criteria, which emphasized the *presence* of abnormalities, until the emergence of the concept of negative symptoms in the 1970s. Negative symptoms—that is, abnormalities marked by the absence of normal function in a particular area, include alogia (absence of thought), apathy (absence of normal affect) and amotivation—could subsume the specific absence of awareness of illness. Although unawareness of illness is not part of the criteria for any psychiatric diagnosis, it is generally understood to be a common feature of conditions on the schizophrenia spectrum.

The continuum from unawareness to insight spans a considerable range from severe anosognosia to denial of the presence of a mental illness to dismissing the significance of symptoms. Less severe instances of "poor insight" do not necessarily reflect a less severe impairment in the same process(es) that produce extreme instances. People with mental illness sometimes present a view of their condition that seems paradoxical to neo-Kraepelinian clinicians. For example, they deny having a mental illness but agree that antipsychotic medication is beneficial to their personal and social functioning. Such patients may actually have a more multidimensional, systemic understanding of their condition than clinicians adhering to a simplistic view of "poor insight" as a negative symptom. As is the case with delusions, impairment in insight may reflect, to some degree, the normal interpersonal dynamics wherein belief, power, and agreement jostle for dominance.

Psychopathology research has only recently begun to unravel the vicissitudes of "poor insight" in people with disabling mental illness. Significant advances in our ability to distinguish problems originating in neurocognitive impairment from problems more associated with psychological and psychosocial factors are likely to emerge in this decade. (For a very accessible and comprehensive discussion of insight in severe mental illness, and implications for treatment and rehabilitation, see Amador & Johanson, 2000; for a review of clinical and scientific literature, see Amador et al., 1994; for analysis of the neurophysiological, neurocognitive, and sociocognitive factors in insight, see Kasapis, Amador, Yale, Strauss, & Gorman, 1995; Mohamed, Fleming, Penn, & Spaulding, 1999; Morgan, Orr, et al., 1999; Morgan, Vearnals, et al., 1999.)

## Social Cognition, Mood and Emotion

What we colloquially recognize as "mood" and "emotion" is a complex mix of neurophysiological, neurocognitive, and sociocognitive processes and processing states. In neo-Kraepelinian psychiatry, affective disorders are conceptualized as illnesses whose expression occurs primarily in the domain of *mood*, especially in balancing euphoria (mania) against dysphoria (depression). Anxiety disorders are illnesses whose expression occurs primarily in the domain of *emotion*, specifically the emotion of fear (anxiety is fear in the absence of a natural, fear-inducing condition, such as physical threat). Emotional disorders (anxiety, in particular) are also associated with other diagnoses, for example, fear of abandonment in childhood separation disorders. Mood and emotion disorders are commonly diagnosed in individuals with severe mental illness (not necessarily as the primary diagnosis; both mood and emotion disorders have high comorbidity with diagnoses in the schizophrenia spectrum). The potentially disabling condition(s) diagnosed as *borderline personality disorder* may involve multiple problems in both mood and emotion regulation. As discussed previously, other psychopathological states may involve significant mood or emotion dysregulation, such as the role of anger (and perhaps also fear) in paranoia.

Even within the neo-Kraepelinian community, there is recognition that mood and anxiety disorders represent interactions of factors at different levels of biosystemic organization. The clinical effectiveness of both pharmacological and psychosocial interventions in treating these disorders is compelling evidence of this complexity (discussed in Chapter 4). Our neurophysiological status influences what we think about, how we evaluate ourselves and other people, how we set and pursue personal goals, and how frequently we feel sad, happy, angry, fearful, or confident. Conversely, those sociocognitive processes influence our neurophysiology and feeling states. Functioning in either domain can be influenced therapeutically by manipulating the other.

Experimental and clinical research has illuminated considerably the types of social cognition processes most pertinent to problems in mood and emotion (Leven, 1992; Piasecki & Hollon, 1987; Simons, Garfield, & Murphy, 1984; Sweeney, Anderson, & Bailey, 1986; Weiner et al., 1971). These include attribution processes, especially attributions about the self, and cognitive *schemas*, which appear to be important in mood and emotion regulation. Schemas are associations and interrelationships between various domains of information stored in memory. These relationships are what we colloquially recognize as "meaning." Sociocognitive processes draw upon schemas in the course of making attributions and performing related functions. For example, when we watch a baseball player engage in a dispute with the umpire, we understand that their conflict occurs within the schematic context of the baseball game. Challenging the umpire has a revered tradition, and a special meaning, within that context. Were we to observe two businessmen in suits interacting in a similar way at a bus stop, we would interpret their behavior and the situation quite differently. However, a person unfamiliar with the schemata of baseball would interpret the two situations as more alike. Thus the structure of a person's schemas can have a pervasive impact on those processes and, ultimately, on the mood and emotional states that the processes influence. This is why schemas are often the target of intervention in CBT and related forms of psychosocial treatment.

## CLINICAL ASSESSMENT OF PROBLEMS IN THE SOCIOCOGNITIVE LEVEL OF FUNCTIONING

The prototype problem set of the integrated paradigm includes four problem titles in the sociocognitive level of functioning:

- Social problem-solving insufficiency
- Symptom-linked attribution problem
- Mood-linked attribution problem
- Achievement-linked attribution problem

*Social problem-solving insufficiency* is a persistent failure to resolve problems encountered routinely in daily life (e.g., interpersonal conflicts) or to develop effective ways to meet basic personal needs (e.g., the need for shelter or social affiliation). It is usually evidenced by a history of such failures that cannot be explained as neurophysiological or neurocognitive problems. Attribution-linked problems are the product of the problematic way in which a person understands states of affairs or causes of events (e.g., a "pessimist"); *symptom-linked attribution problems* are those in which the attributions represent psychotic symptoms (e.g., delusional beliefs). Mood-linked attribution problems are those in which the attributions are associated with distinct mood states (e.g., the self-deprecating attributions, remorse, and guilt associated with depression, or the grandiose attributions associated with mania). *Achievement-linked attribution problems* are those in which attributions and their associated schemata are associated with failure to formulate and pursue ordinary life goals (e.g., sustaining a job, contributing to the rent, pursuing aesthetic interests). An explicit or implicit belief that abject dependence on others is the only feasible strategy for interpersonal functioning, that one cannot possibly function more independently, or that institutionalization represents the best of all possible worlds potentially reflects an achievement-linked attribution problem.

## Step 1: Identifying Persisting Sociocognitive Problems

Inclusion of one or more of these as problems in a rehabilitation plan reflects the treatment team's working hypothesis that sociocognitive factors constitute significant barriers to optimal functioning, and that these problems cannot be resolved with interventions that target either more molecular (neurophysiological or neurocognitive) or more molar (sociobehavioral) levels. Such a hypothesis typically would be entertained when there is sufficient data to establish that the behavior suggesting the presence of the problem persists after resolution of acute neurophysiological dysregulation. This identification is a significant diagnostic step, as the effects of acute psychosis often extend to the sociocognitive level, and resolution of the acute state often eliminates these effects. On the other hand, qualitatively similar sociocognitive impairments often persist.

## Step 2: Considering Tonic Neurophysiological Factors

The next step is to consider the role of a *tonic* neurophysiological problem. There is considerable evidence that mood disorders and related clinical conditions are associated with tonic neurophysiological states that can be manipulated pharmacologically. These states are known to produce effects at the sociocognitive level. For example, in the integrated paradigm, the choice of an antidepressant drug to treat a mood disorder such as depression reflects a hypothesis that the depression can be treated most successfully as a tonic neurophysiological dysregulation. This hypothesis would be represented by including "tonic neurophysiological dysregulation" as a problem title on the rehabilitation plan. It is important to note here that choice of the neurophysiological problem title and a pharmacotherapeutic intervention does *not* negate the presence of a sociocognitive component in the clinical presentation of depression. In the integrated paradigm, it is assumed that neurophysiological and sociocognitive processes are ultimately linked by reciprocally causal mechanisms. The selection of the problem title reflects the hypothesis that intervention at the neurophysiological level (i.e., pharmacotherapy) will contribute uniquely and independently to resolution of all the functional problems associated with the dysregulation (i.e., the clinical picture of depression), in a manner that benefits the recovering person. All the sociocognitive problems in the prototype problem set are potentially linked to tonic CNS dysregulation.

Including a tonic neurophysiological problem associated with clinical expression at the sociocognitive level does not obviate including a complementary problem within the sociocognitive level. Including two problems associated with a single clinical presentation reflects a hypothesis that interventions associated with the separate problems will contribute uniquely, but in complementary ways, to rehabilitation. A decision to provide pharmacological and psychosocial treatment for depression reflects such a hypothesis (the sociocognitive problem title probably would be "mood-linked attribution problem"). Again, the choice of problem title reflects not only hypotheses about the psychopathology of the clinical picture, but also the technological assessment and intervention options available to the treatment team and the various consequences of these choices for the recovering person.

A two-problem joint intervention approach may be optimal when circumstances limit opportunity for separately testing the separate effects of medication versus psychotherapy for severe depression. Often there is an imperative to resolve presenting problems (e.g., an insufferable and potentially dangerous depressive state) that outweighs the advantages of specifically determining the unique contributions of separate interventions. A one-problem-at-a-time approach may be optimal only when circumstances permit separate evaluation of the treatments to further inform the rehabilitation plan. Some individuals would opt for medication alone or psychotherapy alone, if they knew that one or the other would be sufficient. Of course, when only one intervention does the job, costs are lower. On the other hand, long-term costs may outweigh shorter-term costs. For example, for some people with depression, the risk of future relapse associated with discontinuing pharmacotherapy outweighs the higher short-term cost of psychotherapy, which has a lower risk of relapse upon completion. These are all factors that must be considered when deciding whether to include a tonic neurophysiological dysregulation problem or a sociocognitive problem or both in an individual rehabilitation plan.

## Step 3: Consideration of Molecular-Level Neurocognitive Impairments

The next step in assessing sociocognitive problems is to determine the degree of involvement of more molecular-level neurocognitive problems. This is not a simple process of elimination, as the mere presence of a neurocognitive impairment does not necessarily limit sociocognitive functioning significantly. On the other hand, severe and pervasive neurocognitive impairment does impose a ceiling on sociocognitive functioning. Although the connection between social problem solving and laboratory problem solving is unclear, neurocognitive impairment in the problem-solving domain is more likely to limit social problem solving than neurocognitive impairment in other domains. In practice, discerning the likelihood that the observed neurocognitive impairment is post-acute, rather than truly residual, affects the decision of whether or when to separate neurocognitive problems from sociocognitive ones in the rehabilitation plan. Earlier in the rehabilitation process, observed neurocognitive impairment is (1) more likely to be post-acute, (2) more likely to respond to neurocognitive intervention, and (3) its resolution is more likely to produce a spontaneous improvement in social cognition. Ultimately, the most convincing evidence that social cognition must be addressed separately is the same evidence that suggests the recovering person has attained maximum benefit from neurocognitive interventions.

## Step 4: Distinguishing between Sociocognitive Problems and More Molar Levels

Sociocognitive problems must also be distinguished from problems at more molar levels of functioning. As with neurocognitive problems, making this discernment is complicated by the indistinct boundaries between social–cognitive processes and those underlying skilled performance of complex activities. The more molar problem domains relevant here are psychophysiological dysregulation and skills deficits. *Psychophysiological dysregulation* involves difficulty in controlling or managing one's own neurophysiological functioning. Mood and anxiety disorders have psychophysiological components. For example, a clinical picture of depression often includes low levels of physical activity reflective of the neurophysiological states associated with depressed mood. Anxiety disorders often include behavioral avoidance, which prevents extinguishing the fear responses that have been conditioned to harmless objects or situations (e.g., fear of cats or fear of social gatherings). Psychosocial interventions for these disorders generally strengthen behavioral skills for managing the psychophysiological responses, which then extinguishes the fear component.

*Skills deficits* are deficiencies in areas crucial to a person's routine daily functioning and/or to rehabilitation and recovery. They include neurocognitive microskills, sociocognitive abilities, a specialized knowledge base (information in long-term memory), and the motivational factors that ensure that the skill is performed when needed. Both psychophysiological regulation and behavioral skills involve significant sociocognitive components. (Psychophysiological dysregulation and skills deficits are discussed in more detail in the next chapter.)

A sociocognitive problem should be distinguished from psychophysiological and behavioral skills problems when there is evidence of difficulties in social cognition that cannot be addressed effectively through the sociocognitive components typically included in psychophysiological and behavioral skills interventions. In practice, such evidence typically comes in the form of an unexpected lack of progress in psychophysiological or skills interventions. For example, an individual with specific problem-solving difficulties may encounter serious difficulty in social skills training. Similarly, a person with persistent poor self-esteem and/or a belief that any interpersonal conflict must be avoided may have difficulty performing assertive social skills, even when the behavioral skills themselves are intact. Symptom-linked attributions (e.g., delusional beliefs) may interfere with skills training that addresses management of one's own mental illness. Achievement-linked attributions (e.g., that social competence is unnecessary) may prevent engagement in any form of skills training. So far, there is no reliable technology for distinguishing specific sociocognitive problems from deficits in more molar levels of self-regulation and behavioral skills, and interventions for the latter often resolve difficulties at the sociocognitive level. Therefore, interventions specific to sociocognitive problems are usually introduced after considerable data has been generated on the person's response to skills training interventions.

As with the relationships between neurocognitive and sociocognitive problems, including a psychophysiological or behavioral skills problem does not obviate inclusion of a sociocognitive problem. In the example of depression, a person's psychophysiological self-regulation deficits may so dominate that neurophysiological and attributional interventions are unnecessary. At the other extreme, a depressed person's neurophysiological, neurocognitive, attributional, and self-regulation problems may be so independent from one another that specific interventions are required for all three. Often, poor social skills contribute to depression by prohibiting gratifying social affiliation, so social skills training is necessary as well. The particular combination of problems used to address components of a clinical presentation such as "depression" reflects the team's hypotheses about the independence of those components and their amenability to domain-specific interventions.

## Tools for Assessing Social Cognition

Four types of data inform assessment of sociocognitive functioning. The first, most familiar to mental health professionals (particularly psychologists) is that generated by conventional psychological testing. A second type comes from more recently developed laboratory tests, specialized for the purpose of assessing the cognitive (and other) aspects of interpersonal functioning in severe mental illness. A third type, also more recently developed, has been generated in the course of providing cognitive and cognitive-behavioral therapy. A fourth, less formal or structured type, comes from the social behavior and verbalizations of the recovering person and people in the recovering person's social environment. Data from all these sources should be integrated into a formulation that characterizes the role of social cognition in an individual's recovery and rehabilitation.

Conventional psychological assessment addresses highly relevant aspects of the sociocognitive domain. Personality inventories, sentence completion formats, and other instruments that elicit people's beliefs, attitudes, and social behavior patterns can be as useful in rehabilitation as they are in other clinical contexts.

Social problem solving is a domain of cognition not directly assessed by conventional psychological measures but of particular importance for rehabilitation. (For a comprehensive discussion of assessing problem solving, see D'Zurilla & Maydeu-Olivares, 1995). Some attention (though not enough) has been given to the development of less conventional laboratory instruments for this purpose. The Assessment of Interpersonal Problem-Solving Skills (AIPSS; Donahoe, unpublished; Donahoe et al., 1990) is an elaborate method for assessing problem-solving abilities in social situations. The instrument includes a set of videotaped vignettes, most of which portray an ordinary interpersonal conflict situation. The assessment subject watches each vignette and then is quizzed to determine what information was apprehended and retained. Next, the subject is asked to suggest ways to resolve the conflict. Finally, the subject is asked to pick the best solution and demonstrate in a role-play with the examiner. The entire process is videotaped and then scored by trained observers. The scored protocol provides a quantitative appraisal of the subject's performance in four domains reflecting apprehension and understanding of the problem, ability to generate effective solutions, and ability to enact them. The AIPSS provides a comprehensive, ecologically valid and detailed assessment of interpersonal problem-solving ability, and has been used effectively in research studies (e.g., Addington & Addington, 1999; Spaulding, Reed, et al., 1999). However, it is ponderous and expensive, and rarely used outside a research context. This is unfortunate, as no other instrument aspires to provide such a complete and detailed assessment of a person's interpersonal problem-solving ability. Materials for using the AIPSS are available from the developer (Donahoe, unpublished).

The Social Cue Recognition Task (SCRT; Corrigan & Nelson, 1998) uses videotaped vignettes to assess individuals' ability to recognize and interpret common social cues and requires less than an hour to administer. A specially trained technician can administer it. Scoring and interpretation are straightforward. Research indicates good reliability and construct validity, but so far there are no reports on clinical use. This book's authors have some clinical experience with the instrument, though limited, and have found that it can provide useful data economically in this domain of social cognition. By itself, it could be used as a measure for tracking recovery—that is, as a key indicator for a short-term goal in the rehabilitation plan. For the purposes of case formulation, the SCRT, used in conjunction with neuropsychological assessment, could help articulate the nature of neurocognitive and sociocognitive impairments, their relationships to neurophysiological problems, and their impact on sociobehavioral functioning.

The Means–Ends Problem Solving procedure (MEPS) uses a more conventional psychological test format to assess performance of the specific steps in problem-solving therapy (discussed below). In the MEPS, scenarios are described to the test subject, who is then asked to construct goals, and tactics for attaining the goals, that would resolve some problem in the scenario. These are then scored for relevance and probable effectiveness. The MEPS appears to measure a relatively unitary aspect of social cognition (Platt & Spivack, 1975), although it also correlates with some other sociocognitive characteristics as measured by conventional instruments (Platt & Siegel, 1976). There is too little research on the MEPS with people who have severe mental illness to be confident of its usefulness, but as the search for better and more practical measures of social cognition proceeds, instruments like the MEPS deserve the attention of clinical researchers (see House & Scott, 1996).

The Bell Object Relations Reality Testing Inventory (BORRTI; Bell, 2001), based on modernized psychodynamic sociocognitive constructs, is an interesting instrument in a conventional questionnaire format. Derived from ego psychology concepts (e.g., reality testing), it provides a psychometrically credible assessment of demonstrable relevance to the experience and social functioning of people with severe mental illness. It should not be surprising that empirically validated psychodynamic constructs might converge with constructs rooted in experimental and social psychology. Research on instruments like the BORRTI is likely to contribute substantially to the clinical technology for assessing social cognition.

A number of instruments that measure parameters relevant to attribution theory, especially the construct of *locus of control*, are associated with therapy strategies based on attributional analyses of mental illness (Bentall, 2001; Bentall & Kinderman, 1998). Locus of control refers to a person's tendency to attribute the cause of events to external (environmental) or internal (personal agency) factors. Locus of control attributions interact with other parameters (e.g., belief in the consistency or inevitability of causal factors) to shape a person's overall functioning. In mental illness, these factors may conspire to influence the content and/or function of problematic attributions, including delusions. Systematic assessment of these parameters is a key part of cognitive-behavioral intervention.

## INTERVENTIONS FOR PROBLEMS IN SOCIAL COGNITION

### Social Problem-Solving Insufficiency

This problem category is directly addressed by the problem-solving approach in cognitive-behavioral therapy (CBT; D'Zurilla, 1988). This is one of the oldest and most established of the modern CBT approaches. A number of specific modalities and manuals have been produced over the several decades of its development. Problem-solving therapy is usually done in a group format, although it works well in a dyadic format as well. In the widely disseminated skills training modules produced by the UCLA Center for Rehabilitation of Schizophrenia (see Kuehnel, Liberman, Storzbach, & Rose, 1990), the problem-solving approach has been thoroughly integrated with behavioral–social skills training.

The problem-solving approach involves didactic teaching of a multi-step algorithm for identifying, analyzing, and solving problems. After participants learn the algorithm, they practice applying it first to prototype problems described by the group leader, then to problems in their own lives.

The algorithm is generally some variation on the following steps:

1. Identify that there is a problem in need of a solution.
2. Articulate the nature of the problem.
3. Generate as many potential solutions as possible, without regard to practicality.
4. Analyze the potential solutions with respect to practicality and probability of solving the problem.
5. Choose the solution having the best potential and determine what action is necessary to implement it.
6. Implement the solution and evaluate the outcome.
7. If the problem has not been resolved, return to step 2 and repeat the process, determining at each step whether the previous analysis was accurate and complete.

After taking participants through a few initial didactic iterations of the steps, homework assignments help them learn how to apply the principles to their own problems in natural settings. In group settings, the participants share their experiences and help each other identify problems. Interpersonal interaction in pursuit of problem-solving objectives is encouraged and facilitated by the group leaders. As problem solutions are articulated, participants role-play the particular interpersonal behaviors and skills necessary to implement the solutions. Role-playing in this context is a structured exercise in which a particular interpersonal interaction is performed by group participants, each of whom assumes a designated character or role. Role-playing is a key tool in social skills training (discussed in the next chapter), so this part of the problem-solving modality overlaps with social skills training. One of the UCLA skills training modules, Interpersonal Problem Solving, interweaves problem solving and more behavioral skills training in a single group format.

Whether treated as a separate modality or interwoven in social skills training, the problem-solving approach immediately creates a new interpersonal context among the participants. In Western cultures, when one person expresses distress over some problem, others in that person's social milieu typically respond by attempting to assist directly in resolving the problem (e.g., offering advice or actually intervening).[1] If the others perceive themselves to be unable to assist in directly resolving the problem, they may respond by offering emotional support (e.g., sympathizing, reassuring, etc.). Social contexts in which there would be no response to the distress include a perception that problem solving or offering emotional support regarding the current situation is inappropriate (e.g., circumstances demand attention to other things, such as getting a job done), or that the individuals involved do not have the appropriate interpersonal relationships for engaging in problem solving ("It's none of my business"). The problem-solving model creates circumstances quite different from any of these. The problem-solving situation is determined not by the person's distress but by the rehabilitation plan. In other words, it is the social consensus that the group members would benefit from engaging in the therapeutic activity, rather than the fact that any one person "has a problem," that gives the problem-solving activity its meaning. Although there are plentiful opportunities for emotional support, that is not the central expressed purpose of the activity. There is no expectation that any of the participants will give good advice, provide emotional support, or claim or disclaim any responsibility for the problem or its solution. Nevertheless, there is an overriding presumption that everyone has problems, and the purpose of the group session is to become better at identifying and solving problems. Participants' problems are identified and analyzed according to a protocol (the algorithm) known to all. This meta-framework gives the problem-solving therapy approach a matter-of-fact tone and a task-oriented quality that most people experience as quite different from their normal experience in problem situations.

People with severe mental illness are often in the role of expressing distress over a problem and the need to solve it, just like anyone else. However, the social role of "mentally ill person" can affect the quality and experience of the social problem solving in which they are engaged. People in the social milieu of a person with mental illness are generally more likely to respond to expressions of distress by giving advice or directly intervening, as opposed to offering emotional support or engaging in problem analysis.

---

[1]No claim is being made here about the cultural specificity of this effect. The authors have no information on cultural differences, but are familiar with use of the problem-solving approach in a Western, Euro-American cultural context.

In this sense, people with mental illness are more likely to find themselves in a social role more akin to that of children, who are generally understood to lack the cognitive capacity to engage in more sophisticated problem analysis and solution generation. However, children are also more generally understood to need emotional support. These social factors conspire to make it especially difficult for people with severe mental illness to engage in productive social problem solving. The unusual context of the problem-solving therapeutic approach is especially salient to such individuals. They often show a surprising affinity for the approach, and they experience its matter-of-fact quality and its assumption that "everybody has problems to solve" as uniquely empowering.

*Example*

Consider the differences between the following two dialogues, in terms of the kinds of social cognition and social role performance they might produce in the recovering person.

DIALOGUE 1

Recovering person (RP): This new medication is making my mouth dry.

Helping person (HP): Sometimes medications will do that, but there are ways to counteract it. Tell your psychiatrist about it, and she'll do something to help.

RP: She never listens to me.

HP: I'll call her and tell her it's a problem for you.

RP: I don't have an appointment until next month.

HP: I'll see if I can get an early appointment for you.

RP: I don't have any way of getting there.

HP: I'll call a taxi for you.

DIALOGUE 2

RP: This new medication is making my mouth dry.

HP: It sounds like it's making you uncomfortable.

RP: I think I'll stop taking my medication.

HP: That would be one solution. Do any other possible solutions come to mind?

RP: Maybe I can get it changed.

HP: How might you do that?

RP: Well, I could talk to Dr. Jones about it, but I don't have an appointment until next month.

HP: You feel that's a long time to be so uncomfortable. Is there some way you could get an earlier appointment?

RP: I could go to another psychiatrist.

HP: That's a possibility. Are there other possibilities?

RP: I could call and see if Dr. Jones could give me an earlier appointment.

HP: Are there any drawbacks to that solution?

RP: I don't have a way of getting there unless the program van takes me.

HP: What are some other ways you could get there?

The various qualities and benefits of the problem-solving approach make it particularly amenable to "export" from the group room to the therapeutic milieu. Family members and direct care staff commonly find themselves in the role of "participant in the recovering person's problem solving." It can be difficult to perform that role without falling into a habitual pattern of giving advice and/or directly intervening but providing little emotional support. This response pattern tends to perpetuate a social relationship in which the recovering person is viewed as incompetent and undeserving of emotional support, for whom decisions must be made and basic tasks performed. (Cognitive dissonance predicts that if we treat others unsympathetically, then we also construct a belief that these others are undeserving of sympathy.)

This state of affairs is very similar to the behavioral construct of "doing for" (Paul & Lentz, 1977). *Doing for* can be operationalized and measured by observational instruments such as the Staff–Patient Interaction Chronograph (SRIC), a powerful instrument for ascertaining the social milieu of rehabilitation environments. A goal of milieu management in the social learning model of psychiatric rehabilitation is to minimize *doing for* behavior and replace it with *doing with* behavior, in which staff and recovering person collaborate, or with greater independence on the part of the recovering person. (This practice is discussed further in Chapter 11.)

The problem-solving therapeutic approach provides a procedural scheme for interrupting this interpersonal pattern. The key individuals in the recovering person's social milieu (including the recovering person) can be recruited into the problem-solving enterprise by teaching them the algorithm and securing an agreement to use it instead of customary responses, at least in specified situations. Practicing the problem-solving algorithm in this manner facilitates use of the algorithm in a naturalistic setting and increases the recovering person's experience of emotional support. The initial steps of the algorithm—acknowledging the existence of a problem and its distressing qualities—are typically experienced as a supportive acknowledgment of the situation and the person's distress. In addition, attributional changes are fostered as the individuals involved begin to view the recovering person as competent and deserving of emotional support. (Use of problem solving and related techniques in the therapeutic milieu is further discussed in Chapter 11.)

The problem-solving approach sometimes provides an alternative way of understanding a complex set of problems, such as those that pervade a mental illness. Many individuals understandably see themselves as victims of a disease. Such attributions, however, can pervade a person's meaning systems to such a degree that the disease makes all aspirations seem futile, all endeavors hopeless. The problem-solving algorithm focuses attention on particular aspects of complex problems, thereby breaking them down into manageable parts. The recovering person learns to understand symptoms and functional limitations as problems to be analyzed and solved, rather than as inevitable consequences of an all-powerful disease. In this sense, the effects of the problem-solving approach are similar to the effects of *reframing*, a key tactic in CBT. People with severe mental illness sometimes experience this particular type of reframing as especially empowering, and their overall engagement in the rehabilitation enterprise may increase in response.

## Symptom-Linked Attribution Problems

Delusions that (1) interfere with personal and social functioning, (2) persist despite resolution of acute psychosis, and (3) are not resolved by education and skills training in management of one's mental illness are appropriate targets for specialized sociocognitive interventions. Delusional behavior was often a target of early behavior modification efforts (Liberman, Teigen, Patterson, & Baker, 1973; Nydegger, 1972; Patterson & Teigen, 1973; Wincze, Leitenberg, & Agras, 1972), which were met with some success, although it remained unclear whether actual sociocognitive recovery occurred or simply a change in overt behavior. The last several years have seen considerable research on use of dyadic CBT specially adapted to address delusions and other attribution problems associated with severe mental illness (Alford & Correia, 1994; Alford, Fleece, & Rothblum, 1982; Bentall & Kinderman, 1998; Chadwick, Birchwood, & Trower, 1996; Haddock et al., 1998; Kinderman, 2001; Kingdon & Turkington, 1991, 1994). The methodology used in this research generally involved a combination of psychoeducation, interpersonal support and validation, and disputational interventions. In disputational interventions, question-and-answer interactions between the recovering person and a therapist are designed to guide the recovering person toward (1) considering the factual basis of the delusion, (2) reflecting on other possible explanations of real events involved in the delusion, (3) testing the validity of the delusion by gathering more information, and (4) examining the consequences of accepting a delusional belief. This approach is similar to traditional individual psychotherapy techniques based on the psychodynamic concept of reality testing. In addition, CBT approaches that make use of cognitive dissonance and related concepts from attribution theory are currently being developed in order to reverse the interpersonal and intrapersonal processes that sustain the delusion. These techniques show promise, but so far there is insufficient data to conclude that sociocognitive interventions contribute uniquely to the resolution of problematic delusional beliefs. Use of these techniques in dyadic therapy requires practice supervised by an experienced clinician. The interested reader should consult the original sources for more detailed elaboration and examples.

## Mood-Linked Attribution Problems

People with severe mental illness are often in situations that would depress anyone. Hence, the role of situational factors in clinical depression must be carefully assessed. Changing the situation may be more important than directly treating the depression. However, situational factors cannot always be resolved. The recovering person may benefit from an intervention that establishes more effective mood-regulating social cognition while coping with difficult circumstances; even when the person's coping would be perfectly adequate in less difficult circumstances, it is an advantageous intervention.

The presence of extraordinary stress also encourages use of pharmacological interventions, under the humane but potentially condescending presumption that "everyone needs chemical help coping with extreme stress." Choosing between a pharmacological and a psychosocial approach to treating mood dysregulation is one of the most debated topics in contemporary mental health. It is a ubiquitous issue in rehabilitation, reflecting the high comorbidity between depression and other psychiatric diagnoses (this was discussed in Chapter 4). In large part, the debate continues because neither pharmacological nor psychosocial approaches have clear superiority. When cost is a manageable factor, joint provision of both is often the safest choice. When a choice of one or the other must be made, the benefits and risks must be weighed for the individual case. As discussed in Chapter 4, the potential benefits of a pharmacological approach include potentially faster clinical response and less demand for the recovering person to engage in the work of psychotherapy. The risks include a higher likelihood of relapse after discontinuing the drug, especially in the presence of sociocognitive vulnerabilities to mood dysregulation. In addition, it is important to consider the implications of depending on a drug, rather than personal agency and a healthy lifestyle, to control one's mood. In the integrated paradigm, inclusion of a mood-linked attribution problem title reflects the team's hypothesis of a significant sociocognitive component in a clinical presentation of mood disorder, even if the clinical presentation is being addressed simultaneously as a tonic neurophysiological dysregulation (i.e., being treated pharmacologically).

Mood-linked attributions are key targets in a variety of CBT approaches (Lewinsohn, Sullivan, & Grosscup, 1982; Rehm, Kaslow, & Rabin, 1987; Williams, 1984), and even more so in schematic forms of cognitive therapy (Beck, Rush, Shaw, & Emery, 1979). *Schematic cognitive therapy* is closely related to CBT but includes more emphasis on particular attributions and systems of meaning that maintain a depressed or manic mood, and less emphasis on performance of relevant personal and social behaviors. *Interpersonal therapy* is procedurally similar to CBT and schematic approaches, although its conceptual roots lie in the psychoanalytic paradigm of Harry Stack Sullivan and his successors, rather than in social learning theory. All three of these related approaches have established effectiveness in resolving mood regulation problems through modifying mood-related social cognition. Attributions about the self (i.e., the self-esteem continuum) are of central concern in all three approaches. Poor self-esteem is often implicated as a persistent vulnerability to both depression and mania. (For a review of treating low self-esteem in severe mental illness, see Fennell, 1998.)

## Achievement-Linked Attribution Problems

As is the case with mood-linked problems, people with mental illness often find themselves in situations that discourage achievement or even aspirations of achievement. First-person accounts of mental illness often include stories of salient events experienced as powerful blows to the recovering person's desire for a productive, meaningful life. These stories typically include accounts of counseling by mental health professionals that focused on the limitations that mental illness is presumed to impose. Although such counseling is probably intended to help the recovering person establish realistic guidelines for personal expectations, it runs a high risk of maintaining or even creating an attributional system wherein meaningful personal achievement is rendered unobtainable. This "glass half empty" mentality is especially true in the medical model, where a person's hopelessness is seen as a rational response to "incurable" illness, and where the purpose of treatment is to make the "patient" as comfortable as possible while awaiting the inevitable. The rehabilitation paradigm offers an intrinsic antidote to the "medical model blues" in its emphasis on recovery rather than cure, and in its various related assumptions about the centrality of the recovering person's engagement in the rehabilitation enterprise. Nevertheless, people inevitably reach their own conclusions about the implications of their mental illness, and it is not uncommon to encounter significant achievement-linked attribution problems in the context of the most progressive rehabilitation.

This condition created by achievement-linked attribution problems is distinct from clinical anosognosia, where neurophysiological and/or neurocognitive problems prevent normal perception and understanding of the mental illness. It is also distinct from a mood-linked attribution problem, where disinterest in achievement is directly associated with a depressive mood state and the neurocognitive impairments that may accompany it. It is less distinct from less severe forms of lack of insight. Ultimately, a perceived lack of insight may be no more than a difference in values; after all, "normal" people exhibit vast variability with respect to the importance attributed to achievement. Similarly, disinterest in achieving greater personal autonomy and independence may reflect a rational apprehension of the risks of autonomy and independence. Many people with mental illness have experienced drastic deprivation and abuse in the world of competent, autonomous adults. Given the effects of their illness as well as the social sanctions and stigma imposed upon people with mental illness, it is more than understandable that, for example, a person might believe that life in a psychiatric institution, where one can at least expect food and shelter, is preferable to the life of a psychotic street person.

Beliefs about personal achievement of people with disabling mental illness who are in their late adolescence or early adulthood should be expected to include the vagaries characteristic of those developmental stages. At the same time, it is in late adolescence and early adulthood that people generally form their core beliefs about personal achievement and what constitutes "a good life." Having a severe mental illness certainly puts this developmental process in a distinct context, but it does not necessarily prohibit the development of adult values and beliefs. In rehabilitation, these values and beliefs require attention even if it is not the mental illness itself that has produced an achievement-linked attribution problem.

The intervention that most focally addresses achievement-linked attribution problems is rehabilitation counseling, a sine qua non in the rehabilitation of people with disabling mental illness. It is the core purpose of rehabilitation counseling to engage the recovering person in the rehabilitation enterprise, and the basic premises of rehabilitation are intrinsically incompatible with an achievement-linked attribution problem. Rehabilitation counseling helps the recovering person identify current values and beliefs, then identify specific steps in the rehabilitation process that could help him or her to actualize those values and beliefs. Achievement-linked attribution problems often stem from a gap between current and desired realities. Once a person apprehends procedural links between action today and desirable consequences in the future, the belief that nothing can or should be done today is weakened. The success of rehabilitation counseling in overcoming achievement-linked attribution problems lies in its ability to elicit and validate a person's existing values and beliefs and link them to specific actions, rather than changing those values and beliefs.

## Example

The following brief excerpt of a rehabilitation counseling session encapsulates the key principles of the approach.

Helping person (HP): If there were one thing about your life you would change, what would it be?

Recovering person (RP): I wish people would just leave me alone.

HP: You feel annoyed or hassled by some people?

RP: Yes—I'm not doing anything wrong or hurting anybody else.

HP: You'd like people to just let you do your own thing?

RP: Yes. Just leave me alone.

HP: What kinds of things would get people to stop hassling you?

RP: I have no idea. I don't know why they do it.

HP: That's a mystery, as you see it.

RP: I guess.

HP: So, if you could figure out why someone is hassling you, you might be able to get the person to stop?

RP: I guess.

HP: Suppose we could identify reasons people might hassle you—might that help?

RP: Maybe.

HP: Suppose we could find something you could do to get people to leave you alone. Would that help?

RP: Maybe.

HP: Would you be willing to spend some time on that—getting people to leave you alone when you don't want to be hassled?

RP: Maybe.

HP: There's a group in this program that might be helpful for that—it's called Interpersonal Skills. How about checking it out to see if it might be helpful?

Ultimately, the best antidote for failure is success. To the degree that a person's lack of interest in recovery is a rational and/or emotional response to past failures (whether or not the failures are due specifically to the mental illness), new successes and achievements are expected to enliven that interest. Recovering people in the first stage of rehabilitation are often "success deprived" and have lost all confidence in their ability to achieve anything. Often, their only recent accomplishment is to immobilize those around them with their bizarre behavior. Such behavior may prevent catastrophic consequences, such as premature hospital discharge or expectations of competence, but it also maintains a pervasive sense of incompetence and futility. As is the case with most people, this sense changes most in response to incompatible events, such as success at a task important to the individual. In the example above, the recovering person's wish to be left alone was potentiated by his experience of constantly being panhandled for cigarettes by other program participants. A few sessions of assertiveness training gave him a simple but effective repertoire for reducing that annoyance. His relief was enhanced by a sense that he had personally implemented a successful intervention that directly affected his own well-being.

The step-by-step nature of rehabilitation is conducive to the systematic facilitation of success experiences. Rehabilitation starts with identifying the person's current ability, then seeks circumstances where that ability can reliably produce some kind of success. For example, people with severe mental illness are often able to engage in, and derive satisfaction from, simple, highly repetitive workshop tasks (e.g., collating and stapling) even when they are unable to engage in more complex work activities. There may be more value in experiencing success at that task, for an extended period of time, than in moving on to more complex tasks. The experience of success can be more beneficial at that stage of recovery than the functional advantages of being able to perform more complex tasks. Similarly, it may be more beneficial to sustain the workshop success experience than to broaden the emphasis of rehabilitation to other domains, such as social skills, at least for a while. Sustained success in the workshop may fortify the person for the more difficult and possibly aversive experience of struggling to acquire social skills. However, this line of thinking presumes that the success in the workshop is highly acknowledged and reinforced.

Much of the task of rehabilitation planning is to anticipate these success opportunities and exploit them. Much of the task of maintaining an effective rehabilitation milieu is to create opportunities for success, then make sure the successes are recognized by the recovering person and acknowledged by his or her social environment. Maintenance of a rehabilitation milieu that is optimized for counteracting problems with achievement-linked attributions is discussed in Chapter 12.

## Chapter 9

# The Sociobehavioral Level of Functioning

The sociobehavioral level of functioning involves the coordination of neurophysiological, neurocognitive, and sociocognitive processes for the purpose of performing behavioral activities in a socially meaningful context. These processes are controlled, to a significant degree, by information stored in the brain's information-processing system. This stored information contains each individual's worldview and responses to it. The information is largely acquired, through learning, throughout life. Its content is therefore specific to each individual's unique experience (although much experience is shared via culture). To understand human functioning at the sociobehavioral level, we must understand not only *how* information is processed (a matter for neuropsychological and sociocognitive analysis) but also the specific *content* of that information.

### THE MANY MEANINGS OF *SKILL*

The enormous complexity of performing behavioral activities in a socially meaningful context is made manageable for scientific study through the concept of *skill*. A skill in the scientific sense is comparable to the colloquial concept, in that both connote ability to perform specific tasks. However, it is important to distinguish carefully between the two concepts in any applications to the field of rehabilitation. In the colloquial version, *skill* usually connotes an ability to perform a nonroutine task (e.g., work tasks such as welding or surgery) or athletic or artistic abilities. Activities that everyone performs daily are not commonly considered to be skills. In addition, in the colloquial usage, *acquired* performance abilities are not clearly distinguished from *native* abilities (i.e., *talent*). In the colloquial usage, the meaning of *skills* tends to be imprecise and even mysterious (e.g., the skill of a virtuoso violinist). In scientific application, any behavioral activity that accomplishes an identifiable purpose and that involves use of acquired information ("knowledge") can potentially be defined, operationalized, measured, studied and manipulated as a skill. In other words, behavioral activity is a skill to the degree that researchers can operationalize and quantify (1) the environmental conditions in which the behavior is performed, (2) the qualities of the behavior, (3) the information required to guide the behavior, and (4) the outcome (accomplishment of some objective or goal).

At a more molar level of organization, skills are associated with particular *social roles*, which are complex informational networks that describe and define the purpose and meaning of performing an aggregate of skills. Our lives are organized around the performance of various social roles— the roles of parent, family member, worker, teacher, student, housekeeper, tourist, religious person, nonconformist, goalie on the soccer team, and so on. Our phenomenological experiences of ourselves and the world are determined, in large part, by the social roles we perform at one time or another. Filling a specific social role generally involves performing skills associated with that role. In addition, beliefs, attitudes, and attributions have important functions in role performance, as discussed in the previous chapter. There is a reciprocal causal relationship between what roles we perform and the beliefs we espouse. Thus the roles we perform and the skills we use in performing those roles are inextricably linked to our beliefs and attitudes about ourselves and the world. For example, we function most effectively as mental health professionals when we perform our technical skills from an inner foundation of believing that our clients really can and do change, and that these changes really do produce a better, happier life. When we abandon those beliefs, we lose effectiveness even while we attempt to go on performing our skills. This absence of affirming belief is the essence of the notorious "burnout" phenomenon.

In some traditional views of mental illness, the "illness" occurs at more molecular levels of human functioning; interventions directed at those levels are "treatment," whereas interventions directed at skill performance are "education" or "coaching." In the neo-Kraepelinian concept of mental illness, interventions directed at the "disease" are "treatment," whereas interventions directed at the developmental or sociobehavioral "consequences of the disease" are ancillary supports (e.g., "psychosocial help"; Klein, 1980). This distinction may serve the economic interests of professional groups whose technologies are limited to the more molecular levels of human functioning, but it does not serve the purposes of rehabilitation. In disabling mental illness, the molecular and molar aspects of disability are too closely linked to put them on difference sides of a diagnostic boundary.

The economic implications of defining any particular human problem as a "medical" condition are significant. Generally, in this culture, practitioners of biomedical technology command higher fees than do practitioners of psychosocial technology. This is true in mental health as well. It is generally expected, therefore, that a practitioner who applies biotechnology to a given problem will command a higher fee than a practitioner who applies psychosocial technology to that problem. This status quo is not expected to create higher costs overall, because biotechnology tends to be seen as more effective and efficient, thereby compensating for the higher practitioner fee. Thus, there is thus a strong incentive for practitioners to use biomedical technology and claim the fees accordingly. Mental health policy tends to reinforce these expectations, although research has certainly not established that higher practitioner costs are indeed offset by greater efficiency and effectiveness. Cognitive dissonance theory accounts for this phenomenon. Mental health administrators are expected to believe that the most expensive technology is the most important, because it is dissonant to believe that one is paying higher fees for ineffective technology. Similarly, individuals who receive high fees for specific practices are expected to strongly believe in the effectiveness and superiority of those practices, even in the face of disconfirmatory scientific evidence. In a humanitarian health care system it would be dissonant to believe that one is using less effective technology because it is more lucrative. Similarly, cognitive dissonance theory accounts for a strong belief that the principles that call for the accoutrements of biomedical technology (e.g., those of neo-Kraepelinian psychiatry) are valid, despite disconfirmatory logic and scientific evidence.

Inability to perform a skill is the result of multiple etiological factors, at various levels of functioning, in different combinations in different people. In the integrated paradigm, skill performance represents one level at which the mental illness is expressed, and it is no more nor less a part of the illness than neurophysiological dysregulation, neurocognitive impairment, or even the social stigmatization to which mentally ill people are subjected. Optimal outcome requires integrated application of technologies, tailored to individual needs, that address the molar- as well as molecular-level problems.

The importance of rejecting the distinction between mental illness and sociobehavioral problems is not limited to clinical conceptualizations. The current preoccupation in Western culture with molecular biology and pharmacology—with "simple" pharmacological solutions to complex human problems—has created a disproportionate investment in medical treatments of disabling mental illness and a neglect of educational or rehabilitative approaches. In the mental health field, the striking but very circumscribed success of psychopharmacotherapy has further encouraged this neglect. In the mental health advocacy community, this neglect is (probably inadvertently) encouraged by a belief, not well supported by research, that viewing mental illness as "a biological disease" reduces stigmatization. (For a systematic scientific analysis of stigma and what to do about it, see Corrigan & Penn, 1999.) The failures of contemporary mental health services, especially for people with chronic, disabling neurodevelopmental conditions, are largely attributable to a simplistic identification of "illness" with the most molecular expressions of those conditions. The prospects for recovery from disabling mental illness rest heavily with development of a new social consensus that recognizes the importance of technologies spanning the entire spectrum of human functioning.

## Declarative and Procedural Information

As discussed in Chapters 5 and 6, skills operate at the neurocognitive level as well as at the level of observable social behavior. Skills involve multiple cognitive and behavioral processes, within and across different levels of biobehavioral organization. *All skills are the product of the interaction of cognitive processes with information that has been acquired and stored.* Generally, skill-related information is stored in long-term memory. Skill-related information is usefully categorized as either declarative or procedural. Declarative information encodes ("declares") facts (and beliefs) about the world, and procedural information encodes behavior sequences ("procedures") associated with performance of the skill. This distinction corresponds to the distinction between two types of learning, explicit/verbal and implicit/procedural, discussed in Chapter 5. Declarative and procedural skill-related information is also organized into (1) *scripts*, which are instructions for analyzing information and responding accordingly in specific situations, and (2) *meta-scripts*, which are instructions on how to select the appropriate script for particular situations.

The declarative and procedural information related to skill performance is used by executive cognitive processes to (1) identify situations demanding a particular skill performance, (2) analyze task demands, (3) activate needed cognitive processes, (4) access further information in memory, and (5) execute the correct behavior sequences ("run the program," in computer argot). In large part, human behavior is comprised of the selection and performance of skills. Many are performed so routinely and with such little impact on conscious experience that they are taken for granted.

## Etiology of Skill Performance Failure

The neurophysiological, neurocognitive, and sociocognitive impairments associated with mental illness compromise acquisition of skills and impair the performance of skills that have been acquired. The social environments in which people with mental illness find themselves may further inhibit skill acquisition and performance. The developmental consequences of mental illness often include deficient declarative and procedural information in critical skill areas. Thus the etiology of a skill performance failure may lie in (1) faulty or absent declarative or procedural information, (2) the executive cognition that processes this information, (3) the environmental circumstances that elicit and/or support the skill performance, or (4) some combination of these three factors.

Often, the compromised skills are those taken for granted by normally functioning individuals, and are therefore deceptively difficult to recognize. These may include skills necessary for basic self-care (e.g., knowing when to change underwear), regulating emotional and behavioral responses to environmental events (e.g., not jumping into the fray when an argument breaks out), and interpreting other people's social behavior and managing interpersonal relationships (e.g., recognizing an opportunity to make a friend).

## The Skill-Role Concept ualization of Mental Illness

One of the most important contributions of the psychiatric rehabilitation paradigm that evolved from social learning theory in the 1970s is the idea of understanding mental illness in terms of sociobehavioral skills and social role performance (Anthony & Liberman, 1986; Goldberg, Schooler, Hogarty, & Roper, 1977; Liberman et al., 1986). The experimental research of the previous decade (e.g., Braginsky et al., 1969) had shown that much of the abnormal social behavior associated with mental illness has the characteristics of a social role. It is not the chaotic result of psychic disorganization so much as a predictable response to contingencies—a purposeful pursuit of a way of life, constrained by the environmental demands of institutions, cultural expectations and stigma, and inability to perform key skills in support of alternative social roles. This view initially competed with that of psychoanalysis, then with reductionistic biological and neo-Kraepelinian formulations. With the emergence of biosystemic paradigms, competition gave way to complementarity. Although preoccupation with neurophysiology and pharmacology in the late 20th century diverted the attention of much of the scientific community, the skill–role conceptualization of mental illness continued to provide a useful understanding of the characteristics of mental illness beyond those associated with neurophysiological dysregulation and neurocognitive impairment.

As the psychiatric rehabilitation paradigm evolved, the skill construct incorporated the cognitive and even physiological substrates of behavioral performance. In the integrated paradigm, behavioral failures can be understood as failures in people's repertoire of skills, in their ability to identify which skills are appropriate for which tasks, in the neurocognitive functions required to control performance of a particular skill, or even in their ability to generate the degree of physiological arousal optimal for a particular task (some tasks require higher arousal and narrowly focused attention, while others require lower arousal and a broader attention focus). To a significant degree, the central goal of rehabilitation is to help people establish timely, reliable performance of key skills, respond to the routine demands of daily living, and be as self-sufficient as possible. Acquiring new skills and/or recovering old skills gives the recovering person a greater range of social role choices. In this sense, the essence of recovery from disabling mental illness is the perogative of choosing roles.

## Psychophysiological and Instrumental Skills

For heuristic purposes, it is convenient to categorize skills relevant to rehabilitation as psychophysiological and instrumental skills. *Psychophysiological skills* are so named because they involve regulation or control of neurophysiological (primarily autonomic) activity by sociocognitive processes that use acquired information stored in memory. *Instrumental skills* are so named because they involve complex behaviors controlled by sociocognitive processes that use acquired information stored in memory to act "instrumentally" on the environment to accomplish specific goals.[1] The distinction is somewhat arbitrary, in that there is commonality and intersection among the neurophysiological and cognitive processes that underlie all skills. It is a useful distinction, however, because the clinical technology for addressing psychophysiological skill development is somewhat different from that for addressing instrumental skill development.

Psychophysiological *skills* should be carefully distinguished from other aspects of psychophysiological functioning. In the experimental psychopathology literature, psychophysiological analysis primarily addresses neurophysiological processes in the central nervous system and their relationships to neurocognition and autonomic activity (e.g., Dawson & Nuechterlein, 1984; Duncan, 1988; Shagass, 1991; Zahn, Frith, & Steinhauer, 1991). Although psychophysiology at this level is clearly important in understanding the etiology and neurocognition of severe mental illness, as a level of analysis and a research paradigm it is distinct from clinical application at the sociobehavioral level. In clinical application the primary focus is on skills (including their sociocognitive components) relevant to activity in the autonomic and peripheral nervous systems, although some CNS processes (e.g., those associated with anxiety) are also of interest.

---

[1]This use of *instrumental* should not be confused with its use in learning theory, "instrumental learning," a synonym for operant learning. Instrumental learning is a set of hypothetical but highly measurable processes that produce acquired instrumental behavior. However, the meaning of *instrumental* as operating upon the environment is common to both uses of the term.

The integrated paradigm's prototype problem set identifies six problems in psychophysiological regulation and six problems in instrumental skill functioning. The different psychophysiological skill problems reflect distinct domains of emotional experience, behavior, and underlying physiology: behavioral activation, mood, anger/aggression, fear/anxiety, appetitive behavior, and sexual behavior. The different instrumental skill problems reflect distinct domains of skill performance: self-care, independent living (housekeeping, cooking, managing a personal budget, etc.), management of one's mental illness, managing recreational/leisure time, occupational functioning, and interpersonal functioning.

Use of skills as the primary units of analysis at the sociobehavioral level is incompatible with the traditional and more pejorative distinction between "normal" and "abnormal" functioning and behavior. One can perform a skill to some measurable degree, from *not at all* to *perfectly*. Repeated failure to perform a skill effectively can be understood as a deficit in the domain of that particular skill. *Deficit* does not mean or connote abnormality. It simply means the person cannot or does not effectively perform the skill. In the integrated paradigm's prototype problem set, the problems associated with instrumental skills are termed deficits in the respective skill domains. Problems in psychophysiological functioning are termed *dysregulations* to emphasize the self-regulatory nature of psychophysiological skills.

The sociobehavioral level includes one additional problem title: that of substance abuse. It is increasingly clear that substance abuse is a major problem among many people with disabling mental illness (Dixon, 1999). Most contemporary theoretical models of substance abuse use a biosystemic frame of reference, acknowledging potential etiological factors at all levels of human functioning. In the integrated paradigm, substance abuse is understood to represent a variety of problems in sociocognitive and sociobehavioral functioning, including deficiencies in the skills required to suppress inappropriate substance use. Each individual demonstrates a unique combination of sociocognitive characteristics and skill failures. This uniqueness is recognized in some theories of substance abuse that discuss how some people self-medicate an anxiety disorder with alcohol while others seek the changes in self-concept that alcohol induces. It should not be surprising that treating substance abuse in people with severe mental illness is currently being approached on multiple levels, including pharmacological (Tsuang, Eckman, Shaner, & Marder, 1999), neurocognitive (Bennett, Bellack, & Gearon, 2001), sociocognitive (i.e., with psychoeducation; Herz et al., 2000), sociobehavioral (Sigmon, Steingard, Anthony, & Higgins, 2000), and socioenvironmental (Sheils & Rolfe, 2000). Systematic multilevel approaches are beginning to emerge (Barrowclough et al., 2001).

Substance abuse is listed as a separate problem on the rehabilitation plan when it is hypothesized that separately addressing contributory factors (e.g., treating dysregulation of fear/anxiety or mood, poor self-esteem) would not fully resolve the problem behavior.

## IMPLICATIONS FOR CLINICAL ASSESSMENT

The skills concept is at the heart of clinical rehabilitation technology in functional assessment. Functional assessment is a formal process of (1) analyzing environmental demands for skill performance, (2) determining the molar and molecular components of the needed skills (neurophysiological, cognitive, behavioral), and (3) evaluating whether those components are present in a person's repertoire. (For a general account of functional assessment, see Nelson & Hayes, 1981; for reviews of functional assessment techniques relevant to severe mental illness, see Anthony, Cohen, & Nemec, 1986; O'Brian, 1993; Yoman & Edelstein, 1994.) Functional assessment technology evolved from the convergence of social learning theory and related technologies as they were incorporated in the psychiatric rehabilitation paradigms of the late 20th century. That era produced voluminous research and materials for training practitioners to use functional assessment to guide skills training in rehabilitation. Increasingly, professional education programs are incorporating functional assessment and skills training in their curricula. Assessment and training tools and materials developed expressly for rehabilitation of severe mental illness are available from Psychiatric Rehabilitation Consultants, P.O. Box 2867, Camarillo, CA 93011-2867. Website: www.psychrehab.com.

Training materials and instruments for guiding functional assessment tend to use a *nomothetic* approach to assessment. Such an approach assumes that there is a discrete number of relevant factors to be measured and evaluated, and that addressing these factors produces a comprehensive and sufficient assessment. In the case of assessing functional skills in people with severe mental illness, some areas are more amenable to this approach than others. Some skills, such as personal grooming and hygiene, cooking, budgeting, and housecleaning, are relatively circumscribed and easily observed in both natural and clinical settings; a standard testing procedure reliably demonstrates whether a person has the competence to perform the needed skills. Similarly, determining whether the person performs the skills in natural settings requires little more than opportunity to observe the person in the natural setting (historical information and the person's self-report may even supplant actual observation). Numerous instruments have been developed for guiding nomothetic functional assessment (e.g., Menditto et al., 1999; Slaton & Westphal, 1999).

Other skills, such as interpersonal and psychophysiological skills, are difficult to measure with nomothetic instruments and usually require a more *idiographic* approach. Idiographic assessment does not assume that there is a discrete number of measurable factors equally applicable to all individuals. To arrive at a valid understanding of a person's repertoire of skills, a preliminary determination needs to identify the particular factors applicable to that person. The assessment then focuses on measurement of those factors. For example, there may be a number of equivalent ways to resolve a particular conflict. People must choose among alternatives, and their choice is based on their own personal characteristics and preferences. Assessing skill performance requires that this complexity be taken into account. People also have unique patterns of autonomic response, and they have to manage unique environmental challenges and demands. To understand a person's psychophysiological dysregulation, it is necessary to understand that person's individual psychophysiological characteristics and environmental conditions.

## Competence versus Performance Deficits

A key clinical issue in functional assessment is determining whether a skill-related failure is due to a problem in competence or performance. In this context, a *competence deficit* means the person lacks the cognitive processing abilities and/or memory information to perform the skill, even under optimal environmental conditions. A *performance deficit* means the person has the ability to perform the skill under special environmental conditions, but does not perform the skill appropriately or when needed under natural conditions. (Caveat: Although the distinction between competence and performance is heuristically useful, it is also somewhat arbitrary. Arguably, the ability to recognize a situation demanding a skill and respond accordingly is part of the skill itself and therefore a type of competence deficit when it is absent. Nevertheless, in the clinical context, competence-based failure has intervention implications quite different from those of performance failures when all other aspects of the skill are intact.) Not knowing how to operate a vacuum cleaner or a dust mop is a competence problem in the domain of living skills. Knowing how to do it but simply not doing it when needed is a performance problem in the same domain. Knowing how to use the equipment but not understanding the importance of periodic housecleaning may account for the performance problem. Expressing a complete understanding of the importance of housecleaning but still not performing the task suggests that a different explanation is necessary. With problems in competence, the recovering person clearly needs to acquire more skill. However, with problems in performance, there is an additional element of motivation. Either the person needs to acquire the particular skills to identify the demand for the housecleaning skill at the right time, or the person's environment needs to provide meaningful consequences for performing or not performing the skill. The latter is less a problem in the sociobehavioral level of functioning than in the interactions between person and environment. (Problems in the person–environment domain are discussed in the following chapter.)

## Functional Behavioral Analysis

Functional behavioral analysis, an idiographic technique for assessing function at the sociobehavioral level (Iwata, Kahng, Wallace, & Lindberg, 2000; O'Brian, 1993), originated in the 1960s as a technological application of learning theory. By the 1980s it had incorporated the cognitive perspective of social learning theory. Functional analysis of behavior is a formal process of identifying the temporal *antecedents* and *consequences* of specific behaviors—those environmental events that occur consistently before or after the behavior being assessed. These events include relevant cognitions and emotions (thoughts and feelings), associated either temporally or through cognitive relationships (e.g., a person's belief that a particular behavior is associated with a particular emotional state). Systematic observation and analysis reveals which behaviors are "controlled" by environmental and organismic antecedents and consequences. This information then can be used to therapeutically manipulate the environment in order to influence expression of the designated behavior. Ultimately, the contribution of functional behavioral analysis to the rehabilitation process is to bring key antecedents and consequences (both organismic and environmental) under the control of the recovering person.

Functional behavioral analysis is used extensively in mental health and educational/developmental settings, because it is extremely helpful for analyzing behavioral problems that demand a systematic and precise understanding of person–environment interactions. There is an important distinction between precise analysis of person–environment interactions and classification. In traditional clinical thinking (e.g., the medical model), classification is expected to emerge naturally from a full understanding of the processes being classified. The natural classifications that functional behavioral analysis produces are categories of psychological processes and events—for example, reinforcement, discriminatory stimuli—not clinical situations. These categories are an advantage in the sense that they do not contain the invalidating flaws of Kraepelinian diagnosis, but they are nevertheless a limitation in clinical application. In discussing this limitation of functional behavior analysis, behavioral psychologists Steven Hayes and William Follette (1992) suggest a number of alternatives, some of which are recognizable components of the problem-oriented assessment model incorporated in the integrated paradigm. In this sense, the integrated paradigm provides a key context for the use of functional behavioral analysis.

A functional behavioral analysis of the antecedents and consequences of particular problems in skill performance is often the key to determining whether the problem is in the competence or performance domain, and whether and how the individual's environment prompts and rewards skill performance. Person–environment interaction data is also helpful (and sometimes crucial) when assessing neurophysiological and cognitive problems and their role in more molar levels of personal and social functioning.

Adding functional, idiographic analysis of skill performance to the assessment and intervention process adds a gradual, trial-and-test quality that reflects the hypothetico-deductive cycles of rehabilitation, and, in many cases, the cycles of assessing and treating cognitive and neurophysiological problems. Data from functional assessments (and elsewhere) and the effects of interventions must be considered in concert when making key decisions about how problems are identified on the treatment plan and which interventions are selected. A sociobehavioral problem title indicates the team's hypothesis that deficient skill performance is contributing independently to some aspect of the clinical picture (i.e., enumerated under the problem description) and is expected to respond to interventions intended to improve skill performance relevant to the problem. Inclusion of sociobehavioral problems does not preclude inclusion of other problems that address related aspects of the clinical picture. The operative consideration is whether the sociobehavioral problem presents an independent barrier to rehabilitation efforts, for which there is intervention technology of known effectiveness.

## ASSESSMENT AND REHABILITATION
## OF PSYCHOPHYSIOLOGICAL REGULATION SKILLS

People use psychophysiological skills to match their mood state and level of arousal to the changing demands of their environment. These skills include becoming aroused, angry, fearful, and so on, when such states are adaptive, and inhibiting those states when they are not adaptive. Psychophysiological skills are closely associated with management of *stress*, which can be understood generally as the product of excessive, inappropriate, and/or inefficient psychophysiological activation.

Psychophysiological regulatory skills are often deficient in people with severe mental illness. Yet psychophysiological dysregulation problems observed in people with disabling mental illness are comparable to problems observed in people without disabling mental illness. The incidence of these problems in people with disabling mental illness has been overlooked, in part, because of the presumption that such problems are part and parcel of the psychotic disorder. The good news is, there are treatment approaches of known effectiveness for these problems, and we have no reason to expect they would not be effective for people who also have disabling mental illness. (This insight is reflected in current interest in the psychiatric community in recognizing comorbid conditions and providing conjoint treatments accordingly.) At the same time, for each individual it is important to consider whether other problems associated with disabling mental illness are interacting with psychophysiological factors or creating complications for intervention strategies.

Many social roles require skillful psychophysiological self-regulation. Deficits in these skills may limit a person's opportunity to perform desired social roles (e.g., the role of reliable employee) or may even nudge a person into performing a social role wherein poor psychophysiological self-regulation is actually part of the role. For example, in any given situation, a person with poorly regulated anxiety is more prone to experience high anxiety and to perform the role of an anxious, brittle, or "high-strung" individual. Repeated experience reinforces the self-perception that "I am an anxious, high-strung person, unable to deal with situations that demand calm and confidence." This cycle of failure causes the person to avoid situations that might require regulation of anxiety; hence, there are no opportunities to develop better self-regulation skills. The person cultivates a social environment that is optimally suited to a persistently anxious individual, however limited that environment may be. Thus the links between skill performance, social cognition, and social role performance also apply to psychophysiological skills.

The recovering person's experience of the problems associated with psychophysiological dysregulation is a critical factor in assessment and intervention. Psychophysiological dysregulation is often, but not always, associated with the experience of distress. But distressful or not, psychophysiological processes are inherently difficult to describe and discuss in the best of circumstances. Nobody, especially people who are already dealing with mental illness, should be expected to articulate these processes without some preparation. Assessing the recovering person's phenomenological experience and his or her beliefs and attributions about psychophysiological functioning is a crucial part of the rehabilitation planning process. Educating the recovering person about psychophysiological processes and their relevance to rehabilitation and recovery is a key component in any intervention. Often, making a change in attitudes and beliefs is more important than acquiring the missing procedural skills. Many people initially do not believe that they have much, if any, control over their psychophysiological functioning, until they are convinced otherwise through education and direct therapeutic experience. There is little motivation to gain control of something in the face of a strong belief that it cannot possibly be controlled. Similarly, once a person's beliefs about the role of psychophysiological self-regulation is incorporated into the performance of a complex social role, changing the beliefs and/or the social role may be as important as acquiring the missing psychophysiological skills. For example, when helping people learn to regulate anxiety, it may be necessary to challenge the self-perception that "I am an anxious, high-strung individual," and help them develop new social roles incompatible with high anxiety. Functional assessment is usefully complemented by sociocognitive assessment when evaluating these possibilities.

Relaxation training and biofeedback were the earliest forms of psycho-physiological intervention used in rehabilitating people with severe mental illness (see Rickard, Collier, McCoy, & Crist, 1993; Spaulding, Wyss, & Littrell, 1990; Spaulding et al., 1986). As rehabilitation technology evolved, these specific techniques were incorporated into more comprehensive modalities. For general purposes, the evidence for any unique efficacy gained by using biofeedback does not justify the additional time and expense, but relaxation training remains a key component in psychophysiological skills training modalities. Because of the close relationship between psycho-physiological self-regulation and the ability to perform complex social roles, contemporary approaches use combinations of techniques that address multiple levels of functioning, such as relaxation training and sometimes biofeedback (the physiological level), cognitive therapy (the socio-cognitive level), and social skills training (the sociobehavioral level). These combined training modalities are variously conceptualized and packaged as stress management, anger control, and emotional skills training. Cognitive-behavioral treatments for mood and anxiety disorders incorporate components of psychophysiological skills training as well. In addition, socioenvironmental interventions (e.g., training friends and family to prompt the recovering person to use a self-regulation skill) are often useful in facilitating development of psychophysiological self-regulation skills.

## Problems in Behavioral Activation

As discussed in Chapter 6, neurophysiological and neuroendocrine mechanisms play an important role in our daily pattern of activity and rest. We experience the consequences of disrupting our diurnal regulation when we struggle with jet lag or a change in work shift. Our sociobehavioral functioning plays an important role in reestablishing and maintaining this regulation. We plan our travel itineraries to allow for jet lag, we seek information on managing the effects of jet travel and implement what we learn (drink fluids, maintain an exercise schedule, eat lightly, take melatonin, etc.). We arrange our personal schedules and other aspects of our lifestyle to accommodate shift changes at work. We engage in many diverse practices, on a routine daily basis, to match our general level of activation to current environmental demands. We may drink coffee in the morning and cocktails in the evening; we may prepare for especially demanding events by either resting or practicing or both; we may do warm-up exercises of various kinds, adapted to various kinds of skill performance. These are complex skills for managing complex circumstances. Everybody experiences variability in the quality of their skill performance and the successfulness of the outcome.

People with disabling mental illness often experience protracted problems in regulating their behavioral activation patterns. They may find themselves unable to achieve a degree of activation appropriate to perform routine daily activities or participate in rehabilitative activities. Sometimes their diurnal cycle is reversed, resulting in drowsiness or sleep when they should be awake and alert, and high activation when they should be sleeping. These problems are often associated with (1) neurophysiological and/or neuroendocrine dysregulation and (2) severe depression, mania, and the negative symptoms of schizophrenia, as discussed in Chapter 4. Sometimes the reversal is iatrogenic, a side effect of medication; sometimes it is resolved solely through neurophysiological intervention (i.e., pharmacotherapy), at least in the short term. However, problems in regulating behavioral activation often involve sociobehavioral factors as well, and if these factors are not addressed, the person likely will experience an enduring vulnerability to recurrent, negative behavioral and phenomenological consequences. Among the more extensively studied of such factors is *learned helplessness* (Flannery, Penk, & Addo, 1996; Seligman, 1975), which refers to the behavioral immobilization that results from protracted frustration and failure to control aversive events—common in the experience of people with severe mental illness. Clearly, learned helplessness likely would lead to a dysregulation of behavioral activation. The multiplicity of neurophysiological, cognitive, and sociobehavioral factors that coalesce to enhance or detract from one's level of behavioral activation makes it useful to conceptualize the problem as one of psychophysiological dysregulation, requiring skill acquisition (perhaps, among other interventions) for effective resolution.

Psychophysiological dysregulation of the behavioral activation type should be considered for inclusion as a problem title when the recovering person experiences significant difficulties maintaining an activation level appropriate to routine daily activities and/or rehabilitation and recovery. Possible expressions of this problem include persistent drowsiness, a desire to remain in bed all day, cognitive and/or behavioral lethargy, or inattention to daily self-care or work tasks. At the other extreme, sleeplessness, agitation, euphoria, and other behaviors associated with mania or hypomania may also indicate a regulatory problem.

The role of neurophysiological factors should be analyzed carefully before attributing problems in behavioral activation to psychophysiological dysregulation. The hypothesis of psychophysiological dysregulation becomes especially pertinent at the point in recovery from acute dysregulation when no further benefits are expected from psychopharmacotherapy. Activation problems remaining in the "optimally medicated" state are often most usefully addressed as a skills deficit problem. This is true even if the activation problem is, in part, a medication side effect, provided there is consensus on the treatment team that this side effect is an unavoidable consequence of an otherwise optimal regimen. Unfortunately, this position between a rock and a hard place, to borrow an expression, is not an uncommon circumstance in rehabilitating people with disabling mental illness.

Other possible sources of the activation problems must be carefully considered. Sleep apnea (a disruption of normal sleep caused by anatomical blockage of breathing), for example, which is at least as common in people with mental illness as in the population at large, can produce severe diurnal dysregulation. Another possibility: Either hypo- or hyperactivation may represent an avoidance response to intolerable circumstances and/or a self-protective attempt to manage neurophysiological dysregulation. Identification of such factors does not necessarily discourage conceptualization of the problem as one of psychophysiological dysregulation, but it may indicate a need for additional interventions to address circumstances that create the "need" for the regulatory failure.

Interventions for behavioral activation problems should begin with educating the recovering person; helping him or her achieve an understanding that there is a problem and that, potentially, it can be brought under personal control is an important intermediate goal. On the other hand, improved regulation can occur without a fully articulated understanding, so this should not be seen as a prerequisite for further intervention. The underlying issue is whether the recovering person can be engaged in an intervention that will resolve the problem effectively.

Barring the contribution of extenuating factors such as sleep apnea or behavioral avoidance, the key element in regulating behavioral activation is adherence to a consistent, routine schedule of activity—necessary for optimal rehabilitation, anyway, so any program of rehabilitation services should have the capability of developing and supporting such routines. A daily personal schedule is a sine qua non; such a schedule will encourage psychophysiological regulation to the degree that it includes regular (1) aerobic exercise, (2) healthful meals, (3) work/rehabilitation sessions, (4) structured leisure activities, and (5) rest periods as needed. The activity and rest components need to be paced in accordance with the recovering person's stress tolerance and physical stamina. Generally, the schedule is expected to be less demanding at the beginning of the rehabilitation process, with increases in demand as the person recovers. Adjusting the demands of daily routines is an ongoing task requiring the collective judgment of the entire rehabilitation team and a comprehensive set of data on the recovering person's functioning.

Once the personal schedule is in place, directly observing the person's activation level in different settings provides the key information about the nature of the regulatory problem. Functional behavioral analysis identifies environmental events and organismic factors that are maintaining the regulatory problem or that could prompt or reinforce activation levels appropriate to circumstances. Achieving the best possible regulation of behavioral activation is basically a process of identifying the barriers to activation appropriate to adhering to the personal schedule. This intervention may involve highly systematic manipulation of environmental conditions, discussed in the next chapter.

## Dysregulation of Mood

A number of group- and dyadic-format therapy modalities have been developed to enhance individuals' regulation of mood, especially of depression. As discussed in Chapter 8, these modalities generally address processes at the sociocognitive level (e.g., attributions and beliefs) as well as sociobehavioral skills. A number of cognitive-behavioral therapy procedures have been developed for major depression, and *dialectical behavior therapy* (DBT; Linehan, 1993) was developed to address mood dysregulation (and other problems) associated with borderline personality disorder. DBT uses dyadic and group therapy formats to instruct the recovering person in adaptive ways of managing emotional distress, eliminating undesirable behaviors associated with distress (e.g., self-injury), and improving interpersonal functioning. Recently, modalities specialized for treating people with severe mental illness have begun to appear (Hodel & Brenner, 1997; Hodel, Brenner, Merlo, & Teuber, 1998). The modalities developed explicitly for people with SDMI are similar in format to other psychoeducational skills training modalities—that is, symptom management training and social skills training, but with emphasis on skills relevant to identifying, understanding, and managing one's mood and emotions. There is no reason to believe that the specific dysregulations associated with various diagnoses really respect categorical boundaries, and in any case, all kinds of specific mood dysregulation problems are to be expected in disabling mental illness. Neither is there reason to expect that modalities effective for mood dysregulation in some categories would be ineffective in others. Applying these modalities in rehabilitation should follow from a systematic assessment of mood dysregulation problems and concomitant features that may moderate the effectiveness of particular modalities. For example, the current cognitive-behavioral therapies for major depression assume (1) relatively intact neurocognitive functioning, and (2) an intact repertoire of the most basic personal care and social skills. Some modification is required for use with people who have severe problems in these domains. Another example: Dialectical behavior therapy may be optimal to the degree that the clinical picture of mood dysregulation is complicated by parasuicidal behavior, dissociation, substance abuse, history of trauma, self-injurious behavior, and other psychophysiological dysregulations (e.g., of anger or fear) because DBT specifically addresses these problems in addition to mood regulation.

## Dysregulation of Anger/Aggression

In recent years, controlling anger and aggression has become a culture-wide issue. Domestic violence and "road rage" (violence associated with minor traffic altercations) are examples of dysregulation problems that have received widespread public attention and discussion. Cultural and socioeconomic factors may create population-wide vulnerabilities to such problems. It is unclear, and it matters little, whether dysregulation of anger/aggression is more or less common in individuals with disabling mental illness compared to the population at large. It is clear, however, that in the context of disabling mental illness, this particular type of dysregulation can be a significant barrier to optimal personal and social functioning.

### Internal and External Dimensions of Anger/Aggression

Aggression and anger are associated with a relatively distinct pattern of psychophysiological activation. Aggression is thought to be one of a few basic behavior patterns, present in most vertebrates, directly supported by relatively specific CNS structures and mechanisms. These basic behavior patterns include fighting (aggression), fleeing (escape), feeding, and sexual behavior. In humans these four patterns are thought to have specific neuroanatomical and neurophysiological substrates in the limbic system and related subcortical structures. In this sense, identification of anger/aggression, fear/anxiety, or appetitive and sexual dysregulation in the integrated paradigm's prototype problem set may reflect basic structural and functional characteristics of the human organism. However, the integrated paradigm's nosology is not driven by this possibility. More pertinent to rehabilitation, these four types of psychophysiological dysregulation reflect different response patterns that produce different kinds of adjustment and recovery problems, and which are effectively addressed by somewhat different clinical technologies.

At the most primitive level, aggression serves to maintain territorial boundaries; in social species, it helps establish and maintain social structures such as dominance hierarchies. In humans, the primitive brain mechanisms interact with more recently evolved mechanisms and more molar cognition to mediate aggressive behavior. Anger and aggression are associated with distinct patterns of respiratory and cardiovascular activity in the autonomic nervous system. Indeed, the emotional state of "anger" represents a complex interplay of autonomic and CNS activation, which interacts with the person's sociocognitive processing. In any situation, for any person, the probability of behavioral aggression is increased by this pattern of activation.

The reality that physical aggression is strongly sanctioned in contemporary cultures creates an imperative for people to learn how to resolve angry emotional states in other ways. Inevitably, an inefficient ability to do so has a definitive impact on a person's social status and autonomy (leaving aside the moral doctrine that physical aggression is "wrong"). Short of physical aggression, there are behavioral alternatives that may have negative, if not catastrophic, consequences. These include verbal aggression (also known as verbal abuse and vituperation), physical intimidation, extortion, and all the other interpersonal cruelties that humans have invented. *The appearance of any of these behaviors in a clinical picture demands consideration of a psychophysiological dysregulation hypothesis.*

Many factors within and across levels of organismic functioning contribute to aggression, whether or not psychophysiological factors play a role. At the neurophysiological level, aggressive behavior may occur only during periods of acute dysregulation, as in episodic psychosis. Some forms of epilepsy produce aggressive behavior in people who otherwise show no aggression. In such cases, assessment and intervention at the *psycho*physiological level focus on the skills necessary to manage the *neuro*physiological dysregulation, as opposed to managing angry emotional states. In some cases the aggression may reflect extraordinary environmental conditions, rather than failure of psychophysiological regulation. Many people who are not aggressive under normal conditions can be provoked to aggression under extreme circumstances. A psychophysiological dysregulation problem should be hypothesized when more molecular interventions (e.g., treatment of neurophysiological dysregulation) or more molar interventions (e.g., resolving extreme environmental conditions) are not expected to be sufficient.

It is also important to note that actual aggression is not the only possible indication of problems in this domain. Some individuals experience frequent, intense episodes of the emotional state of anger, even if they do not manifest the anger as overt aggression. The frequency may be so high, or the person may be so sensitive to eliciting stimuli in the environment, that the clinical picture is of a continuous state. This continuity of state dysregulation is traditionally associated with Krapelinian and neo-Kraepelinian diagnostic categories, including paranoid disorder, paranoid schizophrenia, paranoid personality disorder, borderline personality disorder, and passive–aggressive personality disorder (the last is no longer in the DSM). In some individuals, an angry, hostile, and/or paranoid state is distinctly linked to episodic psychosis, although the mood state and its behavioral expressions may also persist, at diminished intensity, long after other indicators of psychosis have been resolved. In other individuals, the mood state does not display episodic fluctuations. The episodic dimension is reflected (more or less) in the different diagnostic categories. It is unknown whether the dysregulation itself is qualitatively different in the different categories, but it is clear that individuals experience and express their dysregulated emotional states in unique ways. Extensive functional analysis may be required to articulate fully the role of persistent, dysregulated anger in an individual's personal and social functioning.

The concept of dysregulated anger not manifested as aggression carries significant baggage from its history in psychoanalysis and biological psychiatry. Psychodynamic treatment approaches historically have focused on encouraging the behavioral expression of anger, on the assumption that this verbal externalization of it "strengthens" the psychic mechanisms that normally suppress overt aggression. Biological psychiatry assumes a neurophysiological basis of the emotional state and seeks to counteract it with pharmacological interventions. There has been much contention between proponents of these two paradigms. However, *both* approaches neglect the skills aspect of psychophysiological regulation—that is, the role of sociocognitive functioning and acquired information—and therefore both have limited effectiveness. Some individuals do respond sufficiently to pharmacological intervention and some to sociocognitive intervention. However, for many individuals, especially those with disabling mental illness, neither pharmacological nor sociocognitive intervention is sufficient without including a substantial skill acquisition component in rehabilitation.

Whether persistent or episodic, and whether associated with any overt behavior or not, psychophysiological arousal of the anger/aggression type conforms to the Yerkes–Dodson law. The *Yerkes–Dodson law* describes an inverted U-shaped relationship between psychophysiological arousal and cognitive and behavioral functioning (Figure 9.1). (Fear, anxiety, and other qualitative variants of arousal also conform to this law.) At extremely low levels of arousal (as observed in behavioral activation problems), cognitive and behavioral functioning are also suboptimal. As arousal increases, cognitive and behavioral functioning improve to a point of peak performance. As arousal continues to increase beyond the performance peak, cognitive and behavioral functioning decline. At extreme levels of arousal, cognitive and behavioral functioning are seriously compromised. Episodic disruption of cognition and behavioral functioning can be a result of dysregulated

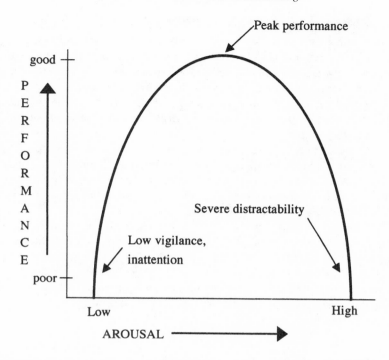

**FIGURE 9.1.** The Yerkes–Dodson function. Performance of any cognitive task is best at a moderate level of psychological arousal. At low arousal, performance is impaired by low vigilance and inattention to the task. At high arousal, performance is impaired by high distractibility.

anger/aggression that is as serious as physical aggression but more difficult to identify.

The recovering person's phenomenological experience of the arousal state is a key issue in assessing and treating dysregulation of anger/aggression. Attributions may range from nonexistent (a complete lack of awareness of any problem) to a detailed awareness of the dysregulated emotional state, and from complete sanguinity to extreme distress and embarrassment. Delusional attributions—for example, the belief that one's anger is the result of intentional provocations—are sometimes present. When the recovering person's understanding of the problem differs from other rehabilitation team members', a careful analysis is necessary. When physical aggression is involved, it is helpful to have a consensus that such aggression is unacceptable. However, other interventions to stop or prevent physical aggression cannot await this consensus. In the integrated paradigm, such interventions are understood to address a problem in the interaction between the person and the social environment—in this case, the person engages in a behavior that the environment will not tolerate (this level of biosystemic functioning is addressed in the next chapter). Even when intervention proceeds without the recovering person's consent, however, efforts should continue to establish consensus that physical aggression is never acceptable.

When physical aggression is not part of the problem, the primacy of team consensus about the nature of the problem must be weighed against the impact the problem has on all aspects of the recovering person's personal and social functioning, rehabilitation, and recovery. In addition, consideration must be given to people in the recovering person's social environment (in some contexts, the rehabilitation team has a responsibility to protect others from the recovering person's aggressive behavior, even when it is short of physical aggression).

Accurately recognizing the causes or triggers of one's anger can be more important for some individuals than managing its autonomic and behavioral components. In such cases, where modifying a person's interpretations of emotional states is expected to be more beneficial than skill acquisition, the problem would be usefully defined as social problem-solving insufficiency (at the sociocognitive level of functioning) rather than a psychophysiological dysregulation.

## Treatment Modalities for Anger/Aggression

Because anger and aggression are almost always associated with interpersonal conflict (real or otherwise), interpersonal skills are inevitably involved in the psychophysiological regulation of anger and aggression. In some individuals, psychophysiological regulation problems may be more attributable to broader deficits in interpersonal skills than to psychophysiological skills. In a sense, one consequence of deficient interpersonal skills is a higher frequency of situations in which anger is experienced and aggression seems an attractive, or at least compelling, option.[2] When a broader interpersonal skills deficit contributes to functional problems associated with anger and/or aggression, social skills training is an important

---

[2]An early form of social skills training, developed in the 1960s, was termed *assertiveness training* to reflect an assumption that emotional problems are the result of deficient social skills, related in turn to a person's conflation of "assertiveness" and "aggression." This perspective reflected a behavioral reconceptualization of the psychoanalytic concept of neurosis and was not particularly informed by cognitive or psychophysiological science. Today, it is possible to draw finer distinctions between the emotional consequences of unassertiveness, social incompetence, and psychophysiological dysregulation, although the techniques pioneered by assertiveness training are recognizably present in contemporary interventions for sociocognitive and sociobehavioral problems.

adjunct to psychophysiological skills training. Sometimes, the concept of a social skills deficit is more consonant with the recovering person's beliefs and attributions than the concept of a psychophysiological dysregulation, and improvement in interpersonal functioning turns out to be sufficient for resolving problems associated with anger and aggression. In such cases identifying the problem as a social skills deficit and resolving it with social skills training finesses the conflict between the recovering person's understanding of the problem and others' on the rehabilitation team. This is an acceptable practice in the integrated paradigm, provided that the goals reflect objective, quantitative measurement of anger and/or aggression. If these indicators fail to show resolution, the team must find another way to reach consensus.

Sociobehavioral intervention modalities for anger and aggression problems have evolved for several decades, and packaged formats are now commercially available. (For a review of sociobehavioral interventions for anger, aggression, and violence, see Crowner, 2001; Howells, 1998). Social learning theory has provided the main conceptual framework for these modalities, with enhancement from experimental psychophysiology. They are usually generically described as *anger management training*. These interventions are increasingly part of training curricula for mental health professionals, in part, because of public concern about aggression and violence. The modalities generally include a combination of sociocognitive and sociobehavioral components (i.e., problem-solving training and social skills training, discussed later in this chapter) specifically focused on regulation of anger/aggression. Behavioral techniques for managing autonomic arousal are often included in these packages, and they may be especially helpful for people with disabling mental illness. In *relaxation training*, the most familiar of these techniques, participants are taught to achieve a deep level of muscle relaxation, which in turn reduces autonomic arousal. It is usually most helpful to train participants to achieve a moderate level of relaxation skill and then incorporate use of this skill in situations known to induce psychophysiological arousal.

*Time out from reinforcement* (TOFR), a technique especially useful for managing and treating dysregulation of anger/aggression, is a milieu-based intervention, and in that sense could be classified as addressing the socioenvironmental level of functioning (the topic of the following chapter). However, one purpose of TOFR interventions is to increase the recovering person's control over psychophysiological arousal, and when used for that purpose, is best classified as a psychophysiological intervention. A TOFR also can be used to control aggressive or otherwise unacceptable behavior independent of its function in skill acquisition. The technique effectively decreases or prevents necessary use of restraint and seclusion, and it lowers the risk of injury—always a plus. However, controlling behavior through environmental manipulation is generally a means to an end in rehabilitation, rather than an end in itself. When any intervention uses environmental means to control behavior (arguably, this includes psychopharmacotherapy), every effort should be made to transfer this control to the recovering person as soon as possible.

TOFR is a *contingency management* technique (contingency management is described further in the following chapter) closely allied with functional behavioral analysis. It is most strongly indicated when the analysis reveals that aggressive or otherwise problematic behavior is consistently preceded by a *ballistic behavior chain*. The behaviors in a ballistic behavior chain typically include increased psychophysiological arousal, increased voice volume, intrusion into others' personal space, and other threatening behavior. This type of sequence is often described in clinical parlance as "escalation." The person engaging in this explosive behavior is oblivious to others' efforts to mollify the escalation or otherwise prevent disaster. The functional analysis provides a detailed description of the circumstances likely to start a ballistic behavior chain and identifies specific behaviors or behavioral qualities (e.g., rising voice tone or loudness) that mark progress toward the target behavior (e.g., a fist fight). In that sense, it is a description of specific episodes of psychophysiological dysregulation.

The TOFR consists of an agreement among relevant individuals—the recovering person and key individuals in the recovering person's environment likely to observe the ballistic behavior chain—that when the initial components of the behavior chain occur, the recovering person will remove him- or herself from the environmental situation, usually to a quiet location, for a specific period of time (from a few seconds to a few minutes). This time-out prevents continued exposure to environmental stimuli (e.g., a person, a task) that otherwise would elicit the ballistic behavior sequence, with its associated psychophysiological arousal, via a reinforcement effect (in colloquial terms, "egged on" to full-blown escalation).[3] Instead the person experiences a reduction of arousal. At the end of the specified period, the person returns to the interaction or task that was interrupted. As arousal level returns to the Yerkes–Dodson performance peak, the person may experience improved cognitive functioning as well. In the context of a broader sociocognitive and sociobehavioral approach to controlling aggression, the recovering person uses this experience to increase awareness of the eliciting stimuli and increasing arousal, bringing both under the control of executive cognition. Additional sociocognitive benefits usually follow, in-

---

[3]The term *reinforcement* reflects the origins of the TOFR in clinical applications of operant learning theory. The TOFR procedure's effect on behavior involves mechanisms other than reinforcement (e.g., extinction of classically conditioned autonomic responses) but for rhetorical economy, these are not included in the term.

cluding development of an internalized locus of control over arousal and aggression, with concomitant improvements in self-esteem and sense of personal efficacy.

TOFR has long been used in special education to control aggression, distractibility, and other undesirable behavioral sequences, and it has well established effectiveness in psychiatric and rehabilitation settings. However, it is underused is such settings. It is unclear why this is so, although recent studies of technology dissemination in mental health venues reveal widespread underuse of many technologies, including psychosocial ones (Lehman, Steinwachs, Dixon, Postrado, et al., 1998). In the case of contingency management, including use of TOFR, possible reasons include a failure to recruit professionals with the relevant expertise, failure of the health care accreditation industry to develop rules and standards for use of contingency management technology in psychiatric settings, and gild conflicts among mental health professionals. Given the increasing public concern about violence and physical restriction in mental health residential settings, the next few years may see increased attention directed toward these possible barriers and an infusion of contingency management technology and expertise.

Unfortunately, TOFR is easily confused with "time-out," a colloquial term that has been incorporated into psychiatric, nursing, and accreditation argot. *Time-out* loosely refers to the use of coercive procedures that require the recovering person to go to a secluded place, in order to avoid further physical restriction (restraint and/or seclusion). Although it is widely used, this type of time-out procedure is not informed by systematic functional analysis, is not expected to contribute to skill acquisition or greater self-control, and is not supported by empirical evidence of clinical effectiveness to the degree that TOFR is supported. Thus, even though time-out is widely accepted as a legitimate technique for controlling aggression, it does not have the scientific support or conceptual integrity necessary for inclusion in the integrated paradigm.

The combination of insufficient expertise and confusion with colloquial and quasitechnical terminology sometimes makes it difficult to provide TOFR and other contingency management technology in rehabilitation settings. Ironically, it is often needed the most in the service settings least prone to use it—that is, institutional settings where aggression is common but the clinical model (neo-Kraepelinian) relies exclusively on pharmacological means to control aggression. This conundrum is discussed further in Chapters 10 and 11.

## Dysregulation of Fear/Anxiety

As with mood dysregulation, considerable development of sociobehavioral therapy modalities for fear/anxiety dysregulation occurred during the late

20th century. These modalities were developed to address the various sub-types of the neo-Kraepelinian diagnosis of anxiety disorder, although their conceptual framework was predominantly that of social learning theory. It is unclear whether the neo-Kraepelinian categories reflect the dysregulation of different psychophysiological mechanisms. However, they do appear to have different sociocognitive and sociobehavioral characteristics. For example, a person who meets diagnostic criteria for panic disorder experiences anxiety and its consequences differently from those who meet the criteria for generalized anxiety disorder or social phobia. As a consequence, the CBT procedures associated with the different diagnoses are somewhat different, but there is controversy as to whether the differences are meaningful. It is possible that the neurophysiological mechanism is the same in all or most cases, and that repeated exposure to the feared object or situation is the key mechanism of treatment. Current research in this area is attempting to determine the critical components of anxiety disorder treatment, and the next several years should see some resolution of this issue. For the time being, dysregulation of fear/anxiety in people with disabling mental illness should be assessed for correspondence to the diagnostic categories and treated with the corresponding intervention modality. Meanwhile, specialized modalities for addressing anxiety in severe mental illness are beginning to appear (Halperin et al., 2000).

## Dysregulation of Appetitive and Sexual Functioning

There is a range of psychophysiological dysregulation patterns associated with appetitive (hunger, thirst) and sexual functioning. Most of these patterns are incorporated under one or another diagnostic category, including eating disorders and psychosexual disorders. These dysregulations, which can cause serious problems in individuals with no other mental illness, add to the disabling effects of other forms of mental illness. It is unclear whether they occur more or less frequently in people with disabling mental illness. Treatments for eating disorders and psychosexual dysfunctions generally include combinations of social skills training, self-regulation skills training, insight-oriented psychotherapy, and socioenvironmental interventions (e.g., marital or family therapy). There is no reason to believe that such approaches would not be effective for people who also have disabling mental illness, although, as with any approach, the interventions must be tailored to individual needs, situations, and problems.

To the degree that psychophysiological regulation plays a relatively minor role, the behaviors associated with appetitive and sexual dysfunction can be the result of neurophysiological dysregulation, cognitive impairment, or social skills deficits. It is important to assess fully the role of medication side effects, neurocognitive impairment, dysfunctional beliefs and attributions, and deficient social skills in the presenting clinical picture.

*Polydipsia* deserves special mention because it occurs frequently in people with disabling mental illness (reviewed by Verghese, De Leon, & Josiassen, 1996). Polydipsia is a psychophysiologically based dysregulation of fluid intake, usually associated with persistent thirst. It occurs along a continuum of severity, with consequences ranging from discomfort to life-threatening disruption of blood chemistry. Polydipsia is poorly understood. It may be a side effect of psychotropic medication, at least in some cases. When it cannot be eliminated through judicious psychopharmacotherapy, psychosocial interventions are sometimes helpful. These interventions generally include combinations of education, skills training, contingency management, or related socioenvironmental interventions (such as training of a family or care provider) (Baldwin, Beck, Menditto, Arms, & Corrier, 1992; Bowen, Glynn, Marshall, Kurth, & Hayden, 1990; Liberman & Marshall, 1993; Shutty & Song, 1997; Waller, Hypde, & Thomas, 1994).

## ASSESSMENT AND REHABILITATION
## OF INSTRUMENTAL SKILL DEFICITS

The technology for assessing and rehabilitating the performance of instrumental skills is extensive and highly evolved. It is also increasingly part of the curricula of professional education and training in a number of disciplines. Materials for training skills trainers are commercially available (see Kuehnel et al., 1990). Packaged skills training materials generally include nomothetic assessment procedures as well. When used along with a broader functional analysis (of performance versus competence problems and environmental factors) and assessment (of neurophysiological, neurocognitive, and sociocognitive factors), it is possible to identify deficits in the performance of instrumental skills in a manner sufficient for most applications in rehabilitation.

In practice, much assessment data on instrumental skill performance comes from the recovering person's social history. Of course, this depends on the quality and completeness of the social history, and whether the historian was alert to indications of deficits in instrumental skills and social role-related problems. Mental health settings based on the medical model do not necessarily encourage or support attention to that level of functioning. Nevertheless, it is not unusual for rehabilitation teams to attempt to deduce skill- and role-related hypotheses from material in historical archives that focuses exclusively on psychotic relapse episodes and medication protocols.

There is a strong tendency among mental health professionals working in traditional psychiatric models to attribute all abnormal behavior to the consequences of neurophysiological dysregulation. This perspective leads to a neglect of information that could illuminate the many other factors relevant to skill and role performance during periods free of acute psychosis. Even when information relevant to skill and role performance is available, it is usually difficult to interpret because so many factors may be affecting performance at any particular time. Assessment of instrumental skills therefore remains heavily dependent on the administration of standardized testing under controlled conditions, and on systematic observation and behavioral analysis in natural settings.

Providing instrumental living skills training is largely a managerial task that includes assembling the human resources for doing nomothetic and idiographic assessment, providing the training, and maintaining rigorous treatment planning and progress review procedures. (For the practical details, see the original sources and the materials commercially available.) The remaining discussion addresses general considerations attendant to providing skills training services to people with disabling mental illness in rehabilitation settings.

## Self-Care and Independent Living Skills Deficits

Self-care and independent living skills cover a broad and heterogeneous array of abilities, from basic personal hygiene to personal budgeting and financial accounting (Wallace, Boone, Donahoe, & Foy, 1985). Deficient performance of *one* of these skills is often a crucial determinant in the level of environmental restriction a recovering person requires for basic safety and a reasonable quality of life. The ability to perform a daily personal hygiene routine can mean the difference between independent living and living in a staffed group home. The ability to perform basic personal budgeting and accounting skills can mean the difference between being recognized as a legally competent adult and having a legal guardian.

These skills are especially vulnerable to disruption by neurophysiological dysregulation, so it is especially important to determine a person's true baseline level of competence and performance. In practice, it may be necessary to postpone some skills assessment until relatively late in the course of rehabilitation. For example, personal budgeting and accounting may continue to be compromised by post-acute neurocognitive deficits for months after resolution of acute positive symptoms. On the other hand, establishing performance of basic hygiene and self-care should not wait for complete return to baseline functioning. Providing training and environmental support for routine daily self-care activities can help the person maintain those activities even during acute psychosis, and may even contribute to post-acute cognitive recovery (this point was discussed in Chapters 6 and 7). Therefore, assessment of self-care skills is an ongoing process in rehabilitation, with a gradual shift in focus from more basic, routine skills (e.g., personal hygiene) to more complex, less routine skills (e.g., making new friends), as recovery proceeds and the recovering person's true baseline deficits are identified.

A special environment is advantageous for providing training in some of these skills, especially in the early stages. In institutional and residential settings, training workshops can be designed to facilitate teaching, coaching, and learning of skills associated with the domestic environment (e.g., simulated kitchens and laundry rooms). However, because these newly acquired skills must be generalized to include natural settings, the trainer must usually follow the trainee into the natural environment to make sure the generalization occurs. The probability of successful generalization is strongly influenced by the similarities between the training environment and the natural setting.

Training in independent living skills has been one of the primary foci of Programs for Assertive Community Treatment (PACT). Although most familiar as an approach to case management, the original PACT programs included a heavy emphasis on rehabilitation, in general, and living skills, in particular. A PACT manual (Allness & Knoedler, 1998) now provides useful guidelines for incorporating training in living skills into a more comprehensive rehabilitation service array. (For a complementary model that combines living skills with case management, see Vacarro, Liberman, Wallace, & Blackwell, 1992.)

## Disorder Management Skills

Materials for assessing and training disorder management skills focus on helping the person (1) gain a conceptual understanding of his or her mental illness, (2) recognize its symptoms and other characteristics, (3) interact effectively with mental health providers, (4) perform personal care activities pertinent to managing the illness (e.g., taking medication on time), and (5) managing environmental conditions that may exacerbate the illness (Eckman et al., 1990; Lecompte & Pelc, 1996). The training is usually conducted in a classroom format with 6 to 10 participants.

Unfortunately, materials on disorder management skills training are generally not sensitive to the vicissitudes of neo-Kraepelinian psychiatry, as discussed in this book. In a mental health system based on the medical model, there is strong tendency to reify diagnostic categories for the purposes of teaching disorder management: for example, "You have schizophrenia, and therefore you must . . . " This approach can deteriorate into a testimonial climate wherein "treatment" becomes little more than persuading people to endorse the DSM and "confess" that they "have" one of its disorders. Such persuasion often leads to arguments about "what is mental illness" and distracts from the more important agenda of rehabilitation: to address functional problems and implement solutions. Even experienced clinicians are sometimes surprised to find that despite fundamental disagreements about whether a person is mentally ill, the discussion can move on to accurate identification of specific symptoms and functional impairments, and then to productive problem solving.

It is possible to explain why people meet specific diagnostic criteria without making unwarranted assumptions about the nature of mental illness: For example, "You have reported having auditory hallucinations, and your behavior is observed by others to show periods of extreme confusion. . . . " Disorder management training in the integrated paradigm acknowledges diagnosis as an accepted convention, but emphasizes that a diagnostic label does not imply anything about the illness or recovery of an individual person. Indeed, it is possible to address all pertinent issues in disorder management training without accepting the validity of the neo-Kraepelinian psychiatric diagnostic framework. Furthermore, the recovering person's beliefs and attributions about mental illness (e.g., I have specific symptoms) may be at variance with neo-Kraepelinian assumptions (e.g., I have a specific mental illness), and the former may be more valid than the latter. Instead, the training focuses on the specific problems associated with mental illness, including the various types and expressions of neurophysiological functioning, and the means of solving those problems. A diathesis–stress model of mental illness is central to this approach, because it not only acknowledges the reality of acute psychosis and relapse but also the organismic and environmental factors that mediate relapse. These factors point directly to the recovering person's role in preventing episodes of neurophysiological dysregulation by performing specific skills.

In recent years *relapse prevention* (Marlatt & Gordon, 1985) has emerged as a useful conceptual framework for offering training in disorder management skills (Birchwood, 1995; Kavanagh, 1992; O'Connor, 1991). First used with substance abuse and problems not particularly associated with disabling mental illness, relapse prevention has proved applicable to a range of situations in which prevention of some episodic state is a central concern. A particularly useful aspect of this approach is the construction of a *relapse prevention plan*, a detailed, written enumeration of vulnerability factors, indications of impending relapse, and procedures for identifying and interrupting the relapse process. Working on the relapse prevention plan is an excellent means of engaging members of the rehabilitation team, and others in the recovering person's social environment, in a common project requiring consensus about existing barriers to rehabilitation and recovery. However, there is more to management of one's disorder than simply preventing relapse. The next few years will probably see important advances in the development of disorder management skills, including integration of new relapse prevention techniques with other aspects of disorder management (e.g., managing residual cognitive impairment).

Gaining an awareness and understanding of one's mental illness is a key factor in disorder management training. Often, didactic education offered by a respected provider in a matter-of-fact manner is sufficient to resolve any beliefs and attributions that would be likely to impede recovery. The instructor's essential message, "This is what we know about mental illness; it's up to you to decide how it relates to you," helps avoid disagreements that would be attributed to lack of insight in traditional models. On the other hand, it is not uncommon that a recovering person masters all the declarative information pertinent to managing his or her disorder without acknowledging any personal relevance or performing the relevant skills. When detrimental attributions and beliefs about the existence of problems and the need for rehabilitation are part of the picture, ongoing assessment is necessary to determine the impact of skills training. Neither acquisition of declarative information nor accurate beliefs are sufficient (or even necessary) for the successful performance of skills.

Stress management skills are widely recognized as important acquisitions for people with severe mental illness, especially with the ascendancy of diathesis–stress theories of schizophrenia (Liberman, 1986). Stress management skills obviously have a significant psychophysiological component, perhaps most directly addressed with relaxation training (see Starkey, Deleone, & Flannery, 1995). However, optimum stress management involves manipulation of the social environment as well as the internal environment. For example, changes in one's daily routines and choice of friends can increase or decrease the stress one experiences. (For a comprehensive account of stress management as a clinical approach, see Woolfolk & Lehrer, 1984.) Stress management skills training is increasingly incorporated into broader curricula for disorder management in rehabilitation (e.g., Falloon, Laporta, Fadden, & Graham-Hole, 1993; Schaub & Liberman, 1999; Tarrier et al., 1993).

## Occupational and Leisure/Recreational Skills

Occupational and leisure/recreational skills comprise the behaviors that people spend most of their time performing. The relevance of social roles to mental illness is clearest in this domain. In the course of institutionalization, people come to spend most of their time occupied with the role of "mental patient." Other occupations, such as work and play, are largely incompatible with that social role.[4] Unfortunately, the deinstitutionalization movement did not eliminate the effects of having lived in an institution. Be-

---

[4]*Occupation* here refers to any behavioral activity, not the colloquial meaning that is synonymous with *vocation, job,* or *career.*

cause people with disabling mental illness often have very limited access to alternative occupations, they become consigned to the role of mental patient in whatever environment they find themselves. Helping the recovering person identify occupations that are incompatible with the mental patient role (e.g., "reliable worker" or "dependable friend"), and making it possible for him or her to spend increasing amounts of time in those occupations, is a central task in the integrated paradigm. There is a demonstrable benefit in helping the recovering person identify, develop, and maintain alternative social roles (Goldberg et al., 1977).

Rehabilitation has traditionally emphasized gainful work as an important goal, and rehabilitation for severe mental illness is no exception, although beliefs about the nature and importance of "work" as an occupation have become polarized within the rehabilitation community (Durham, 1997; Faulkner, 1986; Ford, 1995; Gervey & Bedell, 1994; Roder, Jenull, & Brenner, 1998). Achievement of gainful employment remains one of the most difficult of rehabilitation goals. Historically, gainful employment has been neglected as a goal in mental health services, despite that when asked, many people with disabling mental illness say they would like to have a paying job. Some argue that these considerations require that gainful employment be regarded as a necessary success criterion for all who participate in rehabilitation. On the other hand, many individuals in our culture do not engage in paid employment, and it is somewhat arbitrary to expect that all people with mental illness should do so. Social welfare policy can inadvertently punish people with work disabilities by withholding benefits, if they work at all. Although people with severe mental illness may say they would like a job, they do not necessarily do what is necessary to get and keep one, even when the opportunity occurs. There are many occupations in our culture that are "job-like" and provide satisfaction and self-esteem (e.g., volunteer charity work, hospital and library volunteers), but that do not constitute gainful employment. In the integrated paradigm, the relevant criterion is not whether the occupation is gainful employment, but whether it complements the recovering person's desires, needs, and capabilities.

Historically, leisure activities, unlike work, have been relatively neglected in mental health services, although the importance of leisure-related skills is increasingly recognized in the rehabilitation field (Corrigan, Liberman, & Wong, 1993; Pestle, Card, & Menditto, 1998; Roder et al., 1998). A colloquial view might conflate *leisure* with *inactivity*. However, a moment's reflection reveals that our highly valued leisure time is the subject of considerable activity, not only during the leisure time itself but in its planning and organization. The skills required to identify and pursue leisure-related interests are among those most likely to be taken for granted—yet they are as likely as any other skill to be deficient in people with severe mental illness. This possible deficiency is particularly problematic because people with disabilities tend to have more "leisure time" (i.e., time to engage in leisure instead of work activities) than people without disabilities.

There are commercially available materials that provide training in work- and leisure-related skills (e.g., Kuehnel et al., 1990). As with other skills training programs, these must be used in conjunction with systematic functional analysis of the neurocognitive, sociocognitive, and environmental factors that may limit or support skill performance in this domain.

## Interpersonal Skills Deficits

Social skills training was the first of the social learning theory clinical technologies to be adapted to the rehabilitation of people with disabling mental illness. Original research studies and a meta-analysis of 27 controlled trials (Benton & Schroeder, 1990) consistently demonstrate that formal social skills training improves personal and social functioning and reduces hospital recidivism in participants with schizophrenia. The basic skills required to provide effective social skills training are also central to the panoply of CBT and related modalities. As a result, some mental health providers receive a considerable amount of training and experience in this domain in their professional education. However, CBT modalities and the professional education related to them are not typically designed for use with people with disabling mental illness. There are commercially available materials for social skills training in the context of disabling mental illness (e.g., Kuehnel et al., 1990), but some specialized training and experience is usually necessary, even for providers with a social learning and CBT background, for optimal effectiveness. (For further discussion of adapting general therapy skills to group-format modalities with people who have severe mental illness, see Upper & Flowers, 1994.)

*Role-playing* is the most important component of social skills training. In contrast to traditional, psychodynamically inspired group modalities in which participants discuss issues, social skills training is more overt in nature and often utilizes rehearsal of specific skills as a methodology. This rehearsal is accomplished by engaging the participants in role-playing exercises, wherein individuals play the part of characters in a contrived interpersonal situation. To create situations in the group that elicit important characteristics of interpersonal situations demanding specific skills requires considerable skill of the trainer. (This is not to say that skill is not required to facilitate and interpret interpersonal processes in psychodynamic modalities, only that the skills are very different. One can expect no transfer of training between the two; indeed, highly rehearsed psychodynamic skills may interfere with the acquisition of social skills training skills, and vice versa.) Obviously, the trainer's ability to engage the participants in the role-play and constructively coach them toward optimal skill performance has a strong effect on outcome. The availability of trainers with well developed role-playing skills is a central concern in the administration and management of rehabilitation services.

As discussed in Chapter 8, social skills training is usefully combined with the problem-solving approach of CBT. Group activity alternates between (1) the analytical process of identifying interpersonal problems and formulating behavioral solutions and (2) rehearsing the behavioral solution in a role-play. In this context, the role-play enacts not only the behavioral skills but also the sociocognitive skills that support an effective selection and execution of the interpersonal skills. Often the behavioral rehearsal reveals a need for further sociocognitive processing. For example, the outcome of the role-play may reveal a circumstance or consideration not anticipated in the group's first problem analysis. Incorporation of this new data in a reiteration of the group's analysis engages the crucial sociocognitive skill of reassessing one's tactics in response to changing circumstances

*Bridging the development of skills* from the group room to the natural environment is an especially challenging aspect of social skills training. The interpersonal situations that demand social skills often occur in fleeting moments that cannot be precisely anticipated. Role-playing in the group room can only faintly emulate these situations. The performance of social skills is especially sensitive to psychophysiological fluctuations, in the manner described by the Yerkes–Dodson curve. These fluctuations may occur in response to natural situations but not role-plays in the group room; when this is the case, regulating the psychophysiological component does not get rehearsed. Generally in CBT approaches, generalization issues such as these are addressed through homework assignments and *in vivo* rehearsal, such as planned participation in social activities, giving systematic attention to levels of physiological arousal. These techniques are equally important when conducting social skills training with people who have disabling mental illness. However, they depend on participants' neurocognitive and sociocognitive functioning to a degree that is not always justifiable when disabling mental illness is part of the clinical picture. One strategy for enhancing generalization is to combine social skills training with other community-based skills training modalities (e.g., family therapy) and case management (Vacarro et al., 1992). In addition, it is important that the rehabilitation team monitor progress in social skills training by using instruments that are sensitive to behavioral changes in the ambient milieu, as well as in the group room. Technology for assessing and intervening at the level of person–environment interactions is the topic of the next chapter.

## SUBSTANCE ABUSE

Approaches to treating substance abuse that are based on biosystemic models are generally compatible with rehabilitation practices used by practitioners of the integrated paradigm. Similarity between such approaches and the skills training approaches used in the rehabilitation of people with disabling mental illness is increasing. As previously discussed, relapse prevention, a psychoeducational and skills training format initially developed for substance abuse, has been adapted to preventing psychotic relapse in people with disabling mental illness. Comprehensive substance abuse programs usually include sociocognitive and sociobehavioral modalities that are practically indistinguishable from those used in mental illness rehabilitation programs—for example, social skills training, self-regulation training, living skills training. Thus addressing substance abuse in a rehabilitation context usually involves these modalities that have a broader utility across the entire participant population (not just those with substance abuse problems). In addition, specialized substance abuse modalities have been developed for use with people who have severe mental illness (Barrowclough et al., 2001; Bennet, Bellack, & Gearon, 2001). So far there is scant scientific research (Barrowclough et al., 2001; Bennet, Bellack, & Gearon, 2001) of the unique contribution these modalities may make to overall rehabilitation success, or even to success in controlling substance abuse problems in people recovering from mental illness. In the absence of evidence that such modalities are actually harmful, an argument can be made that rehabilitation programs should generally have the capacity to provide them.

One of the most widespread approaches to substance abuse—the 12-step programs that originated with Alcoholics Anonymous, is not based on a theoretical model of substance abuse so much as on a set of prescriptions for using self-talk and a social support system. There is considerable controversy about the effectiveness of this approach, especially for people with disabling mental illness. There is no clear scientific evidence; anecdotal reports and clinical experience suggest that it is helpful for some individuals and not others. This is probably true for people without mental illness as well.

When confronting a substance abuse problem, a rehabilitation team must apply their functional assessments and formulations to determine which combination of services would be ideal for a particular recipient. The sheer availability of services is unfortunately a factor in many venues. Twelve-step programs are not highly standardized, and they are subject to local perspectives. Some local groups may be especially well suited to the social and interpersonal needs of people with disabling mental illness. However, some are known to espouse a radical approach that places psychopharmacotherapy and alcohol abuse in the same category; these probably would not be suitable. Similarly, some groups develop an atmosphere of confrontation and testimonial-giving that many people with mental illness would find intolerable. Nevertheless, a supportive 12-step group is often an effective means of helping people with severe mental illness maintain abstinence after a course of more intensive sociocognitive and sociobehavioral interventions. As always, the team must take a hypothetico-deductive approach to evaluating the success of interventions, using reliable, objective, and quantitative measurements of key features of the problem.

# Chapter 10

# Person-Environment Interactions

Human adaptation is a continuous interplay between meeting environmental demands and modifying the environment to complement our limitations. Colloquially, we tend to think of environments in terms of their physical features, but the *social* environment is also critically important. As individuals we seek out and create physical and social environments that best complement our temperaments and interests. Because of the complexity of human social environments, the factors that determine whether a particular environment is optimal for a particular individual can be quite complex.

Sometimes extraordinary needs demand extraordinary environments. Engineering extraordinary environments to address extraordinary needs represents a key technology in rehabilitation that tends to be associated with extraordinary *restrictiveness*. Restriction of mobility, independence, and autonomy is always implicated, to some degree, when environments are engineered to support extraordinary needs. Extraordinary environmental support is justified only when its restriction of a person's freedom is less than the restriction that would be likely to result without the environmental support. For the purposes of rehabilitation, careful and systematic analysis of the benefits and the restrictions must accompany every aspect of environmental engineering.

## SUPPORTIVE AND THERAPEUTIC MILIEUS

Severe mental illness often creates a need for extraordinary environmental conditions, sometimes temporarily, to serve the purposes of rehabilitation, and sometimes more permanently, to compensate for irreversible limitations. The special environmental needs of people with disabling mental illness are traditionally understood to fall into two categories: therapeutic and supportive. A therapeutic environment, or *therapeutic milieu*, is one intended to counteract psychopathological processes and promote healing or recovery. A *supportive milieu* is one intended to provide for universal human needs, from nutrition to social affiliation, with the understanding that the people in that milieu are unable to meet those needs themselves. A supportive milieu is provided to compensate for this inability, either temporarily, pending recovery, or permanently, in the case of irreversible disabilities.

Neo-Kraepelinian psychiatry draws a fine distinction between therapy and support, because it also draws a fine distinction between molecular and molar levels of dysfunction. If a "disease" is being "treated," it is therapy; if the "consequences" of the disease are being addressed, it is support (the economic implications of this were noted in the previous chapter). In other paradigms (e.g., some psychodynamic approaches and operant behaviorism) the distinction between therapy and support is acknowledged to be somewhat arbitrary, and the boundary of "disease" is not a worthy criterion for distinguishing between types of intervention. The concept of "supportive therapy" is a ubiquitous example of the ambiguous distinction between therapy and support. Rigorous adherence to the semantic distinction being made in this discussion would render supportive therapy an oxymoron. The term is used because it reflects the general idea that social support in a group therapy format has a generalized beneficial impact on the person's functioning outside the group. Supportive therapy is understood to replace the social support that a person might normally have, were it not for the circumstances of mental illness. There is some evidence that supportive therapy does provide such a benefit. On the other hand, research on psychosocial treatment often uses "supportive therapy" as a control or placebo condition. Supportive therapy is generally seen as a low-cost intervention available in most mental health systems, and for methodological reasons, it is a better experimental control than "no treatment" or "treatment as usual." In the context of research on the treatment of disabling mental illness, "treatment as usual" generally means maintenance of psychopharmacotherapy and case management.

In the integrated paradigm the distinction between therapy and support is meaningful to the degree that it signals a change in the recovering person's functioning. A therapeutic environment is intended to facilitate recovery, whereas a supportive environment is intended to provide for needs without the expectation that it will facilitate recovery. By definition, *recovery* involves ongoing positive functional change. There are circumstances in which lack of functional improvement nevertheless may connote progress in rehabilitation—for example, when a person manages to avoid relapse or hold a job, and each day of "no change" is actually an achievement. Indeed, such circumstances are often listed as short-term goals in rehabilitation plans (e.g., the goal is to remain free of acute neurophysiological dysregulation for 6 months). Reaching such goals is often a key landmark of progress. However, this type of situation is distinct from *recovery*, as used in the integrated paradigm. Two identical environments may be therapeutic for one person, because it is expected to produce therapeutic effects for that person, and supportive for another person, because it is intended to compensate for that person's deficits without the expectation of change. In fact, the same environment may be therapeutic at some points in the course of one person's illness, and supportive at other points.

The distinction between therapy and support is important when weighing the benefits and disadvantages of environmental interventions. The expectation of functional improvement has value that potentially weighs against the cost of the intervention, in terms of money and in terms of restrictions on personal freedom that may result from the intervention. If there is an expectation of change, greater cost and greater restriction may be more justified. Similarly, a supportive but restrictive environment is justifiable to the degree that it reduces the risk of catastrophic developments, such as the dangerous behavior associated with the recurrence of acute psychosis.

The history of rehabilitation for mental illness includes two relatively distinct types of therapeutic environments: therapeutic communities and social learning milieus (both are discussed in Chapter 1). A *therapeutic community* provides a structure and format for conducting the business of everyday life in a communal group. There are many variants, but they generally include frequent community meetings whose purpose is to identify, and make collective decisions about, issues in daily living that affect members of the community. Therapeutic community approaches are often used in group living situations, whether or not the people involved are undergoing rehabilitation. Although therapeutic communities have some demonstrated effectiveness in helping people lead stable lives and avoid hospitalization, the mechanism of this effect is not known, nor is it presumed to address specific problems associated with mental illness.[1] In the integrated paradigm, the unknown territory makes it difficult to characterize a therapeutic community as an intervention for a specific problem. The environment of a therapeutic community may be desirable for a recovering person who prefers or needs a communal lifestyle, and in this sense it may be un-

---

[1] It also should be noted that in Paul and Lentz's (1977) controlled trial, a therapeutic community approach produced an outcome distinctly inferior to a social learning approach, though distinctly superior to standard medical model treatment. However, this finding does not mean that a social learning milieu is always preferable to a therapeutic community, as a supportive or therapeutic environment. Different individuals are expected to respond optimally to different environmental characteristics, and this differential response must be evaluated in a comprehensive functional assessment.

derstood as a supportive environment. Similarly, a therapeutic community may be instrumental in helping people cope with other problems associated with mental illness, especially episodes of neurophysiological dysregulation and post-acute recovery. However, these benefits potentially characterize a variety of environments. Because of these gray areas, *therapeutic community* is generally not characterized as a specific intervention in the integrated paradigm.

The social learning therapeutic milieu includes two relatively discrete components—skills training and contingency management—that can be distinguished as specific interventions for specific problems. Contingency management originally took the form of a *token economy*, and current variants are equally compatible with a social learning milieu (these are described later in this chapter). In the integrated paradigm, contingency management programs are understood as specific interventions for addressing problems in person–environment interactions. Skills training, a key modality in rehabilitation (discussed in Chapter 9) is understood to address specific problems at the sociobehavioral level of functioning.

Social learning therapeutic milieus involve other procedures that cannot be distinguished as an intervention for a specific problem. For example, providers (staff) are systematically trained to avoid interactions in which they are doing things *for* the recovering person; instead they engage in interactions *with* the recovering person, for example, helping the recovering person perform a certain task. These behavioral strategies are enacted not because they are prescribed in an individual's rehabilitation plan, but because they are part of the milieu and apply to everyone in it. In this sense, some aspects of social learning milieus are comparable to therapeutic communities. Similarly, individually tailored interventions are not necessarily incompatible with communal or collective values; group-oriented contingencies have distinct roles and advantages in some environments (Davis & Blankenship, 1996). (For an approach based on communal values and group contingencies, but not on formal contingency management, see Fairweather, Sanders, Maynard, & Cressler, 1969.)

Both therapeutic communities and social learning milieus can be extremely beneficial in rehabilitation, not as specific interventions but as facilitative environments in which specific interventions are enacted. In this sense, rehabilitation is often most effectively conducted in a specialized environment that is *both* supportive and therapeutic. Rehabilitation services are usually provided in the context of a *program*, that is, a distinct collection of providers, services, participants and physical facilities, operating under a single administrative and fiscal auspice. Therapeutic communities and social learning milieus provide organizational principles for the environments of rehabilitation programs. As such, they contribute to successful outcomes but do not function as specific interventions. The design and management of a rehabilitation program's supportive/therapeutic environment—central issues in running a program—are discussed in the final chapter of this book.

One of the rehabilitation team's tasks is to determine the type of physical and social environment that would be optimal for the recovering person. This determination must be based on a comprehensive functional assessment of the person's abilities and the environment's features. Some features of the optimal environment may be identified as specific interventions pertinent to specific problems in the rehabilitation plan. For example, a contingency management agreement, wherein access to spending money is contingent on participation in skills training, may be a key feature of an optimal environment. Others are general features associated with the particular environment—be it a particular therapeutic community, social learning milieu, or other living situation—such as a residential program. In the integrated paradigm, these features are identified and described as the narrative formulation of the rehabilitation plan (discussed in Chapter 3).

A major change in environment, such as discharge from a hospital or moving from a residential facility to independent living, is often an important landmark in rehabilitation progress. In such cases, the narrative formulation describes the necessary features of the destination environment and the recovering person's functional characteristics that make those features necessary. In contemporary medical records conventions, the repository of information on destination environments and related issues is often a separate component of the treatment or rehabilitation plan (e.g., a "discharge plan" section). The integrated paradigm requires that such information be systematically addressed and documented but does not specify where (e.g., in a narrative formulation vs. a special discharge plan section).

## SOCIAL CONTRACTS AND THE SOCIAL ENVIRONMENT

*Social contracts*—explicit or implicit agreements between individuals and groups of individuals—are key features of the human social environment. We tend to associate *contracts* with the law, but legal contracts constitute just one type of social contract. Many, if not most, social contracts are implicit agreements that are maintained not by formal written documents but by cultural traditions, personal relationships, and unspoken understandings. For example, a friendship is, among other things, a set of implicit understandings concerning trust, loyalty, affection, autonomy, and dependability between two people. Implicit social contracts are part of the elemental fabric of our personal phenomenological experience as well as our society. Like basic living skills and social skills, we often take them for granted.

The rehabilitation enterprise involves, among other things, a social contract between the various members of the rehabilitation team. In mental health services, this idea is generally reflected in the concept of a *therapeutic contract* between a provider and a recipient of services. A therapeutic contract articulates (1) the nature of the problems being addressed, (2) the nature of the activity that will address the problems, (3) the goals to be pursued in the course of resolving the problems, and (4) the roles of providers and recipients in pursuing those goals. In this sense, a rehabilitation plan is a highly operationalized therapeutic contract.

People with disabling mental illness sometimes have difficulty apprehending, accepting, and/or adhering to social contracts. This difficulty can be associated with multiple etiological factors, including neurocognitive impairments, sociocognitive characteristics, and sociobehavioral skills deficits. Sometimes this problem is associated with acute psychosis or post-acute neurocognitive impairment and is therefore temporary or reversible. Sometimes it is associated with baseline residual neurocognitive impairment and therefore irreversible. Contingency management is usefully understood as a technology for identifying and articulating implicit social contracts in a manner understandable by people with mental illness. Ideally, this understanding promotes acceptance and adherence. In a therapeutic context, contingency management plays a key role in helping people recover from post-acute neurocognitive impairment (discussed in Chapters 6 and 7), in part, by making the contingencies in social contracts more concrete and immediate in relation to targeted behaviors. In a supportive context, contingency management can make implicit social contracts more accessible to people who cannot respond to them otherwise and may thus enable them to live in a less restrictive environment than would otherwise be the case. Because of this, contingency management skills are potentially useful for families as well as professional providers (Zelitch, 1980).

Token economies involve an intensive degree of operationalization and systematization of natural environmental contingencies. (For the most comprehensive account of a token economy-based rehabilitation program, see Paul & Lentz, 1977; for details on component assessment and data management technologies, see Paul, 1988a, 1988b, 1988c; for an updated review of the outcome of such programs, see Paul & Menditto, 1992.) Severe mental illness sometimes compromises a person's ability to respond to the most fundamental contingencies of life, for example, that basic health is contingent on performance of basic self-care. These contingencies are normally exercised as social contracts: personal autonomy as contingent on adequate self-care; access to economic resources as contingent on performance of socially useful behavior (i.e., work). For people whose mental illness creates an inability to respond to such basic contingencies in a natural environment, including basic social contracts, a token economy environment provides the conditions in which they can respond. For some individuals, the most crucial steps in recovery are responding to basic contingencies, first in a therapeutic token economy and then in more natural environments. As rehabilitation progresses, the concrete reinforcers and carefully scheduled antecedent events of the token economy are gradually replaced by verbal agreements and symbolic and social reinforcers, gradually approximating the normal qualities of social contracts.

Token economy is a useful technology for organizing and administrating contingency management in institutional settings, but it is less applicable in other settings (Glynn, 1990). The concept of a *token* is somewhat paradoxical outside an institution, given that, in normal life we are all participating in a giant token economy, the monetary system. The institutional qualities that make token economy attractive as a contingency management approach include insulation from the external monetary system, pervasive administrative control of the institutional monetary system, and a relatively homogenous participant population with respect to level of adaptive functioning and rehabilitation needs. When these factors do not apply, individualized contingency management programs are better suited. Instead of using a common artificial currency (tokens) as universal reinforcers, an individualized contingency management program identifies reinforcers specific to the individual and builds a contingency system around those (although this system often involves the government-sanctioned "tokens" for which we all work). Similarly, individualized contingency management identifies target behaviors on the basis of individual needs, whereas a token economy generally identifies a range of target behaviors applicable to all participants (Hunter, 2000; Wong & Woolsey, 1989). However, whether token economy or individualized program, the ultimate purpose of contingency management is to help people participate in the social contracts of everyday life to a more normal degree.

## CONTINGENCY MANAGEMENT, REHABILITATION, AND THE LAW

As noted, there are many kinds of social contracts other than legal ones; still, the law does have a way of bringing person–environment problems into sharp focus. People with disabling mental illness often become involved with the law through civil commitment, competence and guardianship proceedings, and even criminal prosecution. These involvements usually constellate some sort of person–environment problems. In a sense, legal proceedings constitute one form of contingency management program, wherein specific punishments (e.g., involuntary commitment) are delivered upon the occurrence of unacceptable behaviors, and rewards (e.g., home visits or day trips) are provided for engaging in treatment and/or progressing in rehabilitation.

However, it is important to distinguish between *punishment* and *reward* as colloquial versus psychological concepts. In both colloquial and legal use, a punishment is an aversive condition that is intended to minimize occurrence of unacceptable behaviors and/or in some views, as retribution. In psychological usage, punishment is defined in terms of its effect on a specified behavior; that is, an event that occurs after the targeted behavior and that produces a decrease in that behavior's frequency. In the psychological sense, punishment and aversiveness are often, but not always, coincident. Clinicians, legal authorities, and others are sometimes misled by exceptional cases wherein events that intuitively seem aversive do not produce reduction in behavior or, in fact, have a seemingly paradoxical reinforcing effect. For example, in some circumstances the effect of such consequences as incarceration, physical restraint, seclusion, or social admonishments is to *increase* rather than decrease the behavior that brings about the consequence. This behavior need not be understood as "masochistic" or some such psychodynamic label. It is more simply thought of as an unfortunate set of anomalous behavior–environmental relationships, often including the longer-term reinforcement available for performing the mental patient social role. Such anomalies occur because reinforcement and punishment are always relative in regard to each person's subjective experience of them and in their effect on behavior. When a seemingly aversive event is part of role performance whose reinforcement value in the long run outweighs the short-term punishment value, the behavior being "punished" paradoxically persists. For example, if a person sees social disapproval as an expected part of the mental patient social role, and performance of the mental patient role as a reliable way to maintain extraordinary social support from caregivers, then the person may purposefully engage in behavior that predictably elicits disapproval or related negative reactions from caregivers. Whereas most people in most circumstances experience social disapproval as punishing rather than reinforcing, it would have a paradoxically reinforcing effect in such a situation. It is also important to note that specific neurocognitive impairments may compromise the processes by which punishment-related information is processed, thus impairing the person's ability to learn from punishing experience. When legal processes are used as contingency management programs, it is necessary to consider reinforcement and punishment in a psychological as well as colloquial perspective. This means applying functional behavioral analysis to identify the effects, precisely and explicitly, of antecedent and consequent events on the behavior of interest rather than making assumptions or taking for granted the reinforcing or punishing properties of the mandated contingencies.

Over the last several years recognition of the parallels between legal processes and clinical techniques in mental health has increased (Wexler & Winnick, 1991). Contingency management is perhaps the clearest example, but there are many areas where legal and clinical concepts are potentially complementary. This recognition has produced *therapeutic jurisprudence*, a new domain of legal scholarship that seeks to optimize the relationship between legal and mental health technologies. Application of therapeutic jurisprudence to the field of rehabilitation for disabling mental illness is an even more recent development. Considering the many legal issues that people with disabling mental illness typically confront, this new application will doubtlessly make important contributions to rehabilitation technology (Elbogen & Tomkins, 1999; Spaulding, Poland, Elbogen, & Ritchie, 2000). Examples include new approaches to civil commitment, guardianship, and court-ordered treatment. These are obviously areas where an integrated perspective of legal and clinical considerations is potentially crucial to recovery and rehabilitation success.

Systematic clinical use of legal contingencies (e.g., conditional release agreements), and technologically informed use of substitute decision makers (i.e., guardians), will become key items in the rehabilitation toolbox. In addition, the principles of therapeutic jurisprudence may resolve some of the most difficult dilemmas in rehabilitation: (1) those that concern conflicts between a recovering person's autonomy and right to consent to treatment and rehabilitation, (2) the humanitarian demand to provide treatment and rehabilitation when it is needed, and (3) the public's interest in the safety and welfare of all citizens.

## ETHICS, PROFESSIONALISM, AND ENVIRONMENTAL ENGINEERING

The complexity of the factors to be considered in designing and creating an optimally supportive and/or therapeutic environment for an individual person demonstrates this is not a task to be undertaken through colloquial conceptualizations, "common sense," or generic clinical training and experience. Extensive functional assessment and analysis of behavior are required to confidently identify the particular behavioral deficits that must be addressed through environmental means. Careful and systematic weighing of cost, restrictions, and potential benefit is necessary to protect the recovering person's right to rehabilitation in the least restrictive environment possible. The recovering person's legal competence to make treatment and rehabilitation decisions must be determined precisely, and the person must be involved accordingly in designing the supportive/therapeutic environment (of course, this applies to all aspects of treatment and rehabilitation). Substitute decision makers must be involved, as needed. In particular, use of contingency management, especially when the recovering person does not have unequivocal veto power over treatment and rehabilitation decisions, requires a sophisticated consideration of legal and ethical, as well as clinical, factors.

The superficial and deceptive similarity between colloquial and psychological concepts of reward and punishment has unfortunately made contingency management vulnerable to abuse by insufficiently prepared providers. Most clinicians today have heard stories of abusive "behavior modification" programs, wherein people are deprived of basic needs to suit the convenience of caregivers. At the other extreme, many mental health professionals lack sufficient knowledge of learning theory principles, functional analysis of behavior, and the law to use contingency management in a responsible and ethical way, and so do not use it and even attempt to disallow its use by qualified professionals. The legal constraints of using contingency management were largely worked out by the mid-1970s (Martin, 1976; Roos, 1974; Stepleton, 1975; Tryon, 1976; Wexler, 1973), and interpretation of those constraints in the clinical and administrative contexts of mental health services followed thereafter (Griffith, 1980; Matson & Kazdin, 1981; White & Morse, 1988).

By the end of the 20th century, debate about contingency management had been supplanted by debate about involuntary treatment, specifically medical model treatment, especially involuntary hospitalization, coerced administration of psychotropic drugs, seclusion, and restraint. At the turn of the century, federal legislation was in progress to curb such practices, and the health care accreditation industry was moving to incorporate new concerns in its guidelines and standards. As of this writing, it remains unclear how issues of involuntary medical treatment will be resolved, as the controversies are becoming increasingly polarized. (For a comprehensive discussion of coercion and involuntary treatment for severe mental illness, see Dennis & Monahan, 1996.) However, controversies over medical model treatments are not necessarily relevant to past controversies about contingency management. The legal scholarship on involuntary use of psychosocial treatment, particularly contingency management, is separate from that on involuntary medical treatment. Continuing confusion about appropriate use of contingency management is somewhat attributable to the controversy about involuntary medical treatment, but the greater factor is widespread ignorance, among mental health professionals, about mental health law, in general, and contingency management technology, in particular.

Confusion and ignorance regarding contingency management and mental health law are exacerbated by guild rivalries among the mental health professions. Neo-Kraepelinian psychiatry implicitly (and sometimes explicitly) devalues technology not conceptually linked to its disease nosology. Nonphysician providers often are not given the professional status and authority necessary to implement contingency management interventions safely and effectively. As with other aspects of social learning-based services, there is an intrinsic conflict between (1) the clinical procedures and decision making necessary for effective contingency management and (2) the traditional administrative and supervisory structures of the mental health medical model (Liberman, 1979; for a comprehensive account of implementing contingency management in medical settings, see Corrigan & Liberman, 1994). Psychologists and other professionals do not experience this conflict outside medical model settings, so it is difficult to interest them in practicing in medical model settings. The implementation of contingency management is historically associated with professional psychologists, who have also been the source of much criticism of the medical model as it has been applied in mental health. Finally, introducing contingency management in institutional settings historically has required a concomitant increase in scrutiny by professionals and paraprofessionals, as well as stronger mechanisms for assuring accountability and quality of care. Scrutiny and accountability are too often resisted by those who practice in traditional institutions.

All these complexities require that use of contingency management in rehabilitation be intensively directed and supervised by specifically trained and experienced professionals. There is considerable disincentive for service agencies to provide contingency management because of the technological difficulties, and also because of guild politics. Historically, the solution has been to avoid it, which accounts for the striking underrepresentation of this technology in services for adults with disabling mental illness. Yet the evidence of the technology's effectiveness, considered in light of the research on socioenvironmental causes of institutionalization, strongly suggests that competent use of contingency management is probably necessary to *prevent* institutionalization. This holds true for any restrictive environment (and "community treatment" environments can be as restrictive as institutions), not just traditional institutions. In other words, a service agency that is not capable of administering contingency management appropriately is at significant risk of *harming* many of its clients who have disabling mental illness. Increasing realization of this risk is part of the ongoing evolution of standards and regulations for mental health services. In the near future, it is likely that simply neglecting contingency management and related technologies will not be a viable solution. Hopefully, agencies will be increasingly constrained to bear the costs, resolve the political disputes, retain qualified providers, and provide competent services in this domain.

## PROBLEMS AT THE LEVEL OF PERSON-ENVIRONMENT INTERACTIONS

A number of serious barriers to recovery from disabling mental illness appears at the level of interactions between individuals and their environments. These problems are often influenced by identifiable factors within and across neurophysiological, cognitive, and/or sociobehavioral levels, but sometimes the causal factors are so many, or so complex, in their interactions, that the problem at the person–environment level cannot be resolved by treating problems only within the more molecular levels. In these cases, it is helpful to identify a person–environment problem and intervene at that level. (As always, this does not preclude intervening at the more molecular levels as well, when it is expected that the various interventions will all contribute separately to rehabilitation progress and recovery.)

Sometimes a causal factor cannot be eliminated, but compensatory tactics can be employed at the environmental level to achieve a similar outcome. For example, if a residual neurocognitive deficit prevents a person from being able to fully manage his or her personal finances, a legal conservator arrangement that ensures timely access to needed funds may be a useful environmental intervention. In some cases, some resolution of the environmental problem must occur before more molecular problems can even be addressed. For example, if there are real or perceived disincentives for participating in rehabilitation (e.g., possible loss of disability entitlements), it may be very difficult to sufficiently engage a person in the enterprise of acquiring better job skills. For these reasons, in rehabilitation it is important to be able to identify problems in person–environment interactions and intervene *at that level*, rather than depend on resolution of intrapersonal problems.

## Baseline Neurocognitive and Sociobehavioral Impairments

At any point in the course of rehabilitation and recovery, combinations of neurocognitive and sociobehavioral problems may render a person incapable of performing activities required for autonomous personal and social functioning. Environmental interventions can serve both supportive and therapeutic purposes at those points. As discussed in Chapters 6 and 7, a social learning milieu, with its contingency management capabilities and intensive structuring of daily routines, facilitates reorganization of microskill hierarchies that have collapsed in the wake of acute psychosis. The rehabilitative success of therapeutic communities, such as the Soteria model, suggests that they too may facilitate recovery from post-acute neurocognitive impairment, although more research is required to confirm this.

Following a period when no further recovery of neurocognitive functioning occurs, despite intensive intervention, remaining impairments must be considered to be truly residual. In the integrated paradigm, this identification of residual impairment is signified by changing the problem title, updating the problem description, revising the goals, and applying supportive/prosthetic interventions rather than therapeutic ones. Neuropsychological assessment provides helpful data for determining (1) when the recovery process has reached a plateau and (2) the role of specific impairments, for example, in memory or executive processes. Sociobehavioral data are also crucial for determining (1) which aspects of personal and social functioning are affected, and (2) which environmental supports are necessary to compensate. Residual neurocognitive impairments must be addressed when they produce persistent failure in acquiring skills or performing them when needed.

Rehabilitative interventions for residual neurocognitive impairments generally operate at the sociobehavioral level by providing environmental structure that supports timely and competent performance of specific skills. In the integrated paradigm's rehabilitation planning procedures, the *problem title* under which the intervention is conducted reflects the affected domain(s) of skill performance (living skills deficit, interpersonal skills deficit, etc.). The *problem description* provides more specific information on the nature of the skills deficits and the role of neurocognitive impairment.[2] The long- and short-term goals are defined in terms of the performance of specific behaviors; a successful environmental intervention is one that makes those behaviors happen, despite the absence of neurocognitive functioning sufficient for more independent skill performance.

As discussed in Chapters 6 and 7, modifying the physical environment is sometimes helpful in compensating for neurocognitive problems such as distractibility and behavioral disinhibition (Goldberg, 1994; Velligan et al., 2000). In addition, contingency management is often a helpful sociobehavioral prosthetic (Heinssen, 1996; Heinssen & Victor, 1994). Applied to neurocognitive and sociobehavioral impairment, contingency management takes advantage of the *immediacy hypothesis* (described in Chapter 6) regarding environmental behavioral control. A superordinate effect of neurocognitive impairment is a loss of ability to respond appropriately to physically, temporally, or conceptually distant contingencies. For example, the prospect of working 2 weeks for a single paycheck may not motivate, or make sense to, a recovering person, even when that person's work skills are otherwise intact. A contingency contract that specifies more immediate reward, however, would be likely to produce reliable work behavior. For another example, a check or money may be too conceptually remote to be salient to a person with severe impairment, whereas the commodities purchased with the money would be salient. A contingency contract that provides for consumatory reinforcement (e.g., food, or an opportunity to en-

---

[2]Note that there is no point in including a separate problem title for the residual neurocognitive impairment itself, because no intervention is expected to affect a residual impairment. When no technology is available to directly address a problem, the problem must be redefined.

gage in a desired activity) would maintain performance where a paycheck would not.

Contingency management programs can also compensate for neurocognitive impairment by translating distant consequences into proximal ones and by strengthening verbal cognition processes. One function of executive neurocognition is to inhibit behavior that has been reinforced under different circumstances. Learning to use verbal cognition (i.e., self-talk) can compensate for executive weakness in this regard. For example, a person may be unable to inhibit impulses to be aggressive or engage in self-destructive behavior due to compromised executive/frontal functioning, and the immediate consequences of such behavior (e.g., gaining social dominance, extortion, recruiting social attention) may further reinforce those behaviors. A suitably crafted contingency management program would translate the long-term consequences of impulsive behavior into more immediate and salient ones and teach the recovering person to verbally rehearse the contingencies (e.g., "If I don't stop this behavior, I won't earn my weekend bonus"), thereby strengthening inhibition processes and reversing the undesirable reinforcement process.

Use of contingency management techniques is commonplace in developmental disability services and, increasingly, in neurological and neurogeriatric services. As discussed earlier in this chapter, it is less commonplace in adult mental health, partly because medical model environments are often professionally inhospitable to the providers most skilled in use of contingency management, usually psychologists. Furthermore, the demands for crafting effective contingency management programs tend to be different in mental health settings. In the population of adults with disabling mental illness, one often encounters residual neurocognitive and sociobehavioral impairment patterns and sociocognitive characteristics that are rare in geriatric or developmental disability populations. Thus there is a lower demand for contingency management prosthetics that systematically prompt or reinforce discrete behaviors in a relatively short time frame, such as those required to support task performance in a workshop or sequences of self-care behaviors in a domestic environment. (Such programs are more frequently helpful early in the post-acute phase, when neurocognitive impairment is more severe and pervasive, independent of the recovering person's residual neurocognitive status. The focus here is on prosthetics for residual impairment.) The task of the provider (the person on the rehabilitation team who takes the lead in designing and evaluating contingency management programs) at this point is less often one of identifying key behaviors whose sequencing comprises skill performance, and more often one of identifying the nature and timing of environmental events optimal to *maintaining* desired social role performance and *suppressing* inappropriate behaviors. Professional training and experience with contingency management do not necessarily prepare the provider for optimal engagement with adults who have severe mental illness. Maintaining sufficient professional expertise and an organizational structure compatible with contingency management is an important issue for running a rehabilitation program (discussed in Chapter 12).

## Rehabilitation Nonadherence

Failure to comply with treatment is one of the most notorious characteristics attributed to people with severe mental illness, especially those with the diagnostic label of schizophrenia. Perhaps more than any other misconception, this attribution is pervaded by unexamined colloquial assumptions, "pop psychology," and social stigma. In our culture "not following doctors' orders" is generally seen as irresponsible, even though everybody does it to some extent. When treatment nonadherence could result in dangerous or unacceptable behavior, as is sometimes the case with mental illness, the public is especially unsympathetic.

In the traditional medical model, nonadherence to treatment is generally assumed to be part of the disorder. "Not following doctors' orders" is irrational, and irrationality is a feature of severe mental illness. "Patients" are not expected to be able to make competent judgments in this domain, and whether or how to participate in treatment is not ultimately up to them. When a reductionist biomedical account of noncompliance is manifestly untenable, colloquial moralistic attributions often substitute. The patient is lazy, unmotivated, dependent, has a personality disorder, or does not want to get better. An unreflective medical model perspective leads to one of two extremes. Either the patient's wishes and perspectives are dismissed and coercion is used to whatever Draconian degree is necessary, or the actual patient is dismissed, deemed undeserving of any assistance.

In the late 20th century, scientific and cultural developments undermined traditional views of treatment nonadherence. In general medicine, there was new awareness that nonadherence to treatment is an issue for all types of patients with all types of illnesses, not just those with mental illness. People often neglect treatment regimens, even when the consequences could be fairly immediate and dire. (An especially striking example is that of ulcerative colitis, a condition that produces episodes of extreme physical discomfort. Recurrence of episodes creates a serious risk for colon cancer. Episodes can be effectively prevented with a simple daily medication regimen, yet noncompliance has been estimated to be as high as 40%.) There was increased public interest in holding health care providers accountable for providing cost-effective services and respecting the rights of service recipients and their families. Consumer and advocacy organizations brought the issue of the rights of people with mental illness into the public arena.

Providers and the public began to become more cognizant of civil rights for people with mental illness, including the right to treatment and the right to refuse treatment. In psychopathology, new understandings of the nature of nonadherence came from the discovery of neurocognitive impairments. Sociocognitive research (e.g., on cognitive dissonance and attributional processes) also suggested new ways of understanding nonadherence. Biomedical research on potentially irreversible side effects of antipsychotic drugs gave new rationality to refusing treatment. Outcome research on traditional forms of psychosocial treatment (e.g., psychodynamic psychotherapy) failed to provide evidence of effectiveness, further reducing justification for coercing people to participate in it. Psychosocial rehabilitation research illuminated the importance of the recovering person's engagement and participation in the rehabilitation enterprise. It became clear that adherence to treatment and/or rehabilitation in mental illness is influenced by many factors at all levels of human functioning.

Modern rehabilitation formats contribute to the complexity of nonadherence issues. It is now well known that the complexity of any treatment regimen increases the risk of nonadherence. Rehabilitation for disabling mental illness is complex, creating many opportunities for nonadherence. The primacy of the recovering person's values and desires are not always compatible with the rehabilitation values of achieving stable personal and social functioning and an optimal quality of life. Assessment of nonadherence is among the most complex and difficult of rehabilitation tasks. Management of adherence problems is usually a central concern of the rehabilitation team, requiring ongoing assessment and reassessment throughout the entire rehabilitation process.

Rehabilitation nonadherence manifests itself in various ways, at different levels of human functioning, and at different points in the course of a person's illness. Ultimately, however, it must be expressed as a failure to perform a particular behavioral activity necessary for recovery, from ingesting a pill to attending rehabilitation team meetings. Disagreements between rehabilitation team members do not, in themselves, constitute nonadherence. In fact, disagreements between team members are to be expected. A problem arises only if the disagreement is about taking a particular action at a particular time (this point is further discussed in the next chapter). It is certainly not uncommon for a recovering person to disagree with other team members about diagnosis, case formulation, interpretation of assessment data, and so on, while still adhering to all aspects of the rehabilitation plan. This is not to say that consensus on these matters is unimportant and does not merit pursuit throughout the course of rehabilitation. It is, and it does. However, if lack of consensus is not expressed as actual nonadherent behavior, it is a problem at the sociocognitive level of functioning (and not necessarily the recovering person's) and should be addressed as such.

Addressing such problems at the sociocognitive level was discussed in Chapter 8.

If there is a behavioral expression of nonadherence, then it is important to determine whether the expression is associated with the recovering person's beliefs and attributions about mental illness and/or the need for rehabilitation. When there is general consensus on the rehabilitation team about the rehabilitation plan and narrative formulation, the nonadherent behavior is usually attributable to neurocognitive impairments and/or absence of necessary sociobehavioral skills. Functional and neuropsychological assessment may trace such problems to memory failure, psychophysiological dysregulation (e.g., inability to tolerate a rehabilitation milieu, associated with uncontrolled anxiety), or specific skills deficiencies (e.g., unable to follow a complex daily schedule). Obviously, each level would need different intervention strategies.

In some cases, the nonadherence appears to be directly related to specific disagreements among treatment team members, including an explicit refusal by the recovering person to participate in some part of (or the entire) rehabilitation plan. In such cases the role of the person's beliefs and attributions must be carefully assessed. The causal influence may be the reverse of our colloquial assumption that beliefs drive behavior (discussed in Chapter 8). A person's rehabilitation adherence may be limited by neurocognitive and/or sociobehavioral problems, but attributional dynamics such as cognitive dissonance may lead to an expressed belief that the nonadherence is due to disagreements between the recovering person and other team members. Struggling with disagreements may be a less productive approach than addressing the limiting factors straightforwardly—the hypothesis being that the person's attributions and beliefs will either change in response to improved functioning or will become independent of actual behavioral adherence.

All equivocations and moderating factors aside, explicit refusal to participate in treatment and rehabilitation is a pervasive barrier to recovery. Rehabilitation providers and recipients often find themselves in situations where some kind of treatment must be undertaken despite the recipient's wishes (*recipient* is preferable to *recovering person* in this context, because people receiving services against their will may object that they do not have a condition from which they need to recover). This situation of enforced treatment occurs when a legal authority (i.e., a court or mental health commitment board) determines that the recipient does not have the legal status to refuse treatment. The legal authority may directly order that treatment be provided or may appoint a substitute decision maker (i.e., a guardian) to make treatment decisions on the person's behalf.

Involuntary treatment is not incompatible with the integrated paradigm, provided two conditions are met: (1) It is the external legal authority, not the team or any of its members, that makes the determination of need for involuntary treatment; and (2) the team has a mandate to provide treatment and rehabilitation according to the recipient's best interests, within the constraints set by the legal authority. Although these may seem like straightforward conditions, they are not. In some legal venues, a passive court all but delegates entire authority to providers. In some mental health settings, it is unclear whether "treatment" is different from "punishment." Recent developments in legal scholarship leave it unclear as to whether a government entity can require functional incarceration (i.e., commitment to a psychiatric institution) without requiring meaningful treatment. The parameters of providing involuntary treatment and rehabilitation to people with disabling mental illness vary considerably according to locale, and the parameters change, over time, at both local and national levels.

The main implication of these various considerations is that providers who serve involuntary recipients must have an ongoing, assertive relationship with the legal system. It is incumbent upon all mental health professionals to (1) thoroughly understand the legal environment in which they provide services, (2) educate judges and prosecutors about the nature of mental illness and rehabilitation technology, (3) ensure that sound scientific principles and technology inform legal decision making, and (4) engage all parties in a rehabilitation plan that is expected to resolve the problems that led to the recipient's loss of the right to make decisions as an autonomous, competent adult. Above all, no mental health professional should fall into the trap of serving as the proxy for a legal authority.

For the purposes of assessment, planning, and intervention, the fact that people are involuntary recipients need not change anything about their role on the rehabilitation team, except that they do not have veto power over team decisions. It bears repeating that even in the special condition of involuntary services compelled by a legal authority, the team should always continue to strive for complete consensus about the rehabilitation plan. Similarly, when a substitute decision maker is involved, that person is to be considered a member of the team as well, but the team should repeatedly assess the factors that necessitate a substitute decision maker and work to resolve those factors, thereby returning autonomy to the recovering person.

Rehabilitation nonadherence must be addressed in terms of specific, observable behaviors relevant to rehabilitation activities. The recovering person's beliefs and attributions are generally not appropriate targets for nonadherence interventions. It would be inappropriate, for example, to construct a contingency management program that selectively reinforces a person for "admitting" to having a mental illness. In contrast, contingency management programs that reinforce people for making self-statements about the nature of their disorder often help recovering individuals overcome memory or impulse control problems (e.g., "If I throw the food, I won't get dessert.") that contribute to treatment nonadherence and other sociobehavioral problems. However, these self-statements operate in the context of the recovering person's appropriate, working understanding of the illness and its characteristics, with general consensus on those elements among team members. Such programs serve to enhance the impact of the recovering person's beliefs on his or her behavioral performance, not to influence his or her beliefs. Attributions and beliefs are generally most appropriately addressed by interventions at the sociocognitive and sociobehavioral levels (as discussed in Chapters 8 and 9).

A key step in assessment, then, is to operationally define the behaviors that represent the recovering person's nonadherence to some aspect of the rehabilitation plan. The team must be especially careful to not mistake mere differences of opinion for noncompliance. Whether a legal authority compels treatment or not, team members must "agree to disagree" about the truth or validity of beliefs and attributions that do not directly constitute *behavioral* nonadherence. The next steps are common to all contingency management interventions. First, in the course of a functional analysis of behavior, a systematic enumeration is conducted of the antecedents and consequences that potentially influence adherent or nonadherent behavior. Next, a survey of the environment is performed to determine who and what might control those antecedents. Next, a process of negotiation is undertaken wherein the recovering person and all parties who control conditions in the recovering person's environment are engaged in the rehabilitation enterprise. This is not a process of finding ways to coerce the recovering person; rather, it is a process of articulating the real and often natural and normal contingencies that the recovering person generally has to manage. This, in turn, requires making the contingencies clear, concrete, and immediate enough to optimally influence the recovering person's behavior. Once the relevant behaviors and contingencies are clear to everyone, it is usually possible to set them down in writing in a way that all concerned parties can understand and endorse. Such *behavioral contracts* (also known as contingency contracts) can be useful tools for the purpose of creating an optimally supportive social environment. (For a focused discussion of how to formulate and use behavioral contracts, see Heinssen, Levendusky, & Hunter, 1995; for a description of a comprehensive manual on writing contracts, see Gewell, Silverstein, & Stewart, 2001.). Figure 10.1 shows an example of a behavioral contract produced by a fictional treatment team.

Contingency management is often seen as impractical, especially outside institutional settings, because clinicians incorrectly believe that the relevant antecedents and consequences must be controlled by the rehabilitation team. We all operate under contingencies that are controlled by individuals or mechanisms in the environment. If we do not show up for work, our boss exercises contingencies. If we do not pay the rent, our land-

# Behavioral Contract

This behavioral contract is an agreement between Joe A, Sally A (Joe A's legal conservator), Agatha Jones (CMHC case manager), and Paul Smith (chief manager, Friendly House residential program).

Paul Smith agrees that Friendly House will provide Joe A a place of residence, and that Joe A has access to the Friendly House housekeeping resources, as long as Joe A is a participant in the CMHC rehabilitation program. Paul Smith also agrees to meet with Joe A once per week for at least 30 minutes to review Joe A's personal budget with him and identify any potential cash-flow problems. Paul Smith also agrees to request a meeting of Joe A's rehabilitation team if he observes any problems with Joe A's cash-flow or with Joe A's observance of the Friendly House rules for residents.

Sally A agrees to act as Joe A's legal conservator. She will receive Joe A's monthly disability and rehabilitation workshop paychecks, pay Joe A's monthly Friendly House bill, and deposit the remainder in Joe A's checking account. She will meet with Joe A once per month for at least 30 minutes to review his personal budget. She agrees to request a meeting of Joe A's rehabilitation team if she encounters budget-related problems that she and Joe A cannot resolve themselves.

Agatha Jones agrees to provide case management and rehabilitation counseling services through the CMHC rehabilitation program. She will meet with Joe A once per month for at least one hour to review his rehabilitation plan, assess progress, and review his relapse prevention plan with him. She will organize a meeting of Joe A's rehabilitation team once per quarter, to be held at the CMHC. The team will review Joe A's rehabilitation plan, make any needed revisions, and update its goals and interventions. Agatha Jones also agrees to organize a meeting of the rehabilitation team upon the request of any of its members, to address problems or other issues not anticipated by the rehabilitation plan.

When this contract goes into effect, the rehabilitation program will include the following components to which Joe A agrees: working 25 hours per week at the rehabilitation workshop, a monthly meeting with Agatha Jones to review progress, two meetings per week with the CMHC AA group, a weekly meeting with Paul Smith to review cash flow, a monthly meeting with Sally A to review Joe A's personal budget, a monthly check-in with the CMHC medication clinic, and membership in the CMHC Young Adults Social Club.

Joe A agrees to live at Friendly House, observe the Friendly House rules for residents, and participate in the CMHC rehabilitation program. He agrees to take his medication(s), as prescribed in the CMHC medication clinic. He agrees to meet with his legal conservator, Sally A, once per month to review his personal budget and conduct any necessary banking tasks. He agrees to keep a list of his money needs, including groceries, clothing, personal care items, and recreation, and an accurate record of his expenditures. He and Sally A will review this record at their monthly meeting and make any needed revisions of the budget. Joe A agrees to notify Agatha Jones immediately if he encounters any problem in participating fully in the rehabilitation program according to this plan.

The signatures below indicate that Joe A, Sally A, Paul Smith, and Agatha Jones all agree to the terms of this behavioral contract.

_____          _____
Joe A                            Sally A

_____          _____
Paul Smith                       Agatha Jones

**FIGURE 10.1.** A sample behavioral contract.

lord takes action. If we do not pay the phone bill, contingencies are exercised by an impersonal but reasonably predictable environmental mechanism, the phone company. The task of the contingency manager is to identify these natural contingencies and engineer their operation to the recovering person's maximum benefit. In a community mental health setting, the only "unnatural" contingency may be the one exercised by the legal authority as a consequence of rehabilitation nonadherence.

A common error in constructing contingencies for nonadherence is to use catastrophic consequences for those contingencies that constitute or bring about termination of treatment or rehabilitation services. An example is, "If you don't come to group, you can't be a participant in this program." This type of contingency is potentially legitimate when used as a criterion for participating in particular activities or programs, when those activities or programs do not represent the person's sole alternative for rehabilitation. For example, participation in community-based therapeutic communities and "clubhouse programs" (described in Chapter 1) is usually contingent on the recovering person's consent and active participation. This consent requirement limits the recipient population to people who can or do give consent and actively participate, which is only a subset of all the people with disabling mental illness who could benefit from rehabilitation. Whether such contingencies are applied on the level of program eligibility or to more limited situations, failure to perform the target behavior must always be seen as a problem that continues to be addressed in the rehabilitation plan, not as a trigger for discontinuing rehabilitation. Most concretely, it is never appropriate to make adherence to *anything* a contingency for the recovering person's membership or participation on the rehabilitation team.

## Socialized Psychiatric Symptoms

Socialized psychiatric symptoms are behaviors that are superficially similar to direct expressions of neurophysiological or neurocognitive impairments, but which can be shown to be under the control of environmental antecedents and/or consequences. Such symptoms are the product of perverse rewards and punishments in mental health institutions and cultures. For example, in many recovering persons' experience, reporting positive psychotic symptoms is the only way to get the attention of mental health professionals. Contingency management is an effective strategy for neutalizing perverse contingencies and eliminating socialized psychiatric symptoms. Ultimately, the hypothesis that a behavioral problem represents a socialized psychiatric symptom is most strongly supported when alteration of its antecedents and/or consequences eliminates the problem.

It can be extremely difficult to detect and assess socialized psychiatric symptoms, especially in those settings overly dependent on a diagnostic medical model and psychopharmacotherapy. It is not unusual to encounter individuals with persistent "symptoms" known to be refractory to any pharmacological intervention, but whose nature and operation have never been investigated. Often, the presence of these symptoms leads to long and fruitless searches for the optimal medication regimen, sometimes resulting in high doses and complex polypharmacy (use of multiple medications) despite persistent ineffectiveness. An unreflective medical model perspective "takes the patient at face value" on the assumption that there is no rational reason for people to "lie to their doctor." Aside from inconsistency with the other medical model tenet that irrationality is intrinsic to mental illness, a careful functional analysis would reveal that, in fact, there are clear environmental contingencies that reinforce expression of symptom-like behavior. These contingencies may even include those created by entitlement programs that require individuals to manifest "diagnosable symptoms" of mental illness in order to qualify for services or monetary benefits.

A more pernicious mechanism of socialized psychiatric symptoms is that associated with performance of a "mental patient" social role. It is pernicious because social roles can incorporate widely dispersed contingencies, involving multiple but subtle reinforcers, any one of which would not sustain role performance by itself. It is their collective effect over time that motivates role performance. For example, one need only consider the ineffable reinforcement and manifest costs attendant to performance of a parental role to appreciate how counterintuitive the desire to perform that role may appear, even to the person performing the role (especially when parenting adolescents). Yet, even given all its travails and precious few overt reinforcements, the role of the parent is one of the most universally desired in our culture. It is fundamental human nature to seek out and perform social roles.

In a mental health system based on the medical model, the role of mental patient may be the only one accessible to a person with disabling mental illness. Despite its obvious drawbacks and limitations, it is a means of getting some security and social affiliation. Even people with severe neurocognitive impairments that limit their ability to abstract and conceptualize are often still capable of associating the performance of symptom-like behavior with the resulting benefits (however limited and qualified). Adapting one's behavior to environmental conditions is part of *learning*, as conceptualized in social learning theory, and in this sense it can be said that the role of mental patient, like other roles, is learned. Discrete aspects of mental patient behavior are learned in various ways, including operant learning through differential reinforcement and observational learning among people in the mental patient role. The human ability to learn through multiple channels is hindered, but seldom completely disabled, by mental illness. In addition, the popular stereotypes and stigma about mental illness in our culture exert strong expectations (*antecedents*, in functional behavioral analysis terminology) about how mentally ill people behave. They are expected to be unmotivated, unreasonable, and prone to violence. We all tend to behave according to expectations, and people with mental illness are no exception.

Functional analysis of behavior can eventually articulate the operative mechanisms that sustain socialized psychiatric symptoms, though this may require time and several iterations of hypothetico-deductive interventions when those mechanisms are dispersed within social role performance. Persistence after resolution of acute psychosis is often an important clue, but other symptoms may also persist this way, such as symptom-linked attribution problems. The most compelling evidence is a demonstration that the symptoms are no longer expressed when identified reinforcers of socialized symptoms are withheld, or when more powerful reinforces are contingent on behaviors incompatible with patient role performance. When the symptoms are part of a broader social role performance, a global shift of contingencies may be necessary to produce a net reduction in the reinforcement value of performing the role compared to the net reinforcement value of performing alternative roles. For example, psychotic behavior in a workshop setting may disappear when keeping a valued job is contingent on an absence of the behavior. The behavior may even persist in other settings where there are no clear adverse contingencies. This is why attention to every quarter of the recovering person's physical and social environment is often necessary, and why every "natural" contingency in the recovering person's environment is potentially part of a therapeutic milieu.

Of course, when engineering such contingencies, great care must be taken to ensure that eliminating undesirable behavior does not compromise detection of psychotic relapse. Even when there is high confidence that certain behavior is socialized and not the expression of an impending relapse, it is advisable to identify at least one person who can monitor the recovering person's phenomenology, so that no planned consequences are applied to reports of psychotic symptoms. At the same time, it is equally important to establish a baseline of such reports before the contingency plan begins. It is not unusual for people with severe mental illness to function well in most settings, apparently free of symptoms or at least free of interference from symptoms, while reporting in a dyadic context that they experience symptoms, sometimes even severe and continuous. Like so many other aspects of mental illness, the nature of residual symptoms and their relationship to baseline functioning and relapse are unique to individuals.

The procedures for addressing socialized psychiatric symptoms with contingency management are generally the same as those that address rehabilitation nonadherence. In fact, rehabilitation nonadherence itself may be part of a generalized mental patient social role performance, and this possibility should be addressed systematically in clinical assessment (including functional analysis) of the behaviors involved.

As with the concept of rehabilitation nonadherence, the concept of socialized psychiatric symptoms often elicits misconceptions about the recovering person's motivation or intent. These misconceptions are particularly likely to surface in medical and colloquial views of illness, wherein feigning a symptom is regarded as dishonest and manipulative. For example, a recovering person who complains of "hearing voices" as a way of getting the attention of care providers and soliciting help when feeling distressed could easily be labeled as manipulative. However, as discussed in Chapter 8, performance of social roles usually involves some particular version of "the truth"—that is, a version adapted to optimal performance of that role. Performing the role of mental patient is no different in that respect. In addition, the neurocognitive and sociobehavioral problems that limit access to other social roles tend to compromise people's ability to articulate why they behave as they do, even when their ability to perform a role is relatively intact. Indeed, as discussed above, many of the roles we perform would be difficult to explain or justify under the most normal of circumstances.

With regard to the pejorative attribution of manipulation as motivation, consider the fact that humans are highly social organisms, for whom manipulation of others is a key social skill. We are not offended by being manipulated, per se, only by being manipulated in an exploitative or disrespectful way. The manipulation skills of people with disabling mental illness are often impaired, making their manipulative efforts more obvious, which may impart the impression of disrespect and exploitation. When clinicians characterize a person as "manipulative," they are, in essence, identifying their ability to apprehend the person's obvious attempts to perform a normal but usually more subtle human activity. In the integrated paradigm, it is not a moral judgment to identify a recovering person's behavior as manipulative or their symptoms as socialized. It is a recognition that multiple factors interact—from neurocognitive impairment to the structure of the mental health system—that coalesce to create a problematic situation.

## Socially Unacceptable Behavior

The problem title of socially unacceptable behavior reflects a need to identify and address specific behavior problems on the grounds of their sheer unacceptability in any social environment. Aggression, stealing, public masturbation, and sexual predation are examples. Such behavior problems in people with severe mental illness are often the direct result of neurophysiological dysregulation, neurocognitive impairment, or sociobehavioral skills deficits, and they resolve once those more molecular-level problems have been resolved. However, sometimes the unacceptable behavior persists after the more molecular-level problems have been resolved as fully as possible. When this reality emerges in the course of ongoing hypothetico-deductive assessment and intervention, the team is compelled to identify the behavior as a separate problem and to assign an environmental level of intervention.

As discussed in Chapter 9, a supportive environmental intervention may be required, in the context of psychophysiological dysregulation of aggression, to protect the recovering person and others from the problem behavior. The intervention plan should include a transition period from a supportive to a therapeutic approach, during which time risks are contained sufficiently to allow a focus on elimination (as opposed to suppression or isolation) of the behavior. To the degree that psychophysiological dysregulation or other skills deficits are part of the picture, the intervention should coordinate contingency management with skills training, including *in vivo* skills training and rehearsal in those situations where the problem behavior is most probable. As with rehabilitation nonadherence and socialized psychiatric symptoms, the unacceptable behavior may be part of a larger social role performance and maintained by environmental contingencies relatively distant from the actual behavior. For example, persistent failure to perform self-care, housekeeping, and personal budgeting may be part of a "dependent mental patient" role, which, in the perception of the recovering person, is what ensures that care providers reliably address his or her needs. To not perform that role or to perform incompatible roles, such as "self-reliant adult" would risk abandonment. Ultimately, the behavior is most effectively and permanently eliminated to the degree that the recovering person successfully performs a highly reinforced social role that is incompatible with the behavior.

## Social-Environmental Conflict

Social–environmental conflict reflects mutually antagonistic interaction patterns involving the recovering person and key individuals in the recovering person's social world. Family members and mental health service providers are often included in these interaction patterns. Research has shown that the presence of such conflict, as measured by such constructs as expressed emotion, is a powerful influence on neurophysiological stability and rehabilitation success (Bebbington & Kuipers, 1988; Hooley, 1985; Kavanaugh, 1992).

The rehabilitation team should consider including social–environmental conflict as a problem when historical data and/or functional assessment indicate specific interaction patterns, repeated over time, that are associated with problem behaviors, distress, exacerbation of baseline symptom levels, or psychotic relapse. Often this data come straight from the recovering person, who can specifically identify the people and/or issues involved in the recurring conflicts. Others in the recovering person's social environment also provide crucial information, usually from quite different perspectives. Often, a third perspective (e.g., that of a clinician) is necessary to fully articulate the nature of the conflict in a way that incorporates all relevant perspectives.

The social–environmental conflicts experienced by people with severe mental illness are often issues familiar to many families; for example, the recovering person's desire for autonomy and independence conflicts with the family's desire to protect the recovering person from his or her own faulty judgments and immaturity. Of course, the involvement of mental illness adds new complexities to such conflicts.

It is sometimes difficult to differentiate the interpersonal conflict itself from the emotional tone and problem-solving processes that the conflict elicits. Whether mental illness is a factor or not, conflicts generally are resolved with greater difficulty when the participants have gone ballistic—when they are psychophysiologically aroused beyond the Yerkes–Dodson performance peak, and/or when cognitive problem solving is not operating optimally. The frustration and anxiety that invariably accompany mental illness tend to exacerbate the tension of not being able to resolve a conflict, and so the people involved (the recovering person and the family) become caught in a spiral of intense distress, ineffective problem solving, and mounting interpersonal conflicts.

Interventions for social–environmental conflict involve combinations of education, skills training, and contingency management. Problem-solving skills are usually the most important in the skills training component, as they have high generalizability and capitalize on the participants' common sense and interpersonal affiliations. It is often useful to teach significant individuals in the recovering person's social environment the rudiments of contingency management, as they are often the individuals who control salient antecedents and consequences. Strengthening psychophysiological skills is also often important. As the term *expressed emotion* implies, people in the social environment of a person with mental illness often find themselves operating at unnecessarily (even counterproductively) high levels of emotional arousal. These emotions generally range from anger and frustration to an overwhelming sense of needing to care for and do things for the recovering person. Bringing these emotions within a more manageable range is often helpful and gratifying for all involved.

All of these principles are incorporated in specially adapted versions of family-based interventions, in particular, behavioral family therapy. Original research studies and meta-analyses confirm that such interventions contribute substantially to rehabilitation outcome (de Jesus-Marie & Streiner, 1994; Lam, 1991). The mechanisms by which family therapy enhances recovery are currently the subject of research. There are probably multiple mechanisms. Family members learn how to reduce the stress associated with their interactions with the recovering person, how to engage in productive problem solving, and how to carry out contingency management programs so as to provide incentives for appropriate behavior and recovery. By participating in contingency management, the family can play a key role in helping the recovering person to generalize to community settings the behaviors and skills acquired in a more intensive treatment milieu.

An extensive literature and continuing educational opportunities are available that facilitate acquisition of the necessary clinical skills (Birchwood & Cochrane, 1992; Falloon, 1990; Falloon, Boyd, & McGill, 1984; Goldstein, 1991; Hogarty et al., 1986; Kuipers, Leff, & Lam, 1992; McFarlane & Cunningham, 1996; Mueser & Glynn, 1995; Snyder & Liberman, 1981). There has been no systematic research on the technical and professional background prerequisites to working successfully with families in rehabilitation for mental illness, but working with family groups in any clinical context is generally understood to require some specialized skills. Until research demonstrates otherwise, it should probably be presumed that a modicum of general training in family interventions is a prerequisite to effectively administering the more specific techniques that have known effectiveness in the rehabilitation of people with mental illness.

## Restrictive Legal Status

Restrictive legal status is a serious and enduring problem for many people with disabling mental illness. Often, changing the behavior of the identified patient is only the first of many steps required to manage this type of problem. Not only must the recovering person change, but a judge or mental health board must accept that the change is meaningful and the original reasons for the person's legal status have been resolved. Achieving this acceptance may require a separate set of skills, including persuasive skills. In addition to the various behavior change techniques previously discussed, the approach of therapeutic jurisprudence provides a systematic way of minimizing conflict and enhancing mutual benefit between an identified patient and the legal system.

The rehabilitation team should consider including restrictive legal status as a separate problem on the rehabilitation plan when there is evidence that the recovering person's behavioral functioning is not the sole determinant of his or her legal status, and that systematic interactions between the recovering person, the rest of the rehabilitation team, and the legal system will be necessary to optimize rehabilitation progress and recovery.

## Unstable Living Conditions

The disproportionate representation of people with mental illness among the homeless population highlights the problematic significance of unstable living conditions. Dealing with such problems is the traditional domain of social work, but special considerations are needed when working with people with disabling mental illness. In recent years, a number of special approaches have evolved in efforts to coordinate access to housing with rehabilitation programs that emphasize development of housekeeping, personal management, and related skills. Similarly, an unstable living condition is often associated with deficient occupational and vocational skills and unavailability of work or other daytime activities. Skills training alone is often insufficient to resolve this problem; special environmental supports (e.g., residential programs capable of applying contingency management) are needed to maintain a stable lifestyle.

The rehabilitation team should consider listing unstable living condition as a problem on the rehabilitation plan when there is evidence that the recovering person's living status cannot be resolved solely through improvements in independent living skills. Typically, the intervention for this problem requires social work consultation and assistance for the purpose of identifying a suitable domestic arrangement and assisting the recovering person in gaining access to that arrangement.

# Part III

## THE ORGANIZATIONAL CONTEXT OF REHABILITATION

Part I described the conceptual framework of an integrated paradigm for assessment, treatment, and rehabilitation of people with disabling mental illness. Part II described the array of assessment and intervention technology necessary to address the heterogeneous needs of recovering people. In this final section, the discussion turns to practical and procedural issues of implementation. Chapter 11 focuses on the rehabilitation *team* and describes the clinical roles and procedural mechanisms by which the team members apply the principles of the integrated paradigm, including the selection and evaluation of rehabilitation interventions. Chapter 12 focuses on the rehabilitation *program* and describes the environmental and administrative conditions that optimize the functioning of rehabilitation teams, and that provide services in the most effective and cost-efficient way.

# Chapter 11

# The Rehabilitation Team

## Structures and Processes

The breadth and complexity of assessment and intervention technology, as described in Part II, demonstrate the importance of a team approach in rehabilitation. Although team approaches have long been an accepted part of mental health services, the particular type of team approach required by the integrated paradigm is different, in rationale and application, from traditional approaches.

### AN OVERVIEW OF ORGANIZATIONAL
### CHANGES IN HEALTH CARE

In the traditional medical model, assessment and decision-making responsibilities ultimately rest with a single person, the *attending physician*. The team members are either consultants, whose opinion the attending physician may seek on particular matters, or extensions of the attending physician, performing assessment and treatment functions under direction. The economic necessity of this type of arrangement is created by the fact that, in many cases, medical care would be prohibitively expensive if the physician were to undertake all needed clinical activities. In this sense, the team is an economically necessary extension of the physician's medical practice.

A corollary concept in this traditional team approach is that the team members' respective knowledge and skills all represent subsets of the physician's. The nonphysician team members, usually identified as *allied health professionals* in medical model argot, are understood to possess some limited repertoire with which they perform functions that the physician would otherwise have to do. Because the nonphysician members have more limited skills, they command lower fees, and services are thus less costly. The quality of care is presumed to be preserved, however, because all key deci-

251

sions are made by the team member with superordinate knowledge, the attending physician.

This most traditional view of treatment teams gradually became less viable across the various domains of health care over the course of the 20th century. As technology became more complex and diverse, it was decreasingly realistic to expect that a single individual could command the technological expertise sufficient to address all of a patient's needs. In response came a proliferation of medical specialties, which continues to characterize the health care landscape today. An important part of this specialization process was the emergence of *primary provider* specialties. A hierarchical system developed wherein certain specialists—family practitioners (formerly, general practitioners), internists, and pediatricians—perform a central, coordinating role of referring patients to other specialists, or *secondary providers*, in response to identification of particular health problems. Neither primary nor secondary provider is subordinate, and clinical responsibilities are passed back and forth, as circumstances demand.

As nonmedical disciplines developed higher and more specialized levels of technological skill, these primary–secondary referral systems increasingly included nonphysician professionals, such as dentists, optometrists, podiatrists, nurse practitioners, pharmacists, physical therapists, social workers, occupational therapists, psychologists, and so on. Current health care services include a variety of treatment team structures, both traditional and nontraditional, sometimes side by side. For example, surgical teams are typically directed by a single physician/surgeon, with the other members performing highly constrained and specified roles. However, surgery also usually includes the participation of a physician specialized in controlling pain and maintaining physiological stability, the anesthesiologist, who is not considered subordinate to the surgeon. In complex surgical situations, different surgeons may preside at different points during a single operation. Family health care typically involves a number of specialized professionals, some operating as subordinates, some operating as independent providers, and some as consultants in collaboration with a primary family physician.

Current practice statutes and regulations create a range of degrees between "subordinate," in the traditional sense, and "independent provider." For example, a variety of professionals are licensed to independently provide services (e.g., psychotherapists or physical therapists), although in some circumstances they do so upon referral by, and/or under the direction of, another professional. Accreditation standards are generally designed to accommodate this degree of local variability; however, doing so is an ongoing task in the rapidly evolving health care communities. A current development in this regard is the concept of *supervising independent practitioner* as a substitute for the traditional status of the attending physician. An independent practitioner is one licensed to provide health care services without supervision or direction. Dentists, optometrists, and pharmacists are among the nonphysician professionals who historically have practiced independently. Increasingly, nurse practitioners and psychologists are accorded this status. There are still substantial differences from one statutory venue to the next. Nevertheless, in regulatory and accreditation language, it is generally proving workable to substitute "licensed independent practitioners practicing within their legal scope" for "licensed physicians."

In psychiatry, and especially in psychiatric institutions, more traditional conceptualizations of the treatment team have tended to persist. Even in settings that ostensibly provide rehabilitation for people with mental illness, the typical team configuration includes a psychiatrist as "team leader," with ultimate authority over all clinical decisions, who directs the other team members to perform assessment, supportive, and therapeutic services. This configuration has been sustained by the infrastructure of health care standards and regulations that historically required a physician to oversee all aspects of a patient's care (especially in hospitals and psychiatric institutions, which are more subject to such regulation). However, the development of the independent practitioner status is changing that reality, even in hospitals. Nonphysicians increasingly perform roles comparable to that of attending physicians, reconceptualized on treatment teams as the role of supervising independent practitioner. Thus neither law nor accreditation practices necessarily require that physicians be "the team leaders" or have comprehensive oversight of mental health services. Nevertheless, guild politics have yielded slowly to changing times, and in many venues, psychiatrists and their professional organizations resist any and all distribution of professional prerogatives to nonpsychiatrists.

A major factor in the evolution of health care team processes has been the issue of legal responsibility and liability. Traditionally, the attending physician is understood to be the individual with whom all legal responsibility lies, because that person exercises control and direction over all aspects of health care. This point often arises in an inverted form in discussions of professional prerogatives. In medical model mental health settings, for example, the argument is often made that a psychiatrist must have superordinate prerogatives over all clinical decisions because the psychiatrist is legally liable for the consequences of such decisions. This is circular logic. The courts have proved quite capable of making fine distinctions between domains of accountability in health care, including mental health. The liability of any professional is determined by the arrangements and agreements that obtain to a particular situation, not the other way around. Even in traditional medical model settings, psychiatrists are not held liable for decisions or events over which they have no control. It is an administrative task to define the boundaries of prerogative and liability in a particular service setting or agency. It is never adequate to simply attribute ultimate liability to *any* individual. The particulars of who is responsible for what must be worked out in detail. Generally, the most stable and cost-effective approach to defining and distributing liability is to take advantage of the full statutory scope of practice of every professional involved in rehabilitation, define responsibility in terms of specific decisions or acts made by individuals, and use a clinical recording and documentation system that clearly shows how decisions are being made and by whom. (This aspect is discussed further in Chapter 12.)

Developments within the medical regulatory and accreditation industry are relevant to rehabilitation to the degree that the boundaries between "health care" and "rehabilitation" are porous or amorphous. The tension between the medical and rehabilitation fields is ubiquitous and longstanding. In a traditional medical model, rehabilitation is generally understood to be a subset of medicine, suggesting that the structures of authority and decision making remain the same. Nonphysician rehabilitation professionals tend to view this issue differently, even as they also recognize the importance of continuity and complementarity between medical and rehabilitative services. When psychiatric rehabilitation was evolving in the late 20th century (discussed in Chapter 1), this issue was the subject of some debate, framed primarily in terms of whether "treatment" is separate from, or part of, comprehensive rehabilitation. In the integrated paradigm, the debate itself is understood as an unhelpful product of neo-Kraepelinian assumptions. There is no real boundary between medical care and rehabilitation, any more than a real boundary exists between schizophrenia and other severe, disabling mental illnesses. The *appearance* of a boundary is created by historical precedents, health care economics, and guild politics. There are both similarities and differences in the medical services required to address, for example, a neurophysiological dysregulation associated with mental illness versus diabetes mellitus. The issue for rehabilitation is not "what is medical and what is not," but which assessments and interventions are required to sufficiently address particular problems, across all levels of human functioning.

A rhetorical distinction is sometimes made between multidisciplinary teams and interdisciplinary teams (Davis et al. 1993; Fordyce, 1982; Mullins, Keller, & Chaney, 1994). Discussions of clinical team processes that do not make this distinction should be interpreted with caution. *Multidisciplinary* teams are ones whose members function relatively autonomously, each pursuing goals identified in the course of separate within-discipline assessments. *Interdisciplinary* teams are ones whose members function in a more integrated and coordinated way, following a treatment plan that incorporates assessment information from all disciplines (and individuals) into a unified set of goals and coordinated provision of services. The traditional medical model assumption of a single physician providing overarching leadership would arguably encourage a more interdisciplinary approach, in that a single leader would be in a position to unify and coordinate all aspects of care. However, in practice, this is very much determined by the personality of the physician team leader. Individuals who respect the contributions of nonmedical professionals encourage interdisciplinary organization, while those who do not tend to preside over a multidisciplinary organization. In the integrated paradigm, team organization is determined by the nature of the problems and the technologies, not by the personality of selected team members. *Interdisciplinary* organization is better suited to the enterprise of rehabilitating people with disabling mental illness.

## REHABILITATION TEAM ROLES IN THE INTEGRATED PARADIGM

As discussed in Chapter 3, in the integrated paradigm the rehabilitation team consists of the recovering person, significant others in the recovering person's social environment (family, friends, colleagues, etc.) and providers of rehabilitation services. The team is usually created when the recovering person, a substitute decision maker, or a legal authority seeks services from an individual provider or agency. As is discussed in Chapter 12, providing appropriate personnel to form individual rehabilitation teams is the central role of a rehabilitation agency or program.

The specific representation of clinical disciplines and specialties on a rehabilitation team will vary over time, as the recovering person's rehabilitation needs evolve. Similarly, the particular activities performed by team members from various disciplines will vary, due to variation in local practice statutes and individual backgrounds. It is therefore unhelpful to define rehabilitation teams in terms of specific professions, disciplines, or individuals (with one exception, discussed below). However, it is possible to identify particular *roles* that generally need to be performed by one team member or another. Team members often perform more than one role, and roles are sometimes passed back and forth, as circumstances change and rehabilitation and recovery progress.

### The Role of the Recovering Person

Obviously, this is the exception to the rule that roles are not isomorphic with individual team members. The recovering person has the most important role on the team: (1) to express the desires and preferences that are critical to the success of rehabilitation, (2) to participate as the recipient of the services, and ultimately to define what constitutes recovery and rehabilitation success for him or her. The recovering person also provides important information on the subjective experience of the mental illness and of the rehabilitation and recovery processes. Finally, the recovering person must make choices and give consent, as the team considers the various clinical decisions involved in the rehabilitation enterprise.

## The Role of Substitute Decision Maker

The nature of disabling mental illness is such that sometimes a legally appointed substitute decision maker is involved in the rehabilitation endeavor. Although terminology and rules vary across legal venues, a substitute decision maker is generally a *guardian*, who has broad purview and responsibilities for making decisions, or a *conservator*, whose purview is constrained to financial decisions. Family members often agree to be guardians or conservators. Attorneys and mental health service providers sometimes function in this role, sometimes for a fee, sometimes pro bono.

Increasingly, the law provides for very specific and circumscribed roles for substitute decision makers. A *limited guardianship* specifies the particular domains in which the guardian is to make decisions on the recovering person's behalf, and in what circumstances. Limited guardianships are relatively new to the field of mental illness rehabilitation. Considerable scholarly work and new application in this area, especially in the approach of therapeutic jurisprudence, are likely to emerge in the next few years. Whatever the particular substitute decision-making provisions in a particular case, it is important for the rehabilitation team to understand, in detail, how the provisions will affect the recovering person's participation in the rehabilitation enterprise. Consultation with the recovering person's attorney or other legal authority should always be considered to ensure accurate and complete understanding of the provisions of the case. (For a review of substitute decision makers and related issues in rehabilitation, see Spaulding et al., 2000.)

Sometimes a recovering person's substitute decision maker is a court or civil commitment board, in the sense that the person's decision to participate in treatment and/or rehabilitation is mandated, to some degree, by that entity. The legal authority typically does not function as a team member, in the sense of participating in the assessment, planning, and implementation of rehabilitation. Rather, it mandates services (usually in some specified setting), reviews and approves treatment and/or rehabilitation plans, and approves changes in the recovering person's legal status, as requested by the recovering person and/or the rest of the team.

Recently, models have evolved that specify more direct participation by courts in mental health services, especially in the area of treatment for substance abuse problems (Belenko, 2002). To the degree that such problems are among the ones associated with disabling mental illness, these models may become important in rehabilitation (Monahan et al., 2001; Watson, Luchins, Hanrahan, Heyman, & Lurigio, 2000). As with limited guardianship, there is considerable interest in, and controversy about, developing this type of substitute decision-making process for use with people who have disabling mental illness. In particular, the concept of *outpatient commitment* is being intensively studied and implemented in many legal venues (reviewed by Ridgely, Borum, & Petrila, 2001). Outpatient commitment allows a legal authority to relax the criterion of "clear and present danger" generally used in inpatient commitment and to compel participation in community-based services. This coercion is justified when clinical data indicate that a "clear and present danger" will develop unless the person participates in services. However, there is much debate about which domains of consent are included under the rubric of traditional commitment, let alone new and modified versions. The next few years will see important developments in this domain, and rehabilitation professionals will have to keep abreast of the developments. Meanwhile, rehabilitation professionals need to become sufficiently informed about how court supervision and other mechanisms of substitute decision making work in their particular practice venues, and to verify that the team processes are congruent with those mechanisms. It is of particular note that the limited amount of empirical evidence available on the clinical impact of outpatient commitment indicates that there is little or no benefit without modern rehabilitation services (Steadman et al., 1999; Swartz et al., 2001).

As of this writing, U.S. Supreme Court rulings suggest that legal commitment does not necessarily confer a right to treatment. In other words, legal authorities may incarcerate people or otherwise abridge their civil rights, on the grounds that they have a mental illness, without the expectation or intent to provide treatment to address the mental illness. The context of this ruling concerns sex offenders found to be mentally ill, so it is unclear how the ruling may apply to people with disabling mental illness. It could have a broad and significant impact on modified forms of mandated treatment (e.g., outpatient commitment), but as of this writing, it is too early to determine exactly what that impact will be. Other Supreme Court rulings, especially concerning the applicability to the Americans with Disabilities Act, appear to affirm that individuals with mental illness or developmental disabilities have a right to live in the least restrictive and most normal circumstances that their functioning permits—which suggests that rehabilitative services must be provided to such individuals.

## The Role of Supervising Independent Practitioner

As noted, the role of a supervising independent practitioner is roughly comparable to the traditional role of the attending physician or the primary provider in a family health care system. The person who performs this role must have comprehensive knowledge and experience specific to the field of mental illness rehabilitation. This expertise must include psycholegal considerations as well as clinical considerations, as traditionally understood (e.g., issues of substitute decision making, as discussed above). The key role of this team member is to provide continuity and context over the course of rehabilitation by taking primary responsibility for the narrative formulation of the rehabilitation plan, which expresses the team's collective understanding of the recovering person's assets and liabilities, the barriers to recovery, and the overall strategy for overcoming those barriers (discussed in Chapter 3). Similarly, the supervising independent practitioner functions as the "institutional memory" of the team by providing the conceptual mortar that maintains the logical integrity of the rehabilitation plan over the (sometimes protracted) course of rehabilitation and recovery.

The primacy of case formulation and planning in the supervising practitioner's role requires that he or she have comprehensive expertise in the assessment modalities central to rehabilitation, particularly functional assessment and functional analysis of behavior. Applying this expertise, the supervising practitioner plays a key role by identifying the clinical issues that need assessment and ensuring that the appropriate assessments are conducted and appropriately interpreted.

Rehabilitation counseling is closely associated with these responsibilities, although the role of rehabilitation counselor is not necessarily performed by just one person. The supervising practitioner is expected to play a central part in rehabilitation counseling, especially early in the process when the most fundamental understandings are being established. However, rehabilitation counseling is an ongoing process. The recovering person's desires and goals often change, and these changes must inform the ongoing development and modification of the narrative formulation and the rehabilitation plan. It is often efficient for a designated team member (not necessarily the supervising practitioner) to assume the primary responsibility for ongoing rehabilitation counseling.

In many contexts, the supervising practitioner also provides professional oversight—that is, he or she provides the assurance, required by health care regulations and accreditation standards, that all aspects of the recovering person's condition and situation are being addressed appropriately. In these contexts, a professional credential recognized as representing the legal status of "independent practitioner" is a prerequisite to performing this role.

The role of supervising practitioner carries much conceptual and emotional "baggage" from its history in traditional medical models of mental health services. Mental health providers often have considerable difficulty integrating the primary–secondary provider concept into team functioning, even when their own health care is managed by a primary provider family physician who works in collaboration with nonsubordinate secondary providers. Because of concerns about liability and responsibility, psychiatrists often feel compelled to exercise superordinate authority at their own personal discretion, and other providers often feel compelled to cede professional prerogatives to the team psychiatrist. This dynamic is enabled by the Kraepelinian assumption that the most important information pertinent to treatment (i.e., the information needed to make a diagnosis) is reliably obtained in limited, interview-based office encounters between the patient and the psychiatrist, who is the only team member qualified to collect and interpret such information (as in the physical examination in medicine). Often, information from the office encounters is the psychiatrist's sole source, and it takes precedence over any information reported by subordinate providers. As nonphysician roles continue to evolve in the health care field, psychiatrists experience a mounting incentive to assert authority by overriding the decisions of other team members. Overriding team members' decisions is incompatible with the integrated paradigm; it creates a risk to the recovering person in the form of exposure to counterproductive and even toxic interpersonal processes.

The phenomenon of "staff splitting" is familiar even in traditional medical model settings. When differences of opinion among team members are "resolved" through the unilateral action of one member, the recovering person is compelled to exercise interpersonal strategies that are seldom useful in more normal social contexts. Instead of engaging in collaborative decision making and striving for a consensual view of treatment and rehabilitation, the incentive is to develop a "special" relationship with the superordinate team member so that team decisions can be subverted. In traditional medical model settings, different team members usually have different information about what is going on with the recovering person, and often the psychiatrist has the least information (again, this is enabled by Kraepelinian assumptions). Most mental health providers with experience in institutional psychiatric settings have observed the results of this situation. Patients develop interpersonal skills that serve short-term purposes, such as getting privileges or avoiding the natural consequences of inappropriate behavior, by concentrating on manipulating the impressions and judgments of the team psychiatrist. These skills serve them poorly in more normative settings, and so a new incentive is created to stay in environments where the skills are more often rewarded (i.e., institutional settings). To stay in such settings, one is compelled to perform the social role of a mental patient. This dynamic of staff splitting is thus a major contributing factor to the "institutionalization" behavior adopted by recovering individuals.

In this context, staff splitting skills have an interesting developmental parallel. Most parents are well aware of the dangers of one parent overruling the decisions of another through private arrangements with a child, or more generally, of failing to communicate with each other to ensure parental consensus. The shorter-term consequences of this dynamic are marital stress, but the longer-term consequence is the child's development of inappropriate and ineffective interpersonal skills. For the most part, a person is better served by skills that support open discussion, negotiation and achieving social consensus, rather than covert manipulation and subversion. In this sense, rehabilitation recapitulates an important developmental process.

Staff splitting and related processes could be reduced (theoretically) through the maturity, insight, and professional integrity of the psychiatrist, even in institutional medical model settings. However, the ubiquity of institutionalized behavior in mental health systems suggests that it is unrealistic to rely on single individuals to counteract such compelling and pervasive environmental forces. Prevention of institutionalization requires a social infrastructure that systematically eliminates opportunities to engage in, and reinforcement of, institutionalized behavior. The presence of this characteristic is doubtless a major factor in the superiority of social learning-based rehabilitation in institutional settings.

It is a crucial aspect of program administration in rehabilitation to create the social infrastructure and staff attitudes most conducive to appropriate performance of the supervising practitioner role (discussed further in Chapter 12). *All* providers, not just psychiatrists, must have a full understanding and appreciation of the vicissitudes of clinical authority, the nature of primary–secondary provider relationships, the potential toxicity of staff splitting, and the importance of precisely delineating the roles and responsibilities of individual providers. The institutional incentives to perform an inappropriately subordinate role can be just as strong as the incentives to perform a toxic, superordinate role. As is discussed later in this chapter, the assessment and decision-making infrastructure of the integrated paradigm plays a key role in supporting appropriate performance of the supervising practitioner's role.

## The Role of Case Manager or Coordinator

Usually the rehabilitation of people with disabling mental illness requires collaboration among a number of individuals, sometimes across multiple provider agencies. The recovering person participates in rehabilitative activities in a number of venues, including clinics, residential settings, work locations, and leisure environments. Information about the recovering person's functioning and progress must be collected from all of these and assembled for analysis by the team. Often, the risk of episodic neurophysiological dysregulation (psychotic relapse) demands close but coordinated monitoring of the person's daily functioning in one or more of these set-tings. Often, too, there are procedural or logistical problems that prevent full implementation of a rehabilitation plan, and these problems must be detected and brought to the attention of the team. Team decision making requires periodic meetings and conferences. All these demands usually re-quire assigning a team member to a clinical and logistical coordinating role. In traditional mental health parlance, this is the role of the case manager.

Considerable research and development on case management in reha-bilitation for disabling mental illness emerged in the last decade of the 20th century (reviewed by Mueser, Bond, Drake, & Resnick, 1998). A number of approaches are now available, some of which are based on traditional medical model treatment concepts and some of which are more suitable for rehabilitation. The case management role in rehabilitation tends to be more complicated, because rehabilitation is more complicated and involves a greater diversity of specific services and processes. However, concepts of case management and rehabilitation are still in a state of flux, and some-times it is difficult to distinguish a case management model from a model for actual treatment and rehabilitation. Terminology has become convo-luted and sometimes meaningless. Programs for Assertive Case Manage-ment (PACT) is the most prominent example (Allness & Knoedler, 1998; Monroe-DeVita & Mohatt, 1999).

PACT originated during the era in which psychiatric rehabilitation was emerging. It was conceived not just as a model for case management but as a comprehensive approach to rehabilitation for mental illness. Community-based services were emphasized, in part, because it was seen primarily as an alternative to institutionalization early in the deinstitutionalization move-ment. A number of contemporary rehabilitation modalities, most impor-tantly, living skills training and social skills training, were considered part and parcel of the PACT approach. PACT has continued to develop in a manner true to its original form, even to the degree that there is now a pub-lished manual that describes in detail how to run a PACT program (Allness & Knoedler, 1998). Unfortunately, however, the PACT concept underwent some degradation in many mental health venues, and was often replaced by a less sophisticated, more medically disposed model. The rehabilitative mo-dalities were often dropped, leaving only the outreach-oriented case man-agement component and psychotropic medication. Despite protests from the original PACT community, downgraded programs proliferated (often labeled ACT programs to distinguish them from the original PACT model). The downgraded programs were seen as cheap ways of maintaining people with disabling mental illness by minimizing hospitalization. The reduced prospects for recovery that resulted from removal of the original rehabilita-tion focus is not important to policymakers focused on fiscal restraint (see discussions in Burns & Santos, 1995; Steinwachs, 1997).

THE ORGANIZATIONAL CONTEXT OF REHABILITATION

There is little evidence that case management, alone or in combination with medical model treatment, facilitates recovery from severe disabling mental illness. The considerable body of research on the effectiveness of PACT shows inconsistent results; compared to no services or traditional medical model services limited to medication and case management, PACT appears to be more effective at reducing hospitalization, which is a worthy end in itself (Mueser et al., 1998). However, it is doubtful that simply reducing hospitalization brings about recovery (i.e., sustained normalization of personal and social functioning) for most people with severe and disabling mental illness. PACT programs that include the original complement of rehabilitative modalities, especially skills training, appear to produce the best prospects for actual recovery. There is thus considerable reason to believe that case management within the PACT model is an important component of comprehensive rehabilitation.

The integrated paradigm does not require or subscribe to any particular case management model. It is assumed that different models are suitable for different settings. Unlike some views of PACT, the integrated paradigm does not assume that rehabilitation can only occur in community (as opposed to institutional) settings. However, the particular skills required of a case manager in an institutional setting (e.g., a state hospital) are not necessarily identical to the skills required in a community-based setting. The specific skills required in a particular setting may determine which professional background is most suitable for the task. For example, a nursing background may be most suitable in a hospital setting, while a social work background may be most suitable in a community setting. The setting in which a person is served generally changes over the course of rehabilitation, so the role of case manager may usefully pass from one team member to another. During transitional periods (e.g., in a hospital admission or discharge process) the case manager role can be divided between two members, reflecting the two settings or environments involved in the transition. Furthermore, the parameters of case management need to be established within the context of specific service programs to accommodate local circumstances (discussed further in Chapter 12). In short, most rehabilitation teams have a need for case management of some kind, and in most cases a specific team member is given that role.

## The Role of Skills Trainer

Rehabilitation of people with disabling mental illness almost always involves considerable skills training across a number of domains (discussed in Chapter 10). Assessment and intervention produce large amounts of clinical data, all of which must be processed in order to ar-

rive at a complete picture of the recovering person's strengths and liabilities, and of progress toward recovery. Usually, multiple team members
have skills training roles and can represent this perspective in team deliberations. Typically, multiple skills trainers are involved in an individual
rehabilitation plan. These skills trainers may be widely dispersed across
the settings in which rehabilitation occurs. Ideally, everyone who provides
any skills training would participate in all team deliberations; the direct
observations of these trainers can contribute important information to
the team's assessment and progress evaluations. However, such routine
participation is often impractical. Teams require frequent meetings to
conduct their business, and scheduling meetings can be prohibitively difficult when too many people are included. It is often efficacious to have liaison mechanisms, as part of a service program's organizational structure,
that ensure communication between team members and skills trainers
who are not routinely present at team meetings.

Providing skills training requires a substantial amount of expertise, although this expertise is not unique to any particular discipline or profession. It is usually not cost-efficient to include skills training activities in the
role of supervising practitioner or psychopharmacotherapist. A central
component of program administration (discussed in Chapter 12) is one of
ensuring that cost-efficient skills training services are available to rehabilitation teams.

## The Role of Milieu Coordinator

One of the most important concepts in social learning models of rehabilitation is recognition of the therapeutic power of the providers who spend the
most amount of time with the recovering person. To emphasize their central role in the rehabilitation process, Paul and Lentz (1977) termed these
individuals *change agents*. In institutional settings, the change agent is the
psychiatric technician or aide. In community-based rehabilitation this may
mean residential staff, workplace staff, family members or others, depending on the particular setting. Change agents generally implement contingency management and other milieu-based interventions and maintain a
supportive or therapeutic milieu. The direct involvement of change agents
in the assessment, planning, and progress evaluation process is absolutely
critical. As with skills trainers, it is usually impractical to include all the
change agents involved in a person's rehabilitation on the team. It is therefore necessary to designate at least one person on the rehabilitation team as
the *milieu coordinator*, whose role it is to facilitate communication between
all the change agents in all the milieus pertinent to the recovering person's
rehabilitation and the rest of the rehabilitation team. Often, it is most effi-

cient for this person to be the clinical supervisor of the change agents as well. The case manager role is complementary to the milieu coordinator role, and often one team member performs both roles.

## The Role of Psychopharmacotherapist

This role is perhaps the most difficult to efficiently manage. Professionals qualified to prescribe medication are generally the most expensive, and their time must be carefully allotted. At times (e.g., during acute psychosis) intensive psychopharmacotherapeutic services are required. In the assessment phases of planning, the psychopharmacotherapist is centrally involved in the evaluation of neurophysiological dysregulation and making distinctions between neurophysiological and other problems. As discussed in several of the preceding chapters, this assessment process often involves protracted sequences of medication trials and functional behavioral analysis. As rehabilitation progresses and neurophysiological stabilization is achieved and the focus turns to skills acquisition, there may be long periods in which minimal participation by the psychopharmacotherapist is needed. However, relapses do occur, and intensive participation may be needed on short notice. Furthermore, as rehabilitation progresses, medication issues must be revisited periodically to ensure an optimal regimen in relation to the recovering person's changing environment and personal functioning. Substantial administrative flexibility is required to ensure the involvement of the psychopharmacotherapist when it is needed while controlling costs when it is not.

As with the role of supervising practitioner, the role of psychopharmacotherapist carries some significant "baggage" from its history in traditional medical models. In some medical model views, pharmacological intervention is the only "real treatment" in psychiatry, because it is believed to be the only one that addresses the biological origins of the disease. In this view, it is inappropriate for nonphysician providers to play a role in psychopharmacological decisions. Medical model ideas about the "doctor–patient" relationship sometimes lead to a belief that medication decisions are a private matter, not subject to scrutiny by, or involvement of, other individuals. In the integrated paradigm's biosystemic perspective, this insulation is unrealistic and counterproductive. Evaluation of psychotropic drug effects cannot be performed on the basis of office-based interviews. Data from all quarters of the recovering person's world must be collected, compiled, and interpreted. No single provider can accomplish this comprehensive task. Effective pharmacotherapy for people with severe and disabling mental illness requires a highly coordinated team effort, in which the psychopharmacotherapist is a central, but not separate, participant.

In the traditional medical model, a psychiatrist performs the dual roles of psychopharmacotherapist and supervising practitioner. As the health care professions evolve and other practitioners develop supervisory expertise, this dual role is decreasingly necessary or cost-efficient. Furthermore, as rehabilitation and psychopharmacological technologies proliferate, it will be decreasingly realistic to expect a single professional to have sufficient expertise in both fields. Advanced nurse practitioners, clinical pharmacists, and psychologists are currently acquiring psychopharmacological expertise and practice privileges. As rehabilitation becomes more widespread in community settings, family physicians become candidates for this role. Short of prescribing practice, many disciplines have increasing knowledge about psychopharmacology; often, other members of the team are able to make contributions to the assessment and progress evaluation process in this domain. Utilizing other team members' expertise is especially useful in cases involving long-term rehabilitation for mental illness, because psychiatrists are increasingly engaged in dealing with special problems (e.g., atypical responses to medications, intractable side effects, and medical complications) rather than routine psychopharmacological issues. The role performed by the psychiatrist in the integrated paradigm will probably evolve into one of providing consultation on special or unusual medical–behavioral complications, rather than serving as an ongoing team member.

The role of psychopharmacotherapist on a rehabilitation team in the integrated paradigm is substantially different from the traditional role in mental health services. The traditional model of psychopharmacotherapy uses office-based assessment of the "patient's" mental status, with a focus on identifying neo-Kraepelinian symptoms as targets for treatment, and typically does not include systematic consideration of information from the person's social environment. When such information is considered, it is usually anecdotal, seldom objective or quantitative. In the integrated paradigm, this type of assessment is insufficient to reliably determine the role of neurophysiological dysregulation in the recovering person's overall functioning. As discussed in Chapter 4, anamnestic information is notoriously unreliable by itself. Ongoing functional behavioral analysis, neuropsychological assessment, and other data sources are crucial to creating successful interventions for people with severe, disabling mental illness. The recovering person's functioning at all levels and in all pertinent environmental settings must be taken into account. The psychopharmacotherapist serves as a full participant in the collective assessment and progress evaluation activities of the team. Even with the dissemination of psychopharmacological expertise to practitioners in other disciplines, service models continue to adhere to a traditional office-interview format. Hopefully, an evolution in the training of rehabilitation-based psychopharmacotherapists will occur over the next few years, so that the special skills and procedures necessary to function as an effective team member will be more familiar to all. Similarly, developments in health care economics may resolve the fiscal barrier that prevents highly paid psychopharmacologists from spending the required time collaborating directly in the team process.

## DECISION MAKING IN THE REHABILITATION TEAM

As discussed in Chapter 3, the decision making in rehabilitation is both a social and a technological process. Even though human problems may have technological solutions, the *meaning* of any problem—indeed, the very fact that a problem exists—is created by social circumstances. Therefore, the specific means by which problems are addressed and the criteria by which their resolution is judged are the products of social processes. The rehabilitation team serves as a crucible in which social and technological considerations are reduced to their elements, then recombined into an integrated and comprehensive plan of action. The mechanisms by which groups of individuals create complex solutions to complex problems are themselves enormously complex, whether the group is engaged in rehabilitation of mental illness or building an airport. Cognitive and social sciences have only just begun to discern the processes and mechanisms of group-based endeavors. Meanwhile, a working understanding of these processes and mechanisms can be achieved by framing them in terms of the specific *decisions* that mark the course of assessment, intervention, and progress evaluation. For the purposes of rehabilitation, a fairly complete account of team functioning can be expressed in terms of the specific decisions the team must make, when they must make them, and the general principles by which the decisions are made.

The most global decisions the team must make—whether to embark on the rehabilitation enterprise, the team's composition, and in what settings or environments rehabilitation will proceed—are often determined by circumstance and/or social policy as much as by actual team decisions. For example, the recovering person may arrive at the rehabilitation option through the actions of a legal authority or a substitute decision maker. The composition of the team may be determined by the resources available under the auspices of a rehabilitation program. If such circumstances do not apply, then the initial steps in the decision making process—that is, committing to the rehabilitation enterprise and assembling the rehabilitation team—are typically taken by the recovering person, the independent supervising practitioner, and a substitute decision maker (when applicable). Otherwise, the fully assembled team may be involved from the outset. Taking these contingencies into account, the rehabilitation process can be formulated as a set of relatively straightforward decisions.

1. *Decide whether rehabilitation is an appropriate approach for enhancing recovery.* The central consideration in this decision is whether a person with disabling mental illness can be expected to enjoy the greatest possible recovery without rehabilitation. The only circumstance that would rule out rehabilitation before it starts would be the person's complete recovery—that is, return of personal and social functioning to premorbid levels. The only way to determine whether rehabilitation will enhance recovery beyond the degree that occurs spontaneously is to commit to it and evaluate its effects. Essentially, this means that anyone with disabilities associated with mental illness should be considered a candidate for rehabilitation until proven otherwise.

2. *Decide which domains of personal and social functioning need to be addressed, and which resources the team will need to address them.* The nature of severe mental illness is such that barriers to optimal functioning may be found in any and all levels of organismic functioning. By the time it is established that a person's mental illness has produced actual disabilities, as opposed to more temporary disruptions of functioning, the case history typically includes information to determine which levels of functioning those disabilities involve. However, the case history provides only preliminary indications. As rehabilitation progresses, the nature of functional impairments becomes more fully understood. Which domains need assessment and intervention must be continually reassessed, and resources brought to the Team accordingly.

3. *Decide which assets and liabilities will be pertinent to rehabilitation and recovery.* This endeavor involves an assessment that is preliminary to actual construction of the rehabilitation plan. A personal liability is not necessarily a problem in the formal sense, though it may have an influence on rehabilitation strategy. For example, illiteracy is not necessarily a consequence of mental illness, but it is expected to require compensatory planning, especially for skills training interventions. Similarly, an asset is not simply the absence of a problem but a special quality that may enhance rehabilitation and/or figure in the formulation of goals. For example, a hobby or similar interest may provide motivating incentives, opportunities to socialize, and a context in which to exercise neurocognitive or sociocognitive skills. A person's case history should include information sufficient for an initial inventory of assets and liabilities, but additional ones are expected to appear over the course of rehabilitation and recovery.

Accreditation and practice standards require a formal inventory of a person's assets and liabilities as part of the treatment or rehabilitation planning process. Some use of this information is also required, such as explicit identification of the assets relevant to particular interventions. However, there is insufficient detail in such standards to ensure that this application is meaningful, logical, or beneficial. In the integrated paradigm, interventions must be operationally defined to the degree that specific assets and liabilities that could affect response to the intervention are logically identifiable. For example, the use of written prompts, instructional posters, and similar aids in social skills training makes evident the implications of illiteracy as a liability. When liabilities do represent formally defined problems, the integrated paradigm's problem prioritization procedures characterize their impact on interventions for other problems (discussed in Chapter 3). There has been insufficient research on the process of formally identifying liabilities and assets to confidently conclude that this identification has a beneficial impact on rehabilitation. It is generally assumed that formally identifying assets helps counteract the tendency of a problem-oriented clinical approach to emphasize negative attributes and neglect a person's strengths. This possibility is arguably sufficient justification for doing an inventory, preliminary to or as part of treatment planning processes, at least pending systematic research.

4. *Decide which problems should be identified and described as the foci of rehabilitation activities.* As discussed in Chapter 3, this is the essential step in translating assessment data into a structured rehabilitation plan. A rehabilitation plan's problem list summarizes the scope and the foci of the interventions.

5. *Decide which long- and short-term goals represent rehabilitation progress.* Ultimately, the long-term goals are operational definitions of recovery and rehabilitation success for the recovering person; the short-term goals identify the landmarks the team will use to judge progress.

6. *Decide which measures will provide reliable, objective, and quantitative indicators of progress toward goals.* The integrated paradigm demands quantification of progress to the maximum degree allowed by current technology. Implementing quantification procedures requires technological judgments about which instruments provide the practical and valid measurement of progress toward the goals.

7. *Decide which interventions will best facilitate attainment of the goals.* This decision obviously requires skilled technological discernment. The team considers its collective knowledge about which available Intervention modalities would be best suited to address the recovering person's problems, taking into consideration the person's unique assets and liabilities.

8. *Decide whether the outcomes of all the preceding decisions are producing progress, as expected, toward recovery.* This decision represents the outcome of the formal progress evaluation process described in Chapter 3: whether to continue to implement the rehabilitation plan, as formulated, or modify its problem list, goals, or interventions to accommodate new information and/or new working hypotheses.

As discussed in Chapter 3, the team decision-making process is iterative; that is, it proceeds in cycles. The initial decisions must be revisited often, as the subsequent decisions generate new data, to determine whether the team's overall formulation continues to be supported by all available information. Lack of progress in rehabilitation and recovery demands revision of one or more points in the process. Chapter 3 also describes how the integrated paradigm provides a system for documenting the decision-making process and its various outcomes in the rehabilitation plan and progress evaluations.

In addition to specifying an explicit series of clinical decisions, the integrated paradigm generates a set of general principles that guide the team's collective decision-making process. It is recognized that no mental health professional commands all the technological knowledge necessary to make all the decisions involved in the rehabilitation of people with disabling mental illness. At the same time, it is acknowledged that some individuals do have special knowledge or skills that other team members do not. Furthermore, it is recognized that all members of a rehabilitation team have a stake in the decisions that the team makes. These three acknowledgments lead to two key principles of team decision making in the integrated paradigm: *decision by consensus*, and the principle of *exclusive professional purview*.

## Procedural Fidelity, Decision by Consensus, and Exclusive Professional Purview

Rehabilitation of people with disabling mental illness takes place in many settings, with the involvement of many professionals. The actions of those individuals can have a definitive impact on the success of rehabilitation. Use of terms such as "change agent" reflects this reality. It is crucial, then, that these individuals proceed with a common purpose and a common understanding of exactly what must be done to realize the rehabilitation goals.

In the integrated paradigm, common purposes and understandings are facilitated, to some degree, by the intervention technology. When the behavioral actions of providers are operative components of the rehabilitation intervention, as in skills training and contingency management, those actions are delineated in systematic procedural protocols. In a well-designed social skills training procedure, for example, a procedural manual delineates the specific skills to be addressed, the procedures for identifying the relevance of the skills to individual group members, the methods by which the skills are demonstrated and practiced, and so on. A well-designed contingency management program leaves no ambiguity about its target behavior and the antecedents and consequences to be controlled by providers. In the integrated paradigm, this level of operational definition is one more means of manifesting the overall priority for objectivity and quantitative measurement. Adherence to objectively defined and measurable procedures is increasingly recognized as necessary for effective mental health interventions.

This adherence, termed *procedural fidelity*, cannot be assured solely by the use of procedural manuals, however. In many rehabilitation interventions the key to effectiveness is not so much the skill involved in carrying out the procedure but a *robust commitment* to carry out the procedure when the time comes. This is not to say that there is no special skill involved in applying rehabilitation interventions. Of course there is, and it is necessary to ensure that the relevant providers have the appropriate skills. At the same time, the ability to carry out a procedure is not the same as the willingness or commitment to do so. As with sociobehavioral skills deficits in mental illness, competence is not the same as performance. When the relevant providers do have the relevant skills, their *commitment* to procedural fidelity is the key source of variance in clinical effectiveness. The key to creating this commitment is a consensus criterion of decision making.

Mental illness generates special challenges to providers' commitment to procedural fidelity. Interventions often seem counterintuitive, especially to inexperienced providers. Contingency management provides an especially salient example. Systematically withholding reinforcement may seem inconsiderate or even inhumane to a provider insensitive to the pernicious effects of reinforcing performance of a dependent or institutional social role. Similarly, not engaging in "doing for" behavior in a social learning-based therapeutic environment may seem insensitive to a recovering person with severe behavioral deficits. When the recovering person is accustomed to a dependency-rewarding institutional environment, this perception can seem especially painful. When the expectation of reinforcement is strong, withholding reinforcement is often experienced as "punishment," even when such reinforcement would be abnormal in a more natural setting. For example, if a person became accustomed to unlimited access to the hospital canteen while a patient in the receiving unit, after transfer to the rehabilitation unit restricted access to the canteen, contingent on participation in rehabilitation, could be experienced as "punishment" for not participating. The recovering person's emotional response often makes it extremely difficult for the provider (the change agent, in this context) to implement the appropriate contingency. If change agents are left to implement a contingency program to which they have not explicitly committed themselves, they will not implement it with sufficient fidelity. This is why a social learning therapeutic milieu—and, in particular, contingency management—is notoriously difficult to provide outside of a social infrastructure that is highly supportive of the specific procedures involved.

Contingency management is not the only area where providers' social cognition can impinge negatively on rehabilitation. For example, social skills training often appears to address abilities taken so much for granted that it seems pointless or even demeaning to proceed as if a person cannot perform them. At the same time, treating a behavioral problem as a skills deficit may sometimes appear to give undue deference to socially unacceptable behavior. In the language of the integrated paradigm, the hypothesis that a particular behavioral problem represents a skills deficit often competes with the hypothesis that the problem represents a motivated choice. For example, intimidating behavior may reflect an inability to perform more acceptable and effective types of interpersonal negotiation, or a choice to use intimidation despite having a sufficient repertoire of alternatives. The latter would probably be conceptualized as some combination of sociocognitive and social–environmental problems. If social skills trainers do not participate in the team decision to understand a problem as a social skills deficit, they are less committed to that view, compared to the inevitable competing hypotheses, and fidelity and effectiveness are compromised.

*Decision by consensus* enhances procedural fidelity by formally generating personal commitments to accept a particular conceptualization of a problem, until further data render that conceptualization untenable. Decision by consensus is yet another kind of social contract, one that explicitly binds the recovering person and the other team members in personal commitments to each other. Implementing an intervention solely because someone else has prescribed it does not produce this commitment.

Decision by consensus must be managed within the practical context of a working rehabilitation team. As discussed earlier in this chapter, it is usually impractical to include every individual who provides any service or has any involvement on the team. The function of the designated skills trainer or milieu manager is, in part, to serve as proxy as well as liaison. Commitment to fidelity is achieved to the degree that all providers and other participants (e.g., the recovering person, a parent or spouse) perceive that their perspectives and interests are represented in the team's consensus.

Decision by consensus essentially means that any member has veto power over any team decision and, hence, over any element of the rehabilitation plan. Such veto power, distributed among all participants, raises alarms in a medical model, wherein it seems highly irresponsible to allow a less qualified or even nonprofessional team member veto "the doctor's decisions." In the context of rehabilitation, it is irresponsible to pretend that de facto veto power does *not* operate. It is well known among experienced mental health professionals that the doctor's decisions can be manipulated by selectively providing information about the patient, or even by ignoring prescriptions when the prescribed actions cannot be monitored reliably. In this sense, the medical model's premise that all key decisions are made by "the doctor" is a myth. With appropriate training in the integrated paradigm, team members learn to respect each others' judgments, to accept collective responsibility for all aspects of rehabilitation, to use their veto power with utmost circumspection, and perhaps most importantly, to speak up when they know that a particular decision would be problematic.

With the infrastructure that effective program administration provides, in our experiences, decision by consensus enhances rather than compromises the decision making of rehabilitation teams, and it does not lead to inappropriate interference with expert judgment. It is important, however, that specific clinical and administrative procedures be in place to follow when a team is unable to reach consensus in a time frame demanded by a particular decision. These procedures should include an appeal to an administrative mediator capable of weighing the risks of not making a decision against the consequences of overriding a team member's judgment (this type of situation is discussed further in Chapter 12). More importantly, it is a central task in program administration to develop rehabilitation teams that efficiently reach consensus through mutual respect and a commitment to procedural fidelity.

Inevitably, one or another member of the rehabilitation team has professional and technological expertise in a particular domain that other team members do not possess. The concept of *exclusive professional purview* makes this reality compatible with the integrated paradigm's other principles of assessment, intervention, and progress evaluation. It defines particular domains wherein the judgment of one team member is to be accepted by the rest of the team; in such a case, that person's decision replaces consensus as the criterion by which decisions become operative. The principle that each team member has veto power over all team decisions does not apply to decisions made in the domain of a member's previously acknowledged area of exclusive professional purview.

When the team is first assembled, members identify and agree upon domains of decision making in which exclusive professional purview pertains. These domains typically include (1) prescription of specific medications, (2) use of specialized psychological or neuropsychological assessment instruments, (3) forensic clinical assessment, (4) management of government welfare, health care subsidy, and related mechanisms, and (5) primary responsibility for the recovering person's safety and routine health concerns. Traditionally these areas are associated with the disciplines of psychiatry, psychology, social work, and nursing, respectively. However, as discussed earlier in this chapter, health care roles are generally in a state of flux. Responsibilities may be delegated in different ways across different statutory venues and different clinical settings. Working out these responsibilities is a key step in establishing a rehabilitation program, or in assembling a rehabilitation team outside the auspices of a program.

Decision by exclusive professional purview differs from decision via physician prerogative in traditional medical models, although it is similar to the arrangements that occur between two physicians who have separate responsibilities in a family health care system. Unlike physician prerogatives in the traditional medical model, the exercise of exclusive professional purview in the integrated paradigm is precisely defined in terms of specific types of decisions and applies only when there are clear statutory or technological boundaries on the various team members' expertise. In other words, no team member has exclusive purview as a result of his or her profession, seniority, or administrative rank (this is the clearest contrast with traditional medical models, where decision-making purviews are based primarily on professional membership). Rather, purview is based solely on specific areas of expertise not shared by other team members. Most importantly, any decision, including those made within a member's exclusive purview, is subject to review and evaluation by the entire team. For example, it is the psychopharmacotherapist's responsibility to select the medication regimen needed to address a particular neurophysiological dysregulation problem, but it is the entire team's responsibility to evaluate whether the regimen produces the desired result. The starting point of this responsibility is the identification and description of the problem, when specific behaviors are hypothesized to manifest the dysregulation. If the intervention accomplishes part, but not all, of what was expected, the entire team reconceptualizes the problem—that is, they construct a new hypothesis consistent with the new data on the problem's responsiveness to the intervention.

## Case Example

The following description of a team decision process illustrates the interplay of consensus building and the exercise of exclusive professional purview (discussed in the material that follows), as it occurred at a key point in the rehabilitation of the hypothetical case described in Chapter 2 (see also Appendix 2).

> After 6 months of gradual progress, Mr. A's recovery was complicated by the emergence of significant depressive symptoms, including thoughts of suicide. All members of the team were alarmed but expressed differing opinions with regard to what the response should be. Some argued that the depression should be viewed as a CNS dysregulation, possibly revealing a previously undetected neurophysiological vulnerability factor related to Mr. A's psychotic disorder, that should be treated primarily with antidepressant medication. Others argued that the depression was probably an inevitable response to Mr. A's increased awareness of his life situation and his confrontation with his chronic illness. It should therefore be treated as a psychophysiological dysregulation of

274 THE ORGANIZATIONAL CONTEXT OF REHABILITATION

mood, with interventions emphasizing positive cognitive reframing, physical exercise, pragmatic problem solving, stress management skills, and planning for the future. In the ensuing debate, the pro-medication team members argued that Mr. A's emotional distress and risk for suicide demanded as rapid-acting an intervention as possible. Whether or not psychosocial treatment were undertaken, medication should be added to increase the probability of a quick response. They also argued that the research on drug versus psychosocial versus combined treatment of depression gives an edge to combined treatment when the severity is high.

The pro-psychosocial team members countered that there was little evidence that Mr. A had a preexisting CNS dysregulation related to affective symptoms, that environmental conditions overwhelmingly militated for a reactive depression, and that the research evidence on combined treatment is not informative when the affective symptom picture is complicated by psychosis. They also argued that in light of Mr. A's history of substance abuse, prescribing yet another drug as a solution for emotional distress would not necessarily be sending the right message. Finally, they pointed out that if a combined approach were used, it would not be clear for future reference whether the drug, the psychosocial treatment, or both were really required.

Mr. A himself remained generally skeptical of drug treatment, not fully convinced that even the antipsychotic was beneficial, and so he argued against a pharmacological approach to his depression. The team psychiatrist happened to be one of the pro-medication team members, but she acknowledged the relevance of the counter-arguments. She claimed exclusive professional purview over medication decisions, and because of Mr. A's commitment status, she could have overruled all the pro-psychosocial team members and ordered an antidepressant. However, the team formulated a plan that was supported by all members. They agreed to a trial of an intensive psychosocial intervention, to which antidepressant medication would be added if there were insufficient progress after 4 weeks (a period not much longer than that required for an antidepressant drug trial). The psychiatrist reserved her prerogative to start the medication before then, if the severity of the symptoms and/or risk for suicide increased, although some pro-psychosocial team members stated they too would support combined treatment under such conditions.

The iterative nature of assessment, intervention, and progress evaluation in the integrated paradigm requires that *all* decisions, including those made within a team member's exclusive professional purview, are decisions about what to do *first*. All decisions are subject to evaluation, based on the data subsequently generated by those decisions. If an intervention does not elicit the response that is consistent with the team's hypotheses, then either a new intervention is selected, or the problem is reconceptualized. For example, the hypothesis that a person's sad mood and lack of motivation result from a CNS dysregulation of the type associated with depression is not supported after several trials of antidepressant drugs have no effect. An alternate hypothesis must be entertained. The clinical presentation represents (or at least includes) a mood-linked attribution problem, psychophysiological dysregulation of activation or mood, or a socialized psychiatric symptom. The new hypotheses imply different interventions. When the ineffective intervention falls within a member's area of exclusive professional purview, that person must decide whether to (1) persist with the same conceptualization of the problem and try an alternative intervention to achieve the expected outcome, or (2) collaborate with the team to modify the problem and adjust goals and expectations accordingly. To continue with the pharmacological example, if a drug intervention is only partially successful, the psychopharmacotherapist must decide whether to try another drug intervention or propose that other problems be defined to address the remaining barriers to better functioning. This process is often how socialized psychiatric symptoms are systematically distinguished from the expressions of neurophysiological dysregulation. As unsuccessful or partially successful medication trials accumulate, there is an increasing imperative to reconceptualize the problem and try a different approach. Although drug intervention for neurophysiological dysregulation provides an especially concrete example, this process applies to every problem and every intervention in the rehabilitation plan.

Successful implementation of the integrated paradigm's team processes obviously requires considerable maturity and professionalism on the part of all team members. Providers with an unrealistic level of confidence in their ability to determine the best conceptualization and the most effective interventions on the first try often have a high emotional stake in "being right." This attitude can create serious problems. Most experienced mental health providers have observed persistent use of ineffective interventions because nobody is willing to confront the fact that "it's not working." Promiscuous exercise of exclusive professional purview exacerbates the problem. Nobody is willing to confront "the doctor," whether the problematic decisions are truly within his or her technological expertise or not. This situation is incompatible with the integrated paradigm, not to mention the imperfect and incomplete state of psychopathology and mental health technology. All the members of the rehabilitation team must accept the two principles of *decision by consensus* and *exclusive professional purview*, and all must accept personal responsibility for vigorously applying objective, quantitative measurement to evaluate the consequences of all the team's decisions.

In addition to maturity and professionalism, rehabilitation teams are usefully guided by formal procedures. As with skills training and related interventions, the team process is explicated in Procedures Manuals that delineate the roles and principles discussed in this and preceding chapters. Recruiting mature professionals committed to the integrated paradigm and developing manuals to guide team decision making are key aspects of program administration. These and related considerations are addressed in the final chapter of this book.

# Chapter 12

# Administration and Management of Rehabilitation Services

In this chapter we discuss how to run a rehabilitation program. In keeping with the integrated paradigm's emphasis on scientific validation, we cite the research literature where applicable. However, in contrast to the extensive research on the effectiveness of individual modalities and of rehabilitation programs, in general, the research provides relatively little data on the most effective administrative policies and management techniques for rehabilitation serving people with disabling mental illness. The largest and most complete research study of rehabilitation outcome, conducted by Paul and Lentz (1977), included careful attention to program policy and management, but program management and administration were included in the entire package of clinical assessment and treatment; they were not evaluated separately. We know from Paul and Lentz (1977) and subsequent work (e.g., Liberman et al., 1979; Magaro et al., 1978; Paul, 1986a, 1986b, 1988a, 1988b, 1988c) that rehabilitation requires particular policies and management techniques, but there has been insufficient research to demonstrate that particular administrative approaches are superior to others, given the availability of the needed clinical resources and technologies. The authors' views of how best to run a rehabilitation program derive, in part, from our understanding of the special administrative requirements of the kinds of programs that show the best clinical outcome, from our understanding of widely accepted general principles of public administration, and from our own experience.

In particular, we draw upon our own experience in the 20-year development of a rehabilitation program, the Community Transition Program (CTP) in Lincoln, Nebraska. The CTP was inaugurated in 1982, in response to a mandate from the Nebraska state health and human services administration. The mandate called for innovative programs to help people who had been left behind in the state's deinstitutionalization movement.

The CTP was originally created from a conventional long-term custodial ward in the Lincoln Regional Center, one of Nebraska's state hospitals. As the recipient population changed—from people stuck in institutions to people stuck in the "revolving door" of the mental health system—the CTP evolved to meet changing needs. In the late 1990s the original hospital-based program was expanded to include a community-based residential component, operated in conjunction with the Lancaster County Community Mental Health Center and OUR Homes, Inc., a privately owned residential services provider.

The product of a collaboration between Lincoln Regional Center and the Psychology Department of the University of Nebraska–Lincoln, the CTP has served as a research site and training center as well as a service provision agency. Research performed at the site includes program evaluation studies that support the CTP's cost-effectiveness. Over the years, the CTP has gained national and international recognition as a model rehabilitation program for people with the most severe and disabling mental illnesses. Our experience thus derives not only from developing the CTP, but also from consulting with clinicians and administrators from other service systems who wish to develop programs of their own. Our discussion in this chapter includes anecdotes and brief illustrations that are a composite of our clinical, administrative, and consulting experiences.

Although the integrated paradigm does not require any particular type of administrative auspices, services provided according to its principles are generally expected to be organized as a program. There are several reasons for this expectation, ranging from historical to technological. Historically, mental health services for people with severe and disabling conditions have evolved mostly in psychiatric hospitals (public and private), community mental health centers, and rehabilitation centers. These settings have a greater tendency toward centralized organization and administration than, for example, general family health care systems, which tend to be comprised of general and specialized clinics providing primary and secondary services. It is important to note, however, that there is considerable diversity within these four settings; any particular setting may have preexisting administrative structures that are either compatible or incompatible with rehabilitation in the integrated paradigm. (For a comprehensive textbook account of human service administration, see Weiner, 1982; for a textbook account of administration and management of human service programs, see Lewis, Lewis, & Souflee, 1991; for a practical guidebook, see Sluyter, 1998.)

As is the case in most health care settings, management of rehabilitation services includes staff development, coordination among agencies, resolving personnel conflicts, maintaining fiscal stability, myriad administrative concerns, and so on. In modern rehabilitation, the management challenge is further complicated by the diversity of instruments, clinical skills, and intervention resources involved in the enterprise. This diversity makes it difficult, often prohibitive, to provide cost-efficient services outside a centralized administrative context. Also, the technological demands associated with rehabilitation team decision-making processes and procedural fidelity are difficult to meet outside a highly organized administrative context.

This does not mean that rehabilitation and recovery are impossible outside the context of a service program. Many individuals with disabling or potentially disabling mental illness have service needs that are manageable by independent practitioners acting in primary and secondary provider roles. This is fortunate, in part, because service programs are not always available where they are needed. Certainly, some individuals have needs and resources that make rehabilitation outside a service program a viable and even preferable option. However, as of this writing, and probably well into the foreseeable future, such a scenario is the exception rather than the rule.

The mere existence of a service program as an administrative entity does not ensure effective and comprehensive rehabilitation services. Unfortunately, *program* has become a "buzzword" in administrative and policy parlance, connoting intrinsic value independent of service provision realities. In the era of managed care, programs are increasingly viewed with suspicion by administrators sensitive to the need for refined cost accounting and clinical accountability. Sometimes the clinical and administrative structure of a program insulates its providers from changing service demands, thereby perpetuating outmoded or unneeded services. The most salient example is the persistence of state institution-based programs (often the entire hospital constitutes a program, as understood in this discussion) that provide no more than custodial "care" to individuals who, with appropriate rehabilitation, could live well in a less restrictive setting. Similarly, clinical accountability mechanisms within programs may serve little more than the interests of the administrators and professionals who operate them. These suspicions are exacerbated to the degree that programs are (implicitly and often inaccurately) associated with public institutions—which are notoriously resistant to fiscal and clinical accountability.

Such problems are not inevitable characteristics of service programs; in fact, they can be avoided altogether through a rigorous application of the principles and technologies of the integrated paradigm. Still, suspicion is legitimate. Without such rigorous application, arguments against the desirability of programs are often valid. For the purposes of this discussion, the issue is not whether programs are a desirable, accountable, and/or cost-efficient context for rehabilitation; rather, we turn our attention to identifying the key characteristics necessary for effective, accountable, and cost-efficient service programs.

## KEY CHARACTERISTICS OF SERVICE PROGRAMS

The key characteristics of rehabilitation programs for people with disabling mental illness are generated by the integrated paradigm's perspectives on psychopathology, mental health and rehabilitation technology, and the nature of clinical decision making. Basic principles of management, common to most collaborative enterprises, contribute additional characteristics that are also reflected in the principles of clinical decision making. Optimal program structure is that which (1) conforms to our scientific understanding of the nature of mental illness, (2) provides access to all technologies, professional resources, and supportive/therapeutic environments needed for maximum recovery of its service recipients, (3) ensures procedural fidelity for all clinical procedures and clinical decision-making processes, and (4) clearly delineates the functions, responsibilities, and accountability of all providers and participants. These four guidelines translate into specific organizational and administrative components:

1. A coherent, operationally defined mission that commits the program to comprehensive rehabilitation of people with disabling mental illness
2. Operationally defined criteria that identify the program's recipient population
3. A program director who has overall administrative responsibility for the program's operation, including budgetary control over program resources, control over personnel resources, and administrative accountability for the program's clinical effectiveness
4. A procedures manual that delineates (a) the functions of all providers and participants, (b) the structure and organization of the rehabilitation teams that operate within the program, (c) the procedures by which the rehabilitation teams and individual providers make clinical decisions, and (d) procedures for maintaining supportive and therapeutic environmental conditions not routinely addressed by individual rehabilitation plans
5. Professional staff resources sufficient to accomplish the program's rehabilitation mission
6. Paraprofessional, clerical, and support staff resources sufficient for the program's operation

7. Staff training mechanisms sufficient to ensure competence in specialized provider skills

8. A clinical data collection and management system capable of providing the rehabilitation team with the large amount of data generated in the course of rehabilitation, in a format amenable to efficient interpretation, for the purpose of assessment, rehabilitation planning, and progress evaluation

9. For the purposes of quality control, a system for monitoring environmental conditions, clinical documentation, and provider activity

10. For the purposes of program development, a system for regularly evaluating the program's mission, utilization of clinical technology, efficiency, and effectiveness

11. Superordinate administrative support that recognizes the value of the program and provides an appropriate fiscal and regulatory environment for the program's operation

## The Rehabilitation Mission

Common sense and basic management principles require that any complex enterprise identify its *mission*, stated briefly and in concrete terms, including clear and unequivocal criteria by which the enterprise's success can be evaluated. An appropriate mission statement serves a number of complementary functions. It communicates to the world (especially to the health care system of which the program is a component) (1) who the program serves, (2) how it serves them, and (3) the expected benefits of those services—all central issues in health care system administration. System administrators do not necessarily appreciate or understand the nature of disabling mental illness, the value of rehabilitation, the availability of effective rehabilitation technology, or its expected outcome. A program's mission statement provides administrators with an accessible conceptualization about why the program is needed in their service systems. Whether or not they understand the disciplines of mental health and rehabilitation, most system administrators justifiably believe that the value of a truly worthwhile service program can be stated in simple language whose meaning and implications are clear to anyone with a modicum of common sense. Theoretically, at least, these are the programs they are most willing to support through funding. Here is an example of an informative and compelling mission statement: *The mission of this program is to provide state-of-the-art treatment and rehabilitation to individuals with severe and disabling mental illness who cannot be safely or effectively served in any less restrictive setting anywhere in the mental health system, and to help those individuals achieve a stable adjustment and decent quality of life in the community.*

## Defining the Recipient Population

The importance of precisely identifying whom a program serves may seem obvious, but criteria for determining who is to be served are often arbitrary or altogether absent in mental health service administration. In large part, this weakness is a legacy of neo-Kraepelinian nosology. In our experience, many administrators and providers unreflectively believe that a psychiatric diagnosis or a list of diagnoses is sufficient for this purpose. As discussed throughout this book, psychiatric diagnosis provides almost no information about the particular treatment, rehabilitation, or other service needs of any individual person. The health care policy and management community has struggled for decades, with limited success, to develop more suitable criteria for rationally inferring the need for specific services. Functional criteria, such as inability to perform routine activities of daily living, are often included as components of a sufficient definition, but they are seldom sufficient by themselves. *Paradiagnostic* terms such as "psychosis" or "major mental illness" are often included.[1] They have the advantage of capturing a broader and more inherently meaningful set of characteristics than diagnostic categories, but they have the disadvantage of conveying highly variable meanings across venues. When used, they usually must be accompanied by more operational definitions. Logically, if the operational terms themselves are legitimate, they should be sufficient. However, logic interacts with tradition, convention, and familiarity to produce our clinical-administrative terminology.

Defining the recipient population is conceptually inseparable from formulating a program's mission statement and is usefully included in mission statements. However, because of the need for brevity and accessibility in mission statements, additional details are usually needed. The value of broad definitions in a mission statement, for the purposes of planning and system administration, is to identify the recipient population in a way that complements prevailing concepts in the larger mental health service system. The value of more precise definitions is to ensure that the people who receive services in a program are those for whom the program is designed and optimized. Detailed, specific, and operationally defined elaborations of the mission statement's definition of the recipient population should be articu-

---

[1]*Paradiagnostic* here means terms that are part of the traditional psychiatric lexicon that, at times, may have been incorporated in actual diagnostic criteria, but currently are not themselves diagnoses. For example, "psychosis" is a condition that may accompany any of several diagnoses but is part of the diagnostic criteria in only a few. "Major mental illness" has been used in the mental health literature to refer to (1) all the disorders listed in the entire DSM, (2) Axis I of the DSM, (3) those Axis I disorders that are especially severe or debilitating, or (4) specific psychotic disorders such as schizophrenia.

lated in the program's Procedures Manual (discussed later in this chapter), where they are linked to procedures for assessing referrals, making decisions as to whether individuals meet the criteria, and making dispositional decisions accordingly.

At administrative as well as clinical levels, recipient definitions have both inclusive and exclusionary functions. For example, in many public mental health systems, a diagnosis of "developmental disability" qualifies a person for developmental services but may disqualify that person for certain mental health services. Terms such as "substance abuse" and "personality disorder" may perform exclusionary functions. Increasingly, service systems use particular combinations of inclusive and exclusionary criteria, with combinations of diagnostic, paradiagnostic, and functional terms. Regulatory distinctions seldom use specific diagnoses; instead, broad colloquial categories or genres are subsumed, without empirical justification, in neo-Kraepelinian nosology. For example, regulations often distinguish between "personality disorder" and "mental illness," the latter meaning *any* DSM Axis I diagnosis, and the former meaning anything else. The conceptual distinction between personality disorder and mental illness is problematic. In neo-Kraepelinian argot, there is "high comorbidity" between severe mental illness and personality disorder. In scientific terminology, the construct validity of the distinction has not been established. Paradiagnostic terms often reflect broad and vaguely distinguishable groups of diagnoses, which accounts for their frequent use in regulatory language.

For example, "borderline personality disorder" may appear in regulations as an exclusionary criterion (independent of its status as an Axis II diagnosis) that disqualifies people with that diagnosis from receiving certain subsidized mental health or rehabilitation services. The salient characteristics of borderline personality disorder, from a managed care perspective, are high use of expensive services and failure to respond to traditional medical–psychiatric treatment. Of course, these characteristics apply to many other diagnoses, but they are statistically concentrated among people with the borderline personality disorder diagnosis. Excluding such individuals thus has prospects for limiting costs in a mental health system. This is a version of the familiar health care underwriting technique of "cherry picking"—formulating policy so as to limit subsidized services to those who need them least. Generally, a definition of the recipient population that would work in most contemporary mental health administrative systems, and which identifies the individuals for whom the rehabilitation approach in the integrated paradigm is most appropriate (assuming there are further operational definitions in the Procedures Manual), is:

> People with mental illness of adolescent or later onset, who do not meet criteria for "developmental disability," and who experience significant dis-

abilities in personal and social functioning not solely attributable to substance abuse or "personality disorder."

*Mental illness* usually means any DSM Axis I diagnosis, although it could also be defined operationally with functional and paradiagnostic characteristics independent of DSM diagnosis. The age of onset criterion usefully excludes people who are likely to be better served in a developmental disability service system. The disability criterion usefully identifies people who need rehabilitation, as opposed to other mental health services, in a way that can be defined operationally in terms of specific assessment procedures.

The recipient definition should include functional criteria that reflect the resources of the particular program in relation to providing for the recipients' basic health and safety. For example, programs that do not include round-the-clock supervision of recipients may need to exclude such individuals during times when they need such services. A residential program that provides round-the-clock supervision may need to exclude individuals during times when they need especially intensive supervision or a high-security physical environment. Such criteria must be precisely tailored, not only to the characteristics of the program itself and the niche it occupies in the service system, but also to the availability of other services and programs in the system. At the level of the mission statement, language such as " . . . who can be safely served in the program's clinical environment" serves to denote such factors. More specific operational criteria, identifying specific risks, should be elaborated in the program's Procedures Manual.

## The Program Director

Organizing services into a program brings many activities under a single mission, a single budget, a single set of policies and procedures, a single staff, and a single group of service recipients. Basic management principles dictate that there be a single individual with responsibility, accountability, and authority for the entire program, a program director. In some mental health service settings, the need for this position is taken for granted. In others, especially institutions operating within a traditional medical–psychiatric model, it is resisted—sometimes fiercely, in our experience. Even in settings where the concept of a program is generally accepted, the concept of a management structure congruent with the program's mission and organizational structure may not be.

Typically in psychiatric institutions, administrative accountability is dispersed throughout the institution, in departments based on professional discipline—for example, the nursing department (which usually subsumes aides or technicians as well as nurses), the social work department, the occupational therapy department, and so on. The director of nursing has authority over, and is accountable for, nursing services across the institution, the director of social work for social work services, and so on. This distribution may work to the degree that the entire institution constitutes a program, with the institution's chief executive officer as the program director. However, with the diverse missions and technologically sophisticated services that state institutions must provide in modern mental health systems, greatest effectiveness and efficiency comes through developing specialized services for the different populations served within the institution. Within the institution these specialized services are most effectively and efficiently operated as separate programs. When separate programs are organized under a medical model departmental structure, there are inherent conflicts between the management imperatives faced by departmental administrators and the missions of the respective programs. The departments compete with each other over issues of interest to the respective disciplines—for example, over how many staff positions are allotted to the various departments in the institution's budget—but they also must cooperate in order to run interdisciplinary programs. Departmental interests inevitably overshadow program interests. The departmental administrators hold direct responsibility, accountability, and authority for their own departments, but not the programs. As a result, effective and efficient pursuit of program missions is a secondary priority throughout the institution.

Certain characteristics of the medical–psychiatric–institutional administrative model make it especially resistant to reform. The model tends to create a cadre of administrators whose salaries are higher than those of the professional ranks from which they were selected, who thus have considerable incentive to preserve the status of departments and department administrators. Diffusion of responsibility and accountability is also a powerful incentive. In addition to administrative accountability, clinical accountability is diffused. Although the traditional medical model theoretically invests all clinical accountability in the psychiatrist, the de facto sharing of program accountability among the various departments greatly reduces the probability that a psychiatrist, or the group of psychiatrists that constitute the institution's medical staff, will ever be held accountable for the institution's overall clinical outcome. Sometimes pressures for reform, and especially pressure to develop effective rehabilitation services, compel institutions to create "compromise" structures, wherein "programs" are identified and program administrators are given *some* of the authority (often along with *all* the accountability) necessary to run the program. However, such compromises inevitably compromise clinical outcome and efficiency as well. There is no escaping the management reality that a single program with a single mission performs most effectively and efficiently under the direction of a single administrative officer with appropriate accountability and authority.

In essence, the authority invested in the program director serves as a criterion of effective program structure. *The program director must have the authority to*

1. Determine the resource needs of the program
2. Hire and fire all staff and all professionals who provide services within the program
3. Control the budget, or that part of the budget that supports essential program operations and clinical services (this purview may exclude housekeeping, maintenance, and related support functions)
4. Collect and analyze data on provision of services for the purposes of quality control
5. Set and pursue management objectives in the form of quality control goals and program development projects
6. Represent the program and its constituents in interactions with system administrators, accreditation agencies, program participants and their families

*The program director is accountable for*

7. Producing clinical and quality control data that show the program is producing the expected clinical outcomes within budget
8. Ensuring the protection of staff and service recipients' physical safety, psychological well-being, and civil rights

Debate about the program director's authority is often protracted by the failure of the medical model (or, at least, some of its practitioners) to make a fundamental distinction between administrative and clinical prerogatives. It is one thing to countermand the clinical decision of a licensed provider, and quite another to insist that a licensed provider fulfill the terms of his or her job description, follow administrative policy, participate in quality control activities, and so on. Nevertheless, in some interpretations of the medical model, the psychiatrist may define *any* decision as a clinical one. Needless to say, a situation in which a psychiatrist's authority is beyond question or scrutiny invites failures in accountability and compromises program functioning. Such a radical interpretation of medical prerogatives is no longer found often outside public psychiatric institutions and private psychiatric hospitals, but it does remain ubiquitous in those settings, and it is inseparable from the other reasons that effective rehabilitation is difficult to achieve in those settings.

The following anecdote illustrates how administrative prerogatives are separated from clinical prerogatives:

A psychiatrist was hired on contract to provide 16 hours per week of services to an interdisciplinary rehabilitation program. Accreditation standards and clinical needs dictate that about 12 hours are required to meet with individual service recipients, assess their pharmaco-therapeutic needs, and prescribe medication. The remaining 4 hours are required for participation in team meetings to share information, review progress, and revise the rehabilitation plan. Participation in specific team meetings was a specified condition of the contract.

After several weeks, it became evident that the psychiatrist was not attending the team meetings. He was seeing people individually, as required, and prescribing medication, but he stated that he was able to get necessary information more efficiently simply by checking with a nurse at his own convenience. When the program director insisted that the psychiatrist participate in team meetings, according to the pro-gram's procedures manual, the psychiatrist invoked his professional status, stating that only he had the authority to decide what his in-volvement in the team process would be. He appealed to the agency's chief psychiatrist, who affirmed that such practice would be in accor-dance with professional standards, but declined to change the pro-gram's procedures manual or the service contract. The program direc-tor claimed no supervisory prerogatives over the psychiatrist's clinical practice, but did exercise her administrative prerogative to enforce the conditions of the service contract. The contract was terminated and of-fered to another psychiatrist, who was agreeable to adapting his prac-tice to the program's team processes.

Of course, administrators seldom have absolute authority—in indus-try, health care, or anywhere else. They usually work within operating parameters that are set by some superordinate body, a board of direc-tors, a chief executive officer, etc. In health care these parameters are of-ten jointly established by multiple bodies, including medical or profes-sional staffs (the group of independent practitioners who provide services within an agency or institution), governing boards, advisory boards, ac-creditation agencies, government funding offices, private managed care entities, and so on. The operating parameters include agreements about the value and cost of the services, the qualifications of providers, licens-ing criteria of various kinds, the nature of the expected outcome data, the criteria for success, personnel policies, and so on. The program di-rector's task is to operate the program within these parameters, and to participate in the formulation and revision of the parameters so that they best serve the needs that the program is intended to address. In the specific case of rehabilitation, it is also part of the program director's task to make sure that the needs of people with disabling mental illness are well represented in the social and fiscal policy of the health care sys-tem in which the program operates. This often means "selling" system administrators on the (1) need for rehabilitation (and advising them on policy and regulations required to ensure accountability in its provision), and (2) the resources required for its successful pursuit.

Within the program, the program director performs the essential function of ensuring that clinical decisions are made within the parameters established by the program's administrative and regulatory environment. This is the juncture where the distinction between administrative authority and clinical authority is most crucial. Clinical practitioners, independent and otherwise, must be allowed to make the decisions they were specifically trained to make. However, such decisions are always made in the context of laws, regulations, standards of practice, and procedural rules. In the integrated paradigm, the structure of the rehabilitation plan and its associated assessment, intervention, and progress evaluation procedures provide a highly specific set of procedures by which decisions are to be made. It is a key part of the program director's job to ensure that the rehabilitation teams follow these procedures by regularly monitoring the fidelity of individual clinicians to the procedures. Deviation from the procedures indicates decisions are not being made according to agreed-upon principles—a potentially fatal breach of the integrated paradigm's governing values. When quality control data indicate a breach in clinical decision-making procedures, the program director must evaluate the breach, determine whether the problem lies in the clinician(s) or the procedure(s), and take action accordingly.

The following anecdote illustrates a typical situation in which a program director must act on information that indicates a problem in procedural fidelity:

In reviewing data on procedural errors in the implementation of contingency management programs, the program director noticed a pattern. Most of the errors occurred when staff implemented programs designed by a particular member of the psychology staff. However, most of that psychologist's programs were without errors. Further study revealed most of the errors were on programs on which the psychologist was collaborating with a particular staff supervisor. In an informal discussion with the program director, the chief psychologist noted that although the psychologist in question was somewhat inexperienced and tended to design overly complex contingency management programs, this problem was usually corrected when implementation details were worked out with staff supervisors. Further investigation revealed interpersonal conflict between the junior psychologist and one particular staff supervisor; they had both been avoiding the interaction required to de-bug new programs. The program director pointed out the error problem to the psychologist and the supervisor, and cautioned them against letting personal conflicts interfere with necessary collaboration. The error problem subsequently dissipated.

In a sense, the program director is the trustee of a complex social contract that incorporates the interests of governments and regulatory agencies, accreditation bodies, professional disciplines, service systems, service agencies and institutions, and service recipients. The parties to the contract are the administrators who support and fund the program, the practitioners who provide its services, and the people who receive the services. The social contract reaches its most specific and operational level of definition in the program's mission statement and Procedures Manual (further discussed in the next section), and it is supported by myriad laws, policies, procedures, ethical standards and standards of practice. It is the program director's job to preside over the practical aspects of comingling all these parameters in a single program, and to hold all parties responsible for fulfilling the terms of the contract.

In the integrated paradigm, the qualifications for performing any particular role are determined by the skills required, not by a degree or professional membership. The particular skills required of the director of a rehabilitation program for disabling mental illness are not unique to, or even necessarily characteristic of, any of the mental health disciplines. The effective program director needs skills in policy analysis, management of health care services, and staff training. In addition, the program director needs to have sufficient clinical training and experience to understand the basics of risk management, patients' rights, and clinical decision-making processes. Specific experience in rehabilitation of disabling mental illness is required to the degree necessary to determine the technological needs implied by the program's mission. Independent practitioner status is not necessary, because the program director does not necessarily make clinical decisions about individual cases. The complete combination of skills is sometimes found in independent practitioners, but independent practitioner skills remain in high demand, and it is usually not cost-efficient to pay an independent practitioner to perform administrative tasks. The complete combination of skills can be found among master's-level mental health clinicians who also have administrative training and experience (for the purposes of this discussion, postbaccalaureate degrees or certifications in health care disciplines are considered "master's level," whether or not they are degrees in the traditional academic sense or include the word *master's*).

## The Procedures Manual

The use of procedure manuals in mental health services evolved along with the evolution of learning and social learning theory. The emphasis on quantitative precision in measurement and intervention associated with social learning theory made procedures manuals a central concept in clinical practice. In the Paul and Lentz (1977) trial of social learning, therapeutic community, and medical model treatment, the procedures manual entered the canon of psychiatric rehabilitation. That study demonstrated that a detailed manual could be constructed, that mental health providers could be trained to follow it with high fidelity, and that treatment and rehabilitation based on the manual's procedures could produce dramatically more effective results than conventional practice. The manuals for Paul and Lentz's therapeutic community and social learning programs were published as appendices in their book.

The decades since Paul and Lentz's pioneering work have seen considerable evolution in assessment and treatment planning practices. The integrated paradigm incorporates these developments, and they, in turn, should be incorporated in procedures manuals. Similarly, a modern procedures manual must address the technologies that have evolved since the 1970s. Thus, while the Paul and Lentz (1977) manuals focus on interactions between providers (especially change agents) and service recipients, modern manuals must also delineate the procedures to be used in (1) constructing an individualized rehabilitation plan and evaluating its success, and (2) implementing the many assessment and intervention technologies in the modern rehabilitation armamentarium.

As previously discussed, creating and updating a procedures manual is a key part of the program director's task. The procedures manual serves not only as a set of guidelines for providing services, but also as a conceptual and operational framework for conducting quality control and ensuring high fidelity.

## Professional Resources

A key function of a service program is to recruit practitioners to fill the various roles on rehabilitation teams (discussed in Chapter 11). Doing so can be a serious challenge. In many parts of the world, mental health practitioners of any kind are in short supply. Even where they are abundant, few have the special skills required for working effectively with people who have disabling mental illness.

In traditional medical model institutions, recruiting professionals and other staff is an important responsibility of the discipline-based departments (e.g., the nursing department, the social work department, etc.). The departments also perform the complementary function of providing oversight and quality control within disciplinary domains. In the integrated paradigm, these continue to be important and useful functions, but they are more directly subject to the needs of the program and the authority and accountability of the program director. The program must specify the types of professional services it needs, while determinations as to whether individuals are qualified to provide those services are generally made within disciplines. In other words, only nurses evaluate the professional credentials of nurses, only social workers evaluate social workers, and so on. Specific departments provide crucial consultation to the program director on matters of professional competence, including ongoing evaluation of discipline-specific competence and dealing with disciplinary problems. In fact, the value of disciplinary departments in this role is a strong argument for adapting this part of the traditional medical model to contemporary service settings. To function effectively, a program director must have access to discipline-specific consulting resources, outside the program, for all the disciplines that are represented within the program.

## Paraprofessional, Clerical, and Support Staff

Like any health care service, a rehabilitation program requires diverse human resources. The precise configuration depends on the nature and scope of the program—for example, whether it is residential or outpatient, whether it operates under the auspices of a larger institution or agency, how many recipients it serves, and so on. The integrated paradigm is not necessarily different from other mental health models with respect to the number of support staff a program may need, but the specific activities of the support staff may differ. For example, change agents have a very different role in rehabilitation than the caretaking role of aids or technicians in a medical/custodial model (this was discussed in Chapter 10). For another example, the involvement of clerical and support staff in management of clinical data is expected to be greater in programs operating according to the integrated paradigm, because of the greater amount of clinical data that such programs generate and process (this was discussed in Chapter 3).

## Staff Training

Most professional staff bring critical skills associated with their respective professional background, but few have all the skills necessary to fully perform needed roles on the rehabilitation teams. Of course, complete parity is not a useful goal—which is one reason why there are teams. However, all team members, including (perhaps especially) professionals, need to share a basic commitment to the integrated paradigm's biosystemic perspective on mental illness and its principles of interdisciplinary decision making. All team members need to be conversant with the specifics of the program's Procedures Manual. The program itself must provide at least part of the training necessary to ensure that all team members have these skills (depending on what kind and how much training is available in the larger service system of which the program is a component).

Rehabilitation services usually include a number of individuals who are hired with little or no professional preparation. They may perform the roles of change agent, skills trainer, milieu manager, and others, under varying degrees of professional supervision. Agencies and institutions usually provide basic training and "apprenticeship" periods for these individuals, which cover the fundamentals of working in health care settings (i.e., ethics and confidentiality), responding to aggressive behavior and medical emergencies, and so on. Implementing contingency management and other skills related to maintaining a supportive/therapeutic milieu are seldom covered in basic training. Rehabilitation programs often have to provide most of the training their paraprofessional staff will ever receive in these domains. The program's resources must therefore reflect its particular staff training needs, based on what the paraprofessionals are expected to do and what skills they can acquire from external training sources.

The Paul and Lentz (1977) study is an exemplar of staff training. The social learning change agents spent hundreds of hours (the exact number was difficult to determine, because classroom training segued into supervised practice) in basic training that included performance assessments designed to objectively confirm that they had acquired the key skills. There has been insufficient research to conclude how much staff training is necessary to maintain an optimally supportive/therapeutic environment. In our experience, the Paul and Lentz training format is all too rare in mental health systems. For that matter, effective, competently managed therapeutic milieus are all too rare. The reality is that commitment to rehabilitation of people with disabling mental illness requires a commitment to staff training at the levels of program, agency, institution, and service system administration. (For an updated, focused discussion of training staff to implement contingency management in a traditional psychiatric setting, see Hersen, Bellak, & Harris, 1993.)

## The Clinical Data Management System

The amount of data generated in the course of assessment, intervention, and progress evaluation in comprehensive rehabilitation demands a powerful yet efficient data management system. Consider that a rehabilitation regimen may involve 40 hours or more per week of counseling, therapy, skills training, and structured or coached occupational activities (e.g., work, leisure activities). Each modality generates several data points, reflecting the recovering person's attendance, participation, adaptive and maladaptive behavior, and progress in that specific modality. In addition, the rehabilitation milieu includes ongoing measures of ambient behavior, neurophysiological status (e.g., measures of psychosis indicators), performance of hygiene and self-care activities, and social functioning. Individualized milieu-based procedures, such as contingency management programs, may add additional key data. Conventional clinical assessments, such as structured interviews, physical examinations, and psychological tests, are also part of the data base. Hundreds of quantitative data points per week, with additional hundreds entered at longer intervals, are typical. Conventional clinical records (e.g., progress notes and activity logs) are usually not quantitative, but they often contain important information to be analyzed in light of the quantitative data.

Computerization is a prerequisite for this level of data management. Software is increasingly available for management of clinical data in mental health settings, though it is often not suitable for comprehensive rehabilitation. As database software become increasingly sophisticated yet user-friendly, the prospects improve for on-site design and development. That is, a staff member with a modest amount of programming skill may soon be able to develop a software system to meet the needs of an individual rehabilitation program. For some programs with limited scope (e.g., specialized work–skills programs), that day may already have arrived. The technical literature provides considerable information on the design prerequisites of clinical data management systems (Buican, Spaulding, Gordon, & Hindman, 1999). Designing, developing, and maintaining a computerized data management system is a key program administration task.

## Quality Control

The need for quality control is perhaps the most universally accepted principle of modern management, reflecting the degree to which management praxis has been influenced by behavioral science principles. (For a textbook account, see Dickens, 1994; for a review in the context of rehabilitation for severe mental illness, see Mason & Soreff, 1996.) Ensuring productivity and efficiency requires ongoing quantitative monitoring of staff behavior, using precise, reliable, and valid measuring instruments. The concept of quality control has undergone many superficial revisions in response to the "management fads" that have passed through industry, as evidenced by the popularization of such terminological variants as "quality assurance," "total quality management" (TQM), and "continuous quality improvement" (CQI). However, the underlying principle has remained largely the same (for this reason the original term *quality control* is used in this discussion).

Quality control is a key management tool of the rehabilitation program director. As previously discussed, programs are based on complex, operationally defined social contracts. The program director's task is to hold all parties accountable for adhering to the terms of the contract. Data collection in the context of quality control is a prerequisite to this accountability.

An important concept in quality control is that it involves monitoring both *outcome* and *process*. This means that some of the data to be collected must address the outcome (e.g., the success or effectiveness of services) and some must address the way in which services are provided. In clinical settings there are several reasons for this dual focus. Of course, outcome is the ultimate measure for determining whether a program is fulfilling its mission, and the program that can show credible outcome data is more competitive for funding and other support. Independent of outcome, however, services usually must be provided in accordance with standards, and providers are increasingly called upon to demonstrate, with objective, quantitative data, that they are meeting those standards. In a complex rehabilitation regimen, data on service provision is necessary to ensure that the entire regimen is being implemented, as planned. In the case of highly structured and/or manualized interventions, effectiveness can only be expected when process data show that the intervention is being correctly implemented.

Setting up and running a quality control protocol is a basic management skill. However, any protocol needs to be tailored to the mission, technology, and operational characteristics of the activity to which it is applied. A working understanding of these parameters, beyond basic management concepts, is required to ensure that the truly critical aspects of program operation are monitored. Generally, the particular parameters monitored for quality control reflect combinations of physical characteristics (e.g., safety of the physical environment) and procedural events (e.g., adherence to clinical decision-making procedures) as well as combinations of considerations internal to the program (e.g., adherence to the program's Procedures Manual) and external (e.g., adherence to institutional policy, adherence to accreditation standards).

Of course, a quality control protocol is only as effective as the management actions that are undertaken in response to its data. It matters not that data reveal, for example, that a particular staff member fails to follow clinical decision-making procedures, if nobody has the accountability or authority to act on the problem. Lack of mechanisms to act upon quality control findings is a common management problem in mental health services. This absence may be especially problematic in medical model settings, where demands for procedural fidelity are sometimes interpreted as violating physicians' prerogatives. Holding physicians accountable in such settings is usually the job of the medical staff, the group of physicians who provide services within the setting. Physicians can be unreliable at holding each other accountable, except perhaps when their collective interests are put at risk by a transgressor's actions. (This area of unreliability arguably applies to any profession, especially those having independent provider status, although physicians are popularly believed to be particularly vulnerable.) In psychiatry, especially in public service settings, individual physicians tend to be insulated from the consequences of each other's actions, and so there may be little incentive for accountability. Furthermore, the authors' experience is that quality control in mental health services often excludes psychiatrists from accountability demands, on the unsupported presumption that "the medical staff will take care of this." Even when quality control monitoring is extended to physicians' behavior, there is often no mechanism for acting upon problems. Basic management principles, as well as those of the integrated paradigm, require that all providers are held accountable.

Interestingly, contingency management technology is as useful in administration and management as it is in rehabilitation, especially as it relates to quality control (Patrick & Riggar, 1985; Reid & Parsons, 2000). Administrators with social learning backgrounds may find this model particularly appealing for rehabilitation programs (Aylward, Schloss, Alper, & Green, 1996; Foster, 1988; Huberman & O'Brien, 1999; McRae & Lutzker, 1982).

Quality control also can be applied to the performance of the entire program, as distinct from its internal elements. Good mission statements are easily translated into meaningful objective measures, especially outcome measures. Outcome measures in the context of program management usually include (1) objective and subjective measures of client functioning before and after services, (2) the cost of providing the services, and (3) the offset of costs by clinical improvement. This is generally known as *cost–benefit analysis*. (For a textbook account of cost–benefit analysis, see Yates, 1996.) Theoretically, cost–benefit analyses can determine (1) what a program provides, in terms of changes in client functioning and quality of life, (2) much that amount of change costs, and (3) how much money is saved over time by the change. However, the analysis inevitably involves estimates, for example, of the costs of providing specific services or support to individuals with disabilities of varying severity. Such estimates are always vulnerable to skepticism, and small variations can profoundly affect the results. Similarly, outcome measures are always vulnerable to the criticism of being either too specific or behavioral, and therefore lacking ecological validity and social meaning, or too general or subjective, and therefore lacking specificity and objectivity. Administrators tend to be skeptical of analyses performed by providers. Nevertheless, in a rational system, a program that can show a reasonable cost–benefit analysis has an important advantage over a program that cannot. Needless to say, providers would derive some satisfaction from this process, because of their ethical obligation to do their best, even if it did not definitively impact their funding prospects.

## Program Development

Program development is an essential part of running a rehabilitation program. Evolving science, technology, and policy must be integrated with existing practice. This integration of the new into, or replacing, the old is generally taken for granted with pharmaceuticals. New medications are disseminated and used more rapidly than psychosocial technologies (although use of new pharmaceuticals is arguably still slower than should be expected; see Lehman, Steinwachs, Dixon, Goldman, et al., 1998; Lehman, Steinwachs, Dixon, Postrado, et al., 1998). Comprehensive rehabilitation requires attention to technological developments beyond those in the neurophysiological domain. This need must be addressed systematically by the program's leadership, and the costs must be reflected in the program's operating budget.

In current management models, program development is inseparable from quality control. Even if there is no new technology, there is always "room for improvement." This perspective certainly seems applicable in rehabilitation, where, in operational terms, it means treating quality control and program development as having considerable overlap. Accreditation standards and other regulatory mechanisms provide mandates for quality control and improvement that are more specific and operational than the "room for improvement" management philosophy. Minimizing coercion (e.g., by reducing use of restraint and seclusion), maximizing procedural fidelity, enforcing standards of timeliness and completeness in record keeping, requiring logical coherence in treatment and rehabilitation planning—all are codified in standards and regulations, and all translate into objective criteria that can be monitored and improved in an ongoing manner.

The distinction between proactive and reactive management provides another means of formulating philosophy and action with regard to program development. *Reactive management* focuses on identifying problems or failures and taking action to correct them. *Proactive management* focuses on anticipating problems, including the problem of obsolescent technology and procedures. Obviously, both styles are required for efficient and effective program operation. However, it is important to guard against overemphasizing reactive management, because current failures and problems tend to crowd out visions of the future.

The management process of analyzing quality control data, cost data, and outcome data within the program's administrative context (e.g., its mission, its bureaucratic environment, changing service provision standards, etc.) constitutes *program evaluation* that, when combined with a vision of the future, provides guidance for program development. (For a textbook account of program evaluation in human services, see Smith, 1990.)

A balanced and complete program development effort thus involves attention to a combination of program operations:

- Meeting minimal standards of service provision
- Improving performance in key areas on an ongoing basis
- Identifying other areas in need of attention and improvement
- Evaluating new technology
- Planning projects to correct problems and make improvements.

The scope of this activity usually requires a "floating committee" management approach, in which a small standing committee (between four and eight members) monitors overall quality control and program development, expanding or creating subcommittees to address specific concerns or implement specific projects. The standing committee meets regularly to review quality control data, monitor ongoing program development projects, and identify new areas for attention.

## Superordinate Administrative Support

The preceding discussion illuminates the importance of obtaining superordinate administrative support for rehabilitation programs. *Superordinate* refers to the administrators of the agency that houses the program, the administrators of the agencies that provide funds for mental health services, the administrators of the agencies that write and enforce health care service regulations, and the politicians that oversee all these agencies. (For further discussion of the dynamics between these administrative and political levels, see Hunter, 1999; Liberman, 1979.) In this regard there is no difference between the public and the private service sectors. Ultimately, there must be a political mandate for rehabilitation services that is strong enough to convince all the relevant administrators and bureaucracies to support the services through funding and regulatory mechanisms. Although the directors of individual programs must participate assertively in this political process, they obviously cannot make rehabilitation happen in a mental health service system by themselves. They need active support from consumer and advocacy organizations, professional organizations, and community interests groups.

Once political support has been secured, the next challenge is securing sufficiently sophisticated technology. As discussed in various contexts throughout this book, rehabilitation requires special technologies at all levels, from biomedical to administrative. For high-level administrators to effectively support rehabilitation, they need a modicum of understanding about its value and the value of administrative and management technology that promotes effective and efficient services. The people that generate the political mandate also must be prepared to teach, inform, and demonstrate to this end.

## CREATING A REHABILITATION PROGRAM
## FOR PEOPLE WITH DISABLING MENTAL ILLNESS

Rehabilitation is increasingly accepted as the service approach of choice for people with disabling mental illness, but implementation lags behind acceptance. At the current pace, it may be decades before rehabilitation services become commonly available. Until then, typically the first challenge to providing rehabilitation is creating a program where there was none.

Service programs originate through the intersection of policy concerns, provider availability, and popular support. These forces are present in different proportions in different systems. Popular support usually comes in the form of activism by consumer, advocacy, and professional groups. These groups have special interests in social policy that involves services for people with disabling mental illness. By lobbying in the legislative and executive branches, they influence social policy through licensing laws, entitlement laws, funding appropriations, and administrative health care regulations. Policy at any of these levels can either enhance or inhibit the availability of rehabilitation services. Social policy, in turn, influences the availability of professionals and other providers, by offering settings and reimbursement mechanisms for their services. Once a community of rehabilitation providers is established, its technological resources and economic influence can then shape popular support and social policy. As is typical in complex systems, the flow of influence between policy, popular support, and resource availability is nonlinear and multidirectional.

Once a group of individuals has formed an alliance for the purpose of developing services for people with disabling mental illness, the following determinations must be considered:

1. Rehabilitation of the kind generally described in the integrated paradigm is the approach of choice for the recipient population in question
2. Existing or potential financial sources are sufficient to fund the necessary human and technological resources
3. Human and technological resources for providing rehabilitation are available locally, or such resources could be recruited and/or developed
4. The recipient population and their needs are sufficiently focused, so that providing services under the auspices of a program would be optimally effective and cost-efficient.

Once the need and desirability of a rehabilitation program are determined, a work group generally forms to attend to the details of implementation. This may be the same group that determined the need for a program, or it may be a different group, responding to the policy consequences of the original group's determination. For example, in mental health bureaucracies, need determinations (often called *needs assessments* in policy argot) often spawn "requests for proposals" (RFPs), which invite providers to submit bids on providing the designated services. RFPs can be tailored to specify that rehabilitation services must be provided in a program format. When the RFP is successful, a combination of entrepreneurial interest and concern for the recipient population inspires providers to assemble a proposal which, upon winning the bidding competition, eventually becomes the rehabilitation program. For another example, a high-level mental health system administrator may issue a directive (perhaps in response to pressure from public interest groups), to publicly funded agencies and institutions for the purpose of developing rehabilitation programs. The funding and other resources for the new program may be derived, in part or in whole, from funding and resources previously invested in obsolete services (e.g., long-term medical/custodial services). It is important to note, in this regard, that under some conditions, such as reasonably funded institutional settings, rehabilitation programs do not cost more than custodial services.

The work group's next steps include identifying and appointing a program director and the key rehabilitation professionals who will comprise the program's leadership. Often, these individuals are already represented among the work group and, in fact, are the nucleus around which the group formed. Whether recruited internally or externally, the program director and the program's professional leadership must reflect the complete scope of skills and technology required for successful pursuit of the program's mission. Therefore, an accurate survey of local and technological resources is crucial to successfully implementing these program development steps. Local professional organizations can be of some help in identifying individuals with the required background. However, the work group should also pursue contacts with national organizations, both professional and advocacy, and cast as wide a recruitment net as necessary.

Understanding the history of the local and regional mental health communities also can be helpful. There are numerous service systems in which rehabilitation programs or their predecessors thrived at one time but perished in the wake of changing politics and social policy. In such settings, there may be no traces of the past program, and services for people with disabling mental illness are limited to medication monitoring. However, such settings may still harbor individuals who participated in historically progressive efforts, who retain what they learned, and who would again be valuable contributors in a supportive administrative environment. The morale and human resources in a system that has been operating in a regressive medical/custodial environment are not necessarily indicators of what they would be in a rehabilitation environment. In short, sometimes creating a new program includes resurrecting abandoned rehabilitation resources.

The next steps in creating a rehabilitation program include developing the program's Procedures Manual, defining the specific services the program will provide, and developing staff training modalities. These modalities will vary with each program's mission. Generally, however, a comprehensive rehabilitation program should have the capacity to provide all the assessments, interventions, and related services discussed in Chapters 4–10. As discussed earlier in this chapter, staff training is expected to encompass those skills necessary to enact the integrated paradigm's prescriptions for team functioning and clinical decision making and for maintaining a supportive and therapeutic environment. Some amount of training will usually be necessary for staff designated as skills trainers (some professionals may already possess these skills, but other professionals and paraprofessionals will generally need training). Training in contingency management is usually necessary for all staff members, because all are involved, sooner or later, in implementation of that intervention. No health care disciplines include contingency management as part of standard professional training, and very few even make it available. Within a program, the focus and scope of contingency management training are different for different staff. Change agents in inpatient or residential settings generally require the most extensive contingency management implementation skills, but all staff in all settings need to acquire a baseline of familiarity with basic principles.

The final steps in creating a rehabilitation program include hiring the staff, performing the initial staff training, inaugurating the mechanisms for processing referrals and accepting recipients, and assembling the rehabilitation teams. At this point the distinction between creating the program and running it becomes obscure. The final steps are also continuing steps. Recruiting and hiring staff is a never-ending issue because of turnover. Staff training is also a never-ending issue, both because of turnover and because the technology evolves and creates new training needs. Of course, admitting and discharging recipients is the heart of the program's life cycle. Eventually, even the earliest steps in program development (e.g., securing administrative support) must be retraced. Much of the continuing challenge of running a rehabilitation program is a reiteration of creating it.

In a related vein, rehabilitation programs do not always have a discrete beginning, nor do they always follow the steps described here in a linear fashion. Administrative support is often ambivalent, wavering over time. Professional and technological resources come and go in response to myriad economic, demographic, and geographic factors. Programs may evolve slowly over time, through periods of rapid development and quiescence, as the mental health system itself evolves. For providers and administrators, effective commitment to rehabilitation is a long-term commitment to pursue opportunities when and where they appear.

## SPECIAL MANAGEMENT PROBLEMS
## IN REHABILITATION PROGRAMS

A myriad of management problems are common to most health care service situations. Some of these take on special characteristics in the context of rehabilitation for disabling mental illness, and therefore deserve discussion here.

### Drift

*Drift* is a general term for a program's tendency to gradually deviate from basic principles and procedures. It is more than a reduction in procedural fidelity, such as incomplete observance of decision-making procedures or skipping components of a social skills training curriculum. However, lapses in procedural fidelity are often symptoms of drift, especially when they are frequent or persistent. Conducting rehabilitation in accordance with the integrated paradigm is an endeavor that is especially vulnerable to drift. There are many reasons for this vulnerability, including the paradigm's technological complexity, its demand for high levels of procedural fidelity, and its interdisciplinary character.

Quality control is the first line of defense against drift. Ongoing monitoring of the procedural fidelity being observed in key areas is essential. The assessment and progress evaluation steps of the rehabilitation plan process are (1) relatively easy to monitor for fidelity, (2) crucial prerequisites to efficiency, accountability, and effectiveness, and (3) useful early indicators of drift. Contingency management fidelity, both in planning stages and in its implementation in the supportive/therapeutic milieu, is another leading candidate for continual monitoring.

In large part, drift is an attitude of complacency among the program staff and leadership. Behavioral indicators such as procedural fidelity provide signs of a problem, but often the solution lies in renewed *commitment* on the part of the people involved. Achieving this commitment is a notoriously difficult problem in mental health services, especially public mental health. Services are often underfunded, providers often overworked, and there is often something less than a supportive administrative environment for quality services. In addition, the social stigmatization associated with mental illness (discussed in Chapters 9 and 10) affects providers as well as service recipients. Some administrators (and the public) assume that public providers "would be working in the private sector if they could," and sometimes providers believe this of themselves. Providers at all levels often confront a reality that their income is lower than that of colleagues who serve other mental health populations in equivalent positions. It is difficult to maintain high morale and an energetic commitment to quality under these circumstances. Because of these obstacles, maintaining a rehabilita-

tion program inevitably requires creativity in finding and exploiting uncommon incentives. Fortunately, the gratification and satisfaction that providers experience in the wake of successful rehabilitation and recovery can
be quite intense, even sufficient to overcome the absence of more material
rewards. However, this source of gratification does not excuse the program
leadership from making a continuing effort to educate mental health administrators and the public about the value of rehabilitation and the importance of appropriate fiscal support for rehabilitation services.

## Managed Care

Managed care is not intrinsically evil, but it is easily attached to purposes
that sacrifice humanitarianism for economic gain and political expedience
(Hurley & Draper, 1998; Searles & Fox, 1998). The managed care principles increasingly permeating public mental health services bring a simplistic, biologically reductionistic, medical model perspective with them. This
perspective may be helpful for controlling unnecessary medical care costs,
but it is incompatible with rehabilitation in the integrated paradigm at a
number of levels. For one, managed care focuses on discontinuing services
as soon as "medical stability" has been achieved—but people with disabling mental illness are often "medically stable" even while living in the
worst possible conditions because of their illness. The main value of rehabilitation lies in the concept of facilitating long-term improvement of baseline personal and social functioning—not a common notion in the world of
managed care.

   The solution to this problem is not to abolish managed care but to ensure that it is appropriately adapted to the realities of disabling mental illness, the values and principles of rehabilitation and recovery, and the nature of the technology. As with so many other aspects of running a
program, achieving these conditions entails a continuous educational process directed at administrators, politicians, and public interest groups.

## Staff Training

The forces of drift, managed care, and the technological demands of rehabilitation interact to make staff training an especially important issue for
program management. Traditionally, training and education in health care
have been partially subsidized through third-party funding (i.e., paying for
student-provided services in teaching hospitals, Veterans Administration
Medical Centers, state hospitals, community mental health centers, etc.). In
managed care, this subsidization is seen as an unnecessary hidden cost. (For
discussions of health care education under managed care, see DeLeon et al.,
1996; Jacobs, Hoge, Sledge, & Bunney, 1997; Meyer & McLaughlin, 1998;
Schuster & Lovell, 1997.) The infrastructure for education of health care

professionals is currently being dismantled because health care underwriters are no longer willing to pay the "overhead" of training the next generation of providers. Although alarms have been raised, no solutions are apparent at this time. Rehabilitation is as vulnerable to this trend as any other health care enterprise. It is difficult enough to find professionals with specialized rehabilitation skills; with the current trend, fewer resources are available for on-the-job training. This is no less true for paraprofessionals.

Compounding this problem is controversy within the rehabilitation community regarding the limitations of staff training. Highly effective programs, such as that reported by Paul and Lentz (1977), require extraordinary training resources—which may be the reason that they have not proliferated, despite their demonstrated superiority. Even when professionals are trained in specific interventions suitable for traditional office practice, such as behavioral family therapy, they do not necessarily use them (Fadden, 1997). Program-wide implementation of token economy or related technologies often requires entire institutions to change their organizational and administrative infrastructures, and brings many professionals and paraprofessionals under new pressure for accountability and procedural fidelity. Staff training is probably not enough to overcome the omnipresent barriers—including public apathy, stigma and prejudice, politicization of health care, professional guild rivalries, staff burnout, misguided unionism, bureaucratic perfidy—to providing cost-effective services for people with severe mental illness.

Corrigan and colleagues at the University of Chicago's Center for Psychiatric Rehabilitation have developed "interactive staff training" to overcome the resistance engendered by this multiplicity of factors (Corrigan & McCracken, 1997a). Their approach uses various principles of organizational psychology to engage staff and administrators in developing rehabilitation capabilities and acquiring skills. An empirical study of the approach suggests it is effective in reducing aggression and defusing staff resistance within institutional settings (Corrigan, Holmes, Luchns, & Basit, 1995). However, similar effects have been reported with only limited interventions that address organizational as well as staff training issues (Gershater, Lutzker, & Kuehnel, 1997; Milne, Gorenski, Westerman, Leck, & Keegan, 2000; Milne, Keegan, Westerman, & Dudley, 2000; Silverstein, Bowman, & McHugh, 1997; Stark & Stutte, 1990; Sullivan, Richardson, & Spaulding, 1991). There is controversy, sometimes rather heated, about what degree of staff training and other resources is necessary for humane, cost-effective, and well-staffed rehabilitation programs (see, e.g., Corrigan & McCracken, 1997b; Morisse, Batra, Hess, Silverman, & Corrigan, 1996; Paul, Stuve, & Cross, 1997).

In any case, it is highly questionable whether quality rehabilitation services can be provided without ongoing training and education resources for both professional and paraprofessional staff. The future viability of rehabilitation, and perhaps other health care services, may depend on increased public awareness of the impending crisis and a responsive moderation of managed care excesses. Providers, administrators, consumers, and advocates face an uphill battle to secure the economic resources and overcome the institutional obstacles necessary to train providers on the job. Nevertheless, advocacy in this domain remains a requisite activity for running a rehabilitation program.

## Brain Drain

Paradoxically, a rehabilitation program's success can become one of its key vulnerabilities. For the reasons discussed in this chapter, a successful rehabilitation program tends to develop special administrative, management, and clinical skills in its providers. These skills are highly valued in health care service systems and bureaucracies, even when rehabilitation itself is not so highly valued. Program directors who have been successful in securing administrative support for their program are coveted by agencies, institutions, and service systems. The leadership of any well-reputed program inevitably experiences pressure to share their skills and resources outside the program. Providers with respected "high-tech" skills (e.g., in psychopharmacotherapy or neuropsychology) who also have practiced successfully in interdisciplinary services, are coveted by other program directors. Paraprofessionals with training and experience in milieu-based interventions are constantly sought for higher salaried supervisory positions. One characteristic of a successful program is the exodus of a large number of key providers, including program leaders, as they move on to more senior roles elsewhere in the system.

The best strategy may be for rehabilitation programs to take advantage of their pioneering status and make their training and education role highly explicit. Establishing affiliations with universities and professional schools is one way of doing this. Even with the current managed care assault on health care education, established education programs can often provide stability that compensates for the turnover problem. Such affiliations bring additional benefits, such as access to grant funds and faculty resources. The down side is that turnover is *increased* when students are involved, and additional resources are needed for the supervision requirements of student-provided services. Nevertheless, the integrated paradigm is especially compatible with the values and priorities of health care education, and educational resources will probably provide a crucial element of support to rehabilitation programs for years to come.

# Appendix 1

# A Prototype Problem Set for Assessment, Treatment, and Rehabilitation of People with Severe Mental Illness

(Authors' note: The elements in this appendix track the discussions in Chapters 4–10.)

## NEUROPHYSIOLOGICAL LEVEL OF FUNCTIONING

**Problem Title: Episodic Neurophysiological Dysregulation of the Central Nervous System**

*Problem Definition*

A neurophysiological condition characterized by episodes of acute psychosis and highly variable clinical expressions, including extreme subjective distress, extreme affective responses (from euphoric to dysphoric), blunted affective responses, hallucinations, disruption of cognitive functioning, bizarre or socially unacceptable behavior, extreme irritability, and explosiveness. Distinct patterns of abnormality within this problem are traditionally associated with schizophrenia, schizoaffective disorder, severe or psychotic depression, delusional disorder, and bipolar disorder. Recent research on medication response in individuals diagnosed with borderline personality disorder has linked that diagnosis to this type of dysregulation. However, specific characteristics vary highly within and across diagnostic categories. The clinical presentation may meet the criteria for multiple diagnostic categories. In addition to discrete episodes, this problem may include an enduring neurophysiological vulnerability requiring continued intervention to prevent recurrence.

The neurophysiological mechanisms involved are incompletely understood, and numerous specific mechanisms are probably involved in different ways in different individuals. Clinical response to medication also is highly variable, and the optimal regimen may prove to be a single compound or a combination of compounds across different drug families. The critical indication is not the effectiveness of any particular type of neurophysiological-level treatment but a clear pattern of positive clinical response to a known regimen. Data relevant to identification of this problem generally come from subjective report of the recovering person, observations by key informants in the natural environment, social history, and ongoing assessment of response to neurophysiological-level interventions (which may include psychosocial and environmental as well as pharmacological modalities). Ongoing assessment of this problem usually includes gradual discrimination between clinical expressions directly produced by the dysregulation and expressions that are behaviorally similar but are not resolved by optimal neurophysiological intervention. The latter must be further evaluated as possibly representing more molar-level problems. A detailed and protracted functional analysis of behavior may be necessary to complete this process.

Evidence of previous positive response to medications in the antipsychotic and/or antidepressant family is highly suggestive of this pattern of dysregulation. Subjective report, observations by key informants, and systematic behavioral observation are key sources of treatment response data. Neurocognitive assessment is often helpful in evaluating response to intervention, although some baseline data is generally required for comparison.

**Problem Title: Tonic Dysregulation of the Central Nervous System**

*Problem Definition*

A neurophysiological condition characterized by continuous (nonepisodic) cognitive, affective, psychophysiological, and/or behavioral dysfunction. Distinct patterns of abnormality within this problem are associated with residual schizophrenia, depression, dysthymic disorder, anxiety disorder(s), and intermittent explosive disorder. However, specific characteristics vary highly within and across diagnostic categories, and the clinical presentation may meet criteria for multiple diagnostic categories. The dysregulation may be iatrogenic—produced by medications—usually by those being used to treat episodic dysregulation, or by the drugs being used to control the side effects of other drugs (especially anticholinergic drugs).

Tonic neurophysiological dysregulation may be difficult to differentiate from episodic dysregulation. Tonic dysregulation should be considered as a separate problem when (1) the clinical picture does not include evidence of episodic fluctuations, (2) there is evidence of iatrogenic effects, or (3) the effective intervention is qualitatively different from the intervention that most effectively controls episodic dysregulation. Indications of tonic dysregulation often occur as residual impairments (i.e., ones that remain after effective control of an episodic dysregulation). Behaviors associated with tonic dysregulation are also associated with neurocognitive, sociocognitive, sociobehavioral, and socioenvironmental problems. Contributions from these domains should be assessed systematically in the course of defining and treating any tonic dysregulation problem.

The techniques and instruments most useful for assessing tonic neurophysiological dysfunction are generally those used to assess episodic dysfunction, in addition to the assessments used to evaluate the role of more molar-level problems contributing to the clinical picture (which serves to articulate the neurophysiological problem through a process of elimination).

## NEUROCOGNITIVE LEVEL OF FUNCTIONING

**Problem Title: Post-Acute Neurocognitive Impairments**

*Problem Definition*

Impairment in cognitive functioning, in the relatively molecular levels generally addressed by neuropsychological assessment, attributable to the lingering effects of one or more episodes of acute psychosis. Post-acute neurocognitive impairment must be distinguished from (1) impairment that is resolved by neurophysiological treatment of episodic or tonic neurophysiological dysregulation, and (2) residual neurocognitive impairments. Post-acute neurocognitive impairment responds to the passage of time and/or psychosocial intervention after optimal neurophysiological stabilization. Post-acute impairment sometimes requires fairly intensive therapeutic intervention, so the passage of time since acute psychosis is not a sufficient criterion in itself. Neuropsychological assessment is generally most useful for evaluating post-acute impairments, when used systematically in a longitudinal frame of reference.

**Problem Title: Residual Neurocognitive Impairments**

*Problem Definition*

Impairment in cognitive functioning, in the relatively molecular levels generally addressed by neuropsychological assessment, that does not respond to any known neurophysiological or psychosocial intervention. This problem must be identified through a process of elimination that establishes the ineffectiveness of all available interventions.

Neuropsychological assessment is generally most useful for evaluating residual impairments, when used systematically in a longitudinal frame of reference. After identifying the impairments as residual, further assessment articulates the nature of the impairment for the purpose of designing prosthetic or compensatory interventions.

## SOCIOCOGNITIVE LEVEL OF FUNCTIONING

**Problem Title: Social Problem-Solving Insufficiency**

*Problem Definition*

Insufficient ability to (1) identify problematic situations, (2) analyze relevant factors, (3) generate a useable range of solutions, and (4) evaluate the effectiveness of chosen solutions; not attributable to the effects of neurophysiological dysregulation or neurocognitive impairment. A wide range of behavioral characteristics may be associated with this sociocognitive problem, ranging from passivity and dependence to belligerence and aggression. The key characteristic is inability to engage in the cognitive processes necessary for managing routine problems in daily living and/or ordinary interpersonal conflicts. Social behavior may show a lack of problem-solving activity or persistent use of an ineffective solution.

The expressions of this problem may have considerable overlap with expressions of other problems. This problem is the better choice when there is evidence and/or expectation that interventions at other levels will not fully resolve the problem-solving insufficiency and its related behaviors. For example, a mood-linked attribution problem should be cited when there is evidence and/or expectation that a psychotherapeutic intervention focused on modification of intropunitive attributions, and a subsequent normalization of mood, would produce optimal social problem solving. Similarly, social skills deficits should be used when the problem-solving insufficiency is limited to interpersonal conflict and is expected to respond optimally to social skills training. The eliminating factors are (1) problem-solving difficulties limited to particular situations, and (2) the expectation of success in response to broadly focused problem-solving therapy.

## Problem Title: Symptom-Linked Attribution Problem

### Problem Definition

Constellations of beliefs, attitudes, attributions, and related sociocognitive characteristics (e.g., locus of control dimensions) that constitute recognized psychiatric symptoms, usually identified as delusions, including delusions of persecution (paranoid delusions), disfigurement, disease or injury (somatic delusions) that include special abilities or powers (e.g., grandiose delusions) and experience of personal guilt or evilness (e.g., mood-congruent delusions in psychotic depression). Particular beliefs may combine these themes; for example, the belief that one is a famous historical figure and is being persecuted because of that special identity. In some cases, it may be unclear whether the beliefs are independent of perceptual anomalies (e.g., the belief that one is hearing the voice of the devil) or ideas of reference (e.g., the belief that one is receiving secret signals from others. Symptom-linked attributions vary in stability, internal consistency, and complexity; they range from vague, intermittent, amorphous allusions to highly stable, logically coherent, and fully articulated narrative accounts.

Symptom-linked attributions are often associated with neurophysiological dysregulation, especially of the episodic type. Some delusions are associated with neurocognitive impairments and/or tonic neurophysiological dysregulation—for example, that familiar people, places, or things have been replaced by substitutes (Capgrass syndrome). When the attributions are so closely linked to neurophysiological dysregulation that resolution of the latter resolves the former, the attributions are subsumed under the neurophysiological problem title and included in its problem description. The symptom-linked attribution problem title should be used when the attribution problem persists after other indications of acute psychosis have been resolved and further neurophysiological and/or neurocognitive interventions are ineffective. The problem title "socialized psychiatric symptom" should be used instead if the problematic attributions are demonstrably linked to the performance of a "mental patient" social role, and/or there is evidence and/or expectation that a contingency management or related intervention would fully resolve the problem.

Symptom-linked attributions are generally best assessed by using a combination of *anamnestic measures* (e.g., structured interviews) that rate the person's expression of the belief, and *functional behavioral analysis* that identifies the *in vivo* antecedents and consequences of professing the belief. This problem is generally expected to respond optimally to specialized cognitive-behavioral therapy interventions that combine interpersonal support, logical disputation, and formulation of alternative attributions.

## Problem Title: Mood-Linked Attribution Problem

### Problem Definition

Constellations of beliefs, attitudes, attributions, and related sociocognitive characteristics (e.g., locus of control dimensions) that function to produce and/or maintain specific affective states whose frequency or persistence poses a barrier to optimal functioning. The most common expression of this problem is fatalistic and intropunitive belief patterns associated with dysthymia and chronic depression. The attributional constellation produces an overall suppression of effective personal and social functioning, and also represents a vulnerability to episodes of severe disruption spanning all levels of functioning (major depression). Often, the attributional constellation is part of a larger picture, including a neurophysiological diathesis, social skills deficits, and psychophysiological dysregulation, which combine to produce both tonic dysthymia and episodic exacerbations.

At the opposite pole of the dysphoric–euphoric dimension, a pattern of unrealistically positive self-perceptions and denial of problems is associated with hypomania, a vulnerability to mania, and eventually to major depression (when the defensive function of the attributions breaks down).

A third possible constellation of beliefs, attitudes, and attributions includes imputations of other people's hostile intentions, personal powerlessness, and compensatory entitlement, and associated angry mood and belligerent interpersonal behavior. This constellation is distinct from a symptom-linked attribution problem to the degree that it is independent of bizarre beliefs, grossly inaccurate perceptions of social situations, and other social cognitions and behaviors associated with psychotic states.

Because of the frequent links between mood-linked attributions and problems in neurophysiological, psychophysiological, and sociobehavioral functioning, careful attention must be given to specification of these links as alternative or additional problem titles. Mood-linked attributions should be identified as a separate problem when there is evidence and/or expectation that a specialized intervention focusing on attributional functioning will contribute uniquely to recovery. Failure of the problem to respond to resolution of psychotic states or psychopharmacotherapy is a key indication (this does not imply that the neurophysiological hypothesis should always be tested before others are entertained). Given that psychosocial interventions for depression generally combine cognitive, psychophysiological, and sociobehavioral components, use of the attributional problem title should be limited to situations in which the attributional component is hypothesized to be an especially powerful or unique contributor, and the optimal intervention is expected to be one almost exclusively focused on self-perception and related social cognition. In many cases, the attributional problem title should be accompanied by a neurophysiological, psychophysiological, or skills-related problem title, indicating a hypothesis of the presence of relatively independent contributions to the clinical picture at multiple levels.

## Problem Title: Achievement-Linked Attribution Problem

### Problem Definition

Constellations of beliefs, attitudes, attributions, and related sociocognitive characteristics (e.g., locus of control dimensions) regarding one's life circumstances, responsibilities, and personal functioning that constitute a barrier to achieving better functioning and a better quality of life. These constellations may include the belief that a restricted, institutional life is the best available, that the responsibilities and benefits of being a competent adult are undesirable, or that a high-risk and/or dissolute lifestyle is unavoidable. These constellations are often associated with specific patterns of behavior, including persistent pursuit of a self-destructive lifestyle, such as that of a "street person," an itinerant religious figure, or a habitual criminal, and may be associated with unrealistic, fantasy-based personal aspirations, such as winning the lottery, becoming a rock star, or running for president.

For the purposes of rehabilitation planning, the most salient consequence of this sociocognitive pattern is a disinterest in treatment or rehabilitation. If the person experiences ambivalence about his or her self-destructive or unrealistic aspirations, engagement in rehabilitation is likely to be partial or sporadic. Worse, the person who feels no ambivalence is likely to actively resist others' efforts to help him or her obtain treatment and rehabilitation.

Assessment of this problem must take into account the accuracy of the individual's beliefs about the nature of the mental illness and expectations for recovery. However, it should be characterized as a disorder management skills deficit if the problem is hypothesized to be primarily the consequence of inaccurate beliefs and/ or lack of skills regarding the nature and management of the mental illness—for example, "I have a disabling mental illness, and I can't do anything about that; therefore, I'm doomed to a dissolute life"), and there is an expectation that education and skills training in this domain would resolve the problem. Providers and others must be especially vigilant about their own stereotypic beliefs, regarding the achievement potential of people with mental illness. A thorough and accurate assessment of the person's true achievement potential is necessary. Similarly, all must be careful to respect each others' values—people do not always agree about the desirability of particular lifestyles. For example, attending college is a sine qua non for some people but an unnecessary waste of time for others.

The criterion of team consensus is the primary evaluation safeguard when weighing these considerations. When the recovering person is strongly resistant to treatment or rehabilitation, intervention by a legal authority or substitute decision maker is necessary to override his or her wishes. In such cases, choice of this problem title must reflect the best possible accommodation of the person's aspirations, within the legal mandate to provide treatment.

Choice of this problem title reflects a hypothesis that the person will develop more realistic and/or more self-serving aspirations in response to (1) rehabilitation counseling, (2) negotiation with providers and substitute decision makers, (3) success in achieving rehabilitation goals, (4) greater knowledge about the nature of the mental illness, and (5) general improvement in personal and social functioning. Given this broad scope, the interventions for this problem may include the entire rehabilitation plan repertoire. Including the attributional problem title serves to ensure monitoring of progress in the sociocognitive domain, but it does ensure the prescription of specific interventions. Assigning a priority 3 to the problem title indicates that specific interventions are not currently being applied (a priority-3 rating does not necessarily indicate that no progress is expected). A specific intervention under the attributional problem title might prescribe individual cognitive-behavioral therapy, similar to that used to address symptom-linked and mood-linked attribution problems, modified to focus on the individual's beliefs about personal responsibility and dignity, personal worth and success, and short- and longer-term life goals.

## SOCIOBEHAVIORAL LEVEL OF FUNCTIONING

### Skills Deficits

#### General Definition of Skill Deficits

Failure to effectively perform behaviors necessary to accomplish a specifiable purpose, when the failure is not wholly attributable to specific problems at more molecular levels of functioning (i.e., neurophysiological dysregulation or cognitive impairment). For rehabilitation purposes, skills are organized into categories of functionally related elements. These categories comprise the specific skills decifits problem titles.

Skills represent complex combinations of abilities, spanning all levels of biobehavioral functioning, plus acquired information stored in memory, in continuous interaction with multitudinous environmental conditions. The acquired information is often extensive and intricate, accumulated over the entire course of human development. Skills deficits represent problems in any or all of these domains. A skills deficit problem title should be identified when it is hypothesized that optimal rehabilitation benefit will be achieved with skills training interventions— that is, interventions designed to establish effective performance by providing information (education), guided rehearsal of key components (role-play), *in vivo* practice, coaching, and related techniques.

Skills deficits have both competence and performance dimensions. A *competence failure* denotes an inability to perform the skill under optimal environmental conditions. A *performance failure* denotes possession of the skill but nonperformance of it under the environmental conditions in which the skill is normally required. Performance failures also may be attributable to insufficient information and/or failure to apprehend the conditions requiring the skill. Performance failures may also be due to prevailing environmental conditions that do not sufficiently prompt or reward performance of the skill. If sufficient skill performance results from making changes in the environmental conditions, without improvement in competence, the skills training intervention may be limited to contingency management or related manipulations of environmental conditions. Often a combination of environmental manipulation and competence-oriented skills training produces optimal skill acquisition.

The intervention logically falls under the skills deficit problem title if environmental manipulations are used to enhance skill acquisition and are expected to lead to better skill performance under natural conditions. However, the rehabilitation plan should identify a separate residual neurocognitive problem if special environmental conditions are thought to be required on a more permanent basis (i.e., as part of a prosthetic environment). The neurocognitive problem should identify inability to respond to antecedents and consequences of normal proximity sufficient for performance of the specified skill(s) in its problem description.

Skills deficits are generally identified through functional assessment that emphasizes direct observation of skill performance under optimal and natural conditions. Case history information usually contributes to identification and characterization of skills deficits. However, historical information is usually anecdotal, not quantitative, and incomplete with regard to environmental conditions that may support or suppress skill performance. Often, careful functional behavioral analysis is required to distinguish between performance failure consequent to low competence and performance failure due to motivational problems. The latter may include sociocognitive constellations of belief that (1) skill performance is not desirable, (2) environmental conditions are insufficient to prompt and reward skill performance, and/or (3) there are stronger incentives to perform incompatible social roles (e.g., the role of an incompetent mental patient). When such factors are hypothesized, the skills deficit problem should be accompanied by additional problems that identify and address those factors, such as achievement-linked attribution problems and/or environmental conflicts.

## Problem Title: Self-Care Skills Deficits

*Problem Definition*

Insufficient competence and/or performance of skills related to personal care, grooming, hygiene, nutrition, and health.

## Problem Title: Independent Living Skills Deficits

*Problem Definition*

Insufficient competence and/or performance of skills related to the demands of routine adult living, including housekeeping, personal budgeting and banking, utilization of public resources (library, public transportation, etc.), maintenance of wardrobe (purchasing clothing, minor repairs, laundry), household shopping and cooking.

## Problem Title: Disorder Management Deficits

*Problem Definition*

Insufficient competence and/or performance of skills related to management of mental illness, including understanding nature and purpose of medication, ability to identify psychotic symptoms and warning signs of psychotic episodes, management of residual symptoms and deficits, and management of stress.

## Problem Title: Leisure/Recreational Skills Deficits

*Problem Definition*

Insufficient competence and/or performance of skills related to planning and managing leisure time.

## Problem Title: Occupational Skills Deficits

*Problem Definition*

Insufficient competence and/or performance of skills related to maintaining a work role or similar social role (e.g., as a volunteer in a service program, a member of a psychosocial clubhouse program, or participant in an activities program). This problem includes skills generally related to all or most occupational functioning, not skills required for particular vocational pursuits. These include skills relevant to job punctuality, self-regulation and pacing, following instructional protocols, appropriately using problem solving in unfamiliar situations, and maintaining interpersonal relationships appropriate to the occupational setting.

## Problem Title: Interpersonal Skills Deficits

### Problem Definition

Insufficient competence and/or performance of skills related to interpersonal interactions, including making conversation, expressing needs, making requests, identifying and resolving ordinary conflicts, establishing and maintaining friendships.

## Psychophysiological Dysregulations

### Problem Definition

Failure to effectively regulate psychophysiological activation, resulting in subjective distress, cognitive impairment, and/or disruption of skill performance. Psychophysiological dysregulation organizes into distinct patterns, reflecting the relatively independent activity of neurophysiological systems, especially patterns of autonomic activation. These patterns comprise the specific problems.

Psychophysiological regulation involves acquired abilities, most generally the ability to produce particular patterns of activation needed for optimal performance of specific skills. Neurocognitive, sociocogitive, and sociobehavioral processes operate in coordination, using information stored in memory, to achieve psychophysiological regulation. Selection of a psychophysiological dysregulation problem title reflects a hypothesis that functional subjective distress and/or behavioral problems are attributable to processes distributed across these levels. The title selection also reflects an expectation that resolution of the distress and/or behavioral problem will be optimally achieved by skills training interventions—that is, interventions designed to improve psychophysiological regulation by providing information (education), guided rehearsal of key skill components (role-play), in vivo practice, coaching, and related techniques.

The highly variable subjective and behavioral expressions of psychophysiological dysregulations are associated with neurophysiological dysregulation, cognitive impairments, and other sociobehavioral skills deficits. The role of neurophysiological dysregulation should be assessed; the psychophysiological problem should not be used if there is an expectation that neurophysiological intervention would resolve the behavioral problems. Similarly, neurocognitive, sociocognitive, skills deficit, or environmental problem titles should be used when there is an expectation that interventions at these levels would resolve the problems.

### Problem Title: Dysregulation of Behavioral Activation

*Problem Definition*

Disruption of normal cycles of behavioral activity and rest or sleep, reversal of diurnal sleep–wake periods—up all night and asleep all day—to a degree causing subjective distress, cognitive impairment, impairment of instrumental skill performance, and/or difficulty adhering to a daily routine of necessary activities. This problem should be identified when data indicate that the dysregulation is functionally independent from neurophysiological dysregulation and cannot be resolved through intervention at the neurophysiological level.

### Problem Title: Dysregulation of Mood

*Problem Definition*

A pattern of behavior and psychophysiological activation that produces extreme mood fluctuations and/or persistence of one or more mood states that normally would be transient and situation-dependent. The clinical picture may be that associated with the diagnostic and paradiagnostic descriptors for mood disorders such as dysthymia, major depression, hypomania, mania, and paranoia (when used to describe a persistent mood of anger or belligerence). This type of problem is often one component of a clinical picture that includes neurophysiological and sociocognitive components. The contributions of all components must be assessed carefully. In many cases, the most effective rehabilitation strategy involves a combination of neurophysiological, sociocognitive, and sociobehavioral interventions. This problem title should be used when sociobehavioral interventions designed to strengthen a person's affective self-regulation skills are expected to contribute independently to overall outcome.

### Problem Title: Dysregulation of Anger/Aggression

*Problem Definition*

A pattern of psychophysiological dysregulation associated with extreme, explosive, and/or socially unacceptable anger and/or aggression. The clinical picture may conform to the diagnostic criteria for intermittent explosive disorder, but it is usually not diagnosed separately when it is observed in the context of severe mental illness. This problem title should be used when (1) data indicate that the relevant behavior is at least partially independent of neurophysiological, cognitive, and socioenvironmental factors, and (2) a sociobehavioral intervention designed to strengthen self-regulation skills is expected to contribute independently to overall outcome.

**Problem Title: Dysregulation of Fear/Anxiety**

*Problem Definition*

Dysregulation of psychophysiological processes associated with fear and/or anxiety. The dysregulation may be expressed as subjective experience of (1) intense psychophysiological arousal, (2) abnormally frequent experience of normal-intensity arousal, (3) behavioral avoidance of anxiety-producing situations, or (4) some combination of these. When avoidance behavior is operative, the anxiety motivating the avoidance may escape direct subjective awareness. Avoidance may be expressed at neurocognitive and/or sociocognitive levels of functioning, when it is often associated with the paradiagnostic concepts of repression, denial, somatization, or dissociation. The clinical picture may conform to the diagnostic criteria for anxiety disorders or dissociative disorders. However, expressions of this type of dysregulation are observed in many individuals who do not meet the criteria, especially when the clinical picture is dominated by sociocognitive avoidance. Borderline personality disorder is increasingly the diagnostic choice in such cases. People with severe and disabling mental illnesses often show this type of dysregulation, although it is often not diagnosed as a comorbid condition. This problem title should be used when the optimal rehabilitation strategy is expected to (1) include a sociobehavioral intervention designed to educate the person about the nature of anxiety and its self-regulation, (2) block avoidance behaviors, and (3) extinguish conditioned psychophysiological responses to feared stimuli.

**Problem Title: Dysregulation of Appetitive Behavior**

*Problem Definition*

Dysregulation of behaviors associated with hunger and thirst. The diagnostic categories of eating disorders incorporate many of these behavior patterns, although the behavior is not always produced primarily by a psychophysiological dysregulation. Polydipsia (i.e., dysregulation of fluid intake) may also reflect a psychophysiological dysregulation. Medication side effects, medical conditions not associated with mental illness, neurocognitive impairments, dysfunctional beliefs and attributions, deficient social problem-solving, and socioenvironmental circumstances may eclipse the role of psychophysiological dysregulation. This problem title should be used when it is expected that a psychophysiological skills training intervention, intended to strengthen a person's ability to understand and manage hunger or thirst, is expected to contribute uniquely to overall rehabilitation outcome.

    *Polydipsia* deserves special mention, as it is especially frequent in people with disabling mental illness. Polydipsia is usually associated with persistent thirst. It occurs along a continuum of severity, with consequences ranging from subjective discomfort to life-threatening disruption of blood chemistry. Polydipsia is poorly understood. It may be a side effect of psychotropic medication, at least in some cases. When it cannot be eliminated through judicious psychopharmacotherapy, psychosocial interventions are sometimes helpful. These interventions generally include education and skills training; sometimes contingency management or related socioenvironmental interventions (discussed in Chapter 10) are also helpful.

**Problem Title: Dysregulation of Sexual Behavior**

*Problem Definition*

Dysregulation of the psychophysiological aspects of sexual functioning, which may include absence of sexual interest, anorgasmia, erectile dysfunction, ejaculatory dysfunction, and paraphilia. Sexual dysfunctions are often associated with neurophysiological dysregulation, neurocognitive impairment, dysfunctional social cognition, social skills deficits, and socioenvironmental problems. This problem title should be used when there is evidence that impairment of specific psychophysiological mechanisms associated with normal sexual desire and/or sexual response are contributing independently to the clinical picture, and that interventions designed to strengthen the person's control over those mechanisms will contribute uniquely to overall rehabilitation outcome.

**Problem Title: Substance Abuse**

*Problem Definition*

A persistent pattern of using alcohol or other drugs to induce an altered state of consciousness, when such use contributes uniquely to other problems or deficits in a person's neurophysiological, cognitive, and/or sociobehavioral functioning. Problems consequent to substance abuse may include increased vulnerability to episodic neurophysiological dysregulation and acute psychosis and socially unacceptable behaviors associated with obtaining substances of abuse. This problem title should be used when an intervention intended to reduce the person's use of substances is expected to contribute uniquely to rehabilitation outcome.

## SOCIOENVIRONMENTAL PROBLEMS

**Problem Title: Rehabilitation Nonadherence**

*Problem Definition*

A persistent pattern of nonadherence to treatment and/or rehabilitation regimens, when such regimens are expected to produce better personal and social functioning and some degree of recovery from disabling mental illness. The nonadherence may or may not be consistent with the person's subjectively experienced and/or expressed desires. This problem title should be used when (1) the nonadherence cannot be attributed solely to neurophysiological, cognitive, or sociobehavioral factors, (2) interventions directed at those factors do not fully resolve the nonadherence, and (3) socioenvironmental intervention is required, at least temporarily, to establish adherence and facilitate recovery.

### Problem Title: Socialized Psychiatric Symptoms

*Problem Definition*

Behaviors that are similar to expressions of neurophysiological dysregulation (e.g., psychotic symptoms) or cognitive impairment, but which function as social operants and effect specifiable environmental consequences or support performance of a mental patient social role. This problem title should be used when evidence indicates that the behavior does not respond to neurophysiological, cognitive, or sociobehavioral interventions, and it is expected to respond to socioenvironmental interventions.

### Problem Title: Socially Unacceptable Behavior

*Problem Definition*

Specific behaviors that exploit or harm others or are not generally tolerated in normal social environments. This problem title should be used when evidence indicates that the behavior does not respond to neurophysiological, cognitive, or sociobehavioral interventions, and it is expected to respond to socioenvironmental interventions. It may be necessary to use this problem title in cases where the behavior is hypothesized to result from some combination of more molecular-level factors, but where intervention at more molecular levels is not expected to produce results quickly enough to prevent harm. In such cases, pending resolution of more molecular-level problems, this problem title should be used in conjunction with socioenvironmental interventions to prevent harm.

### Problem Title: Social-Environmental Conflict

*Problem Definition*

A problem involving conflict between the recovering person and others in the recovering person's social environment, wherein changes in the recovering person's neurophysiological, cognitive, or sociobehavioral functioning are not expected to fully resolve the conflict. The goals of interventions under this problem title are expected to include changes in the recovering person's behavior and the behavior of

others in the recovering person's social environment. The conflict may be unrelated
to rehabilitation processes, or it may center on the behaviors of others (e.g., hostility, emotional overinvolvement, or any behavior inconsistent with the recovering
person's abilities and autonomy) that do not serve the best interests of the recovering person. This problem title should be used when it is expected that interventions
intended to change the behavior of others as they interact with the recovering person will contribute uniquely to overall rehabilitation outcome.

**Problem Title: Restrictive Legal Status**

*Problem Definition*

Conflict between the recovering person and a legal authority, wherein the legal authority imposes restrictions on the recovering person's rights, due to past determinations of risk, dangerousness, or lack of legal competence. The restrictions may be
anachronistic, reflecting conditions that have changed since their original imposi-
tion. Alternatively, the restrictions may reflect a continuing appraisal by the legal
authority that despite changes in the recovering person, the existing risks are such
that safety demands continued precautions. In either case, changes in the recovering
person's personal and social functioning are insufficient to remove the restrictions.
This problem title should be used when it is expected that socioenvironmental intervention will be required. The intervention would either convince the legal authority
to change the restrictions, or it would create an environment in which the recovering person could pursue rehabilitation and optimal personal and social functioning
within the constraints of the restrictions.

**Problem Title: Unstable Living Situation**

*Problem Definition*

Environmental circumstances that prevent establishment of a stable living situation,
which may include financial limitations, unavailability of suitable housing, or unavailability of necessary support services. Such circumstances are usually associated
with problems in the recovering person's personal and social functioning. This
problem title should be used when improvements in functioning are not expected to
fully stabilize the person's living condition, or when more molecular-level interventions are not expected to produce stabilization quickly enough to provide for the
person's safety and comfort. In both cases, a socioenvironmental intervention is required, on either a temporary or permanent basis.

*Appendix 2*

# Rehabilitation Plan and Progress Evaluation Documents

(Authors' note: The elements in this appendix track the hypothetical case described in Chapter 2.)

The rehabilitation plans and progress evaluation documents in this appendix are designed to demonstrate the principles of assessment and planning discussed in Chapter 3 by using a fairly representative clinical picture of disabling mental illness, and a fairly representative response to intensive rehabilitation. The details of assessment findings and intervention procedures are not included here; they would normally be documented extensively in separate sections of the clinical record (e.g., "Database," "Progress Notes," etc.). Various other clinical documents, often required by recording standards, are omitted because they are not crucial to demonstrating the elements and principles of the integrated paradigm.

The first document is the initial plan, formulated upon admission to the inpatient rehabilitation program at Central State Mental Health Center, a hypothetical state-operated treatment facility.

### MASTER REHABILITATION PLAN (6/01/02)

Rehabilitation client: Joe A
Date of formulation of this plan: June 1, 2002
Date of next progress review: July 1, 2002

Problem title index:

| | |
|---|---|
| Problem 1. Episodic CNS dysregulation | Priority Level: 1 |
| Problem 2. Disorder management skills deficit | Priority Level: 2 |
| Problem 3. Occupational skills deficit | Priority Level: 2 |
| Problem 4. Leisure/recreational skills deficit | Priority Level: 2 |
| Problem 5. Substance abuse | Priority Level: 3 |
| Problem 6. Unstable living situation | Priority Level: 3 |

**Problem 1**

*Problem Title*: Episodic CNS dysregulation
*Priority Level*: 1
*Problem Description*: History of periods of acute psychosis characterized by confusion, agitation, auditory hallucinations, and beliefs that various people are persecuting him; history indicates reliable resolution of the acute episode within 4–6 weeks of antipsychotic medication; duration of episodes without medication intervention is unknown, but history shows no evidence of spontaneous remissions.
*Long-Term Goal*: Establish stable CNS regulation, prevent recurrence of acute psychotic episodes, determine optimal regime for long-term maintenance.
*Short-Term Goal (1)*: Resolve current acute psychosis, eliminate confusion, agitation, and psychotic symptoms.
*Short-Term Goal (2)*: Identify optimal regime, with minimal side effects, for preventing relapse.
*Interventions*: Psychopharmacotherapy, behavior management programs 1 and 2.

1. *Psychopharmacotherapy, intervention parameters*: Scheduled meeting with team psychiatrist, once per week for 30 minutes, for assessment and counseling regarding medications (for current medication regime, see "Physicians Orders" section of medical record).
2. *Behavior management program (1), intervention parameters*: Individualized contingency management program (a) targeting escalating agitation and threats of aggression, and (b) providing staff cues for time-out-from-reinforcement procedure; level-1 privileges contingent on absence of escalation or cooperation with TOFR.
3. *Behavior management program (2), intervention parameters*: Individualized contingency management program targeting adherence to daily schedule, including self-care activities, social/occupational/recreational activities, and scheduled treatment/rehabilitation activities.

*Key Indicators*:

1. Weekly progress note from team psychiatrist, reporting objective and subjective reductions of psychotic symptoms.
2. BPRS: Disorganization, Excitement, and Paranoia items.
3. NOSIE-30 PSY and IRR subscales.
4. Behavior management program data: Records frequency of need for TOFR and cooperation with procedure.
5. Behavior management program data: Records frequency of performing routine activities and adherence to personal schedule.

**Problem 2**

*Problem Title*: Disorder management deficit
*Priority Level*: 2
*Problem Description*: History of repeated hospitalizations following discontinuation of antipsychotic medication. In interview, does not express awareness of psychotic periods or fluctuations in personal and social functioning; does not acknowledge history of medication effects; attributes current hospitalization to conspiracy of police and courts; expresses no understanding of problems in terms of a mental illness or personal dysfunction and has no awareness of techniques for controlling or managing disorder.
*Long-Term Goal*: Reliably perform skills pertinent to managing disorder, preventing relapse, and overcoming disabilities, including medication administration, monitoring for warning signs, stress management, and participating in rehabilitation.
*Short-Term Goal (1)*: Express awareness and understanding of his episodic psychosis; that is, identify psychotic symptoms as such, identify other cognitive and behavioral characteristics of psychosis, and accept the elimination of psychosis as a meaningful goal.
*Short-Term Goal (2)*: Acquire an awareness of having a chronic illness that requires long-term management; that is, comprehend the role of episodic psychosis, the existence and nature of enduring vulnerabilities, and the need for maintenance medication and disorder management skills.
*Short-Term Goal (3)*: Develop and follow a relapse prevention plan.
*Interventions*: Medication counseling, rehabilitation counseling.

1. *Medication counseling, intervention parameters*: Scheduled meeting with team psychiatrist, once per week for 30 minutes, to include individual counseling regarding purpose and use of medication.
2. *Rehabilitation counseling, intervention parameters*: Scheduled meeting with treatment coordinator once per week for 30 minutes, to include discussion of reasons for hospitalization, purpose of treatment and rehabilitation, and progress in resolution of psychotic episode.

*Key Indicators*:

1. Weekly progress note from team psychiatrist, reporting awareness of symptoms, understanding of purpose of medication, and appraisal of medication's effectiveness.
2. Weekly progress note from treatment coordinator, reporting understanding of reasons for hospitalization, purpose of treatment and rehabilitation, appraisal of overall progress, and changes in mental status.

**Problem 3**

*Problem Title*: Occupational skills deficit

*Priority Level*: 2

*Problem Description*: History of sporadic, unsuccessful employment, no evidence of specific vocational skills, expresses no interest in any major occupational role or activity.

*Long-Term Goal*: Reliable performance of a meaningful, gratifying occupational role based on personal preferences, needs, and interests.

*Short-Term Goal (1)*: Identify and describe areas of interest relevant to a possible occupational role.

*Short-Term Goal (2)*: Adhere to a daily schedule, including 2–4 hours per day of occupational activities selected from program menu.

*Interventions*: Rehabilitation counseling, activity schedule.

1. *Rehabilitation counseling, intervention parameters*: Scheduled meeting with occupational therapist once per week for 30 minutes, to include discussion of occupational activities available on program menu, importance of having daily activities, and assistance in construction of a personal daily schedule.
2. *Daily occupational activity schedule, intervention parameters*: Daily schedule of 2–4 hours occupational activities selected from program menu.

*Key Indicators*:

1. Weekly progress note from occupational therapist, reporting on ability to identify and select occupational activities from program menu, specific activity choices, and level of interest in performing activities.
2. Behavior management program data: Records adherence to personal daily schedule of occupational activities.
3. Therapy/activity/class data system: Records attendance, participation, and appropriate/inappropriate behavior in scheduled occupational activities.

**Problem 4**

*Problem Title*: Leisure/recreational skills deficit

*Priority Level*: 2

*Problem Description*: Describes no leisure/recreational interests; no evidence in recent history of any interests or related behavior; expresses very limited knowledge of leisure/recreational opportunities or resources.

*Long-Term Goal*: Reliable pursuit of leisure/recreational interests, based on personal interests, abilities and preferences.

*Short-Term Goal (1)*: Identify and select from program menu leisure/recreational activities suitable for current levels of personal and social functioning and risk management factors.

*Short-Term Goal (2)*: Adhere to a daily schedule, including 1–2 hours per day of leisure/recreational activities selected from program menu.

*Interventions*: Rehabilitation counseling, activity schedule.

1. *Rehabilitation counseling, intervention parameters*: Scheduled meeting with recreation therapist once per week for 30 minutes, to include discussion of recreational activities available on program menu, importance of having recreational interests, appropriate selection of activities, and assistance with construction of a personal leisure/recreational schedule.
2. *Leisure/recreational activity schedule, intervention parameters*: Weekly schedule to include 1–2 hours per day of leisure/recreational activities selected from program menu.

*Key Indicators*:

1. Weekly progress note from recreation therapist, reporting on ability to identify and select leisure/recreational activities from program menu, specific activity choices, level of interest in performing activities, and socialization during activities.
2. Behavior management program data: Records adherence to leisure/recreational activities on personal schedule.
3. Therapy/activity/class data system: Records attendance, participation, appropriate/inappropriate behavior, and social interaction in scheduled leisure/recreational activities.

## Problem 5

*Problem Title*: Substance abuse

*Priority Level*: 3

*Problem Description*: History of indiscriminate use of illicit drugs and alcohol, often associated with aggression and psychotic relapse.

*Long-Term Goal*: Maintain a lifestyle free of substance and alcohol use.

*Short-Term Goal (1)*: Demonstrate an understanding of the risks of substance and alcohol use and the necessity of abstinence.

*Short-Term Goal (2)*: Construct and adhere to a relapse prevention plan that includes abstinence, avoidance of situations that create a risk for use, and recognition of relapse warning signs.

*Interventions*: No interventions at this time (problem is a level-3 priority; problem 1 is preemptive to progress).

*Key Indicators*:

1. Progress report of substance abuse group leaders and therapists.
2. Program log data indicating no substance or alcohol use.
3. Therapy/activity/class data system: Records attendance, participation, and

appropriate/inappropriate behavior in scheduled substance abuse groups and activities.

**Problem 6**

*Problem Title*: Unstable living conditions
*Priority Level*: 3
*Problem Description*: History of homelessness; has no domicile or means of support at this time.
*Long-Term Goal*: Has a place to live suitable for personal needs, with stable means of financial support.
*Short-Term Goal (1)*: Identify housing resources and means for financial support.
*Short-Term Goal (2)*: Establish stable income source sufficient for supporting a domicile.
*Short-Term Goal (3)*: Select a living situation and establish a personal household.
*Interventions*: No interventions at this time (problem is a level-3 priority; problem 1 is preemptive to progress).
*Key Indicators*: Progress report of social worker, reporting housing, financial situation, and arrangements.

## NARRATIVE SUMMARY OF MASTER
## REHABILITATION PLAN (6/01/02)

Mr. Joe A was referred to the Inpatient Rehabilitation Program on 5/22/02 by the Receiving Unit. He was admitted to the Receiving Unit on 4/1/02, under a mental health commitment order. He was referred for inpatient rehabilitation in response to a history of mental health hospitalizations, usually under a commitment order, associated with acute episodes of severe psychosis. The risk of aggression, associated with continuing psychosis with disorganized and paranoid features, indicates that the inpatient program is the least restrictive environment required for safety and effective rehabilitation at this time.

The precipitating events of two previous hospitalizations have been physical altercations. The others have resulted from law enforcement interventions in response to an apparent inability to care for his basic needs (grave disability). Mr. A has been persistently nonadherent to treatment and aftercare plans when he is outside a highly structured (inpatient) environment. Based on this history, Mr. A. is now assessed to be at continuing risk to himself and others, beyond immediate resolution of acute psychosis. A meaningful reduction of the continuing risk will require comprehensive assessment and resolution of the factors associated with his pattern of psychotic relapse.

Assessment of Mr. A's neurophysiological status upon arrival at the rehabilitation program indicates that he has experienced a significant reduction in agitated and aggressive behavior since beginning his current antipsychotic medication regimen in the Receiving Unit. However, he continues to complain of "voices" that sometimes form an incomprehensible cacophony and other times impart vague instructions to leave the hospital and trust no one. During the interview, he demonstrates a moderate degree of odd posturing and grimacing and a generally suspicious demeanor. He states that he was sent illegally to the hospital, has no mental illness or any other problems, and demands to be released immediately. When informed of his rights and access to legal representation, he states he will not do anything because "the lawyers are in on it." At this time he is assessed to be in partial and unstable remission of his acute psychosis.

Mr. A's neurocognitive functioning is substantially and pervasively impaired. Neuropsychological testing indicates impairment in attention, short-term and working memory, and executive functioning. The overall level of impairment is sufficient to interfere significantly with his personal and social functioning and to inhibit his responsivity to psychosocial interventions. The pattern of impairment is generally consistent with partial recovery from an acute psychotic episode. Post-acute and residual neurocognitive impairment cannot be further assessed until further resolution of the acute state, although the social history suggests that significant impairment may remain.

All available data indicate that Mr. A is not interested in treatment and rehabilitation at this time. The history suggests his engagement improves, to some degree, with resolution of acute psychosis. However, there is no evidence that he has ever acknowledged having a mental illness or the continuing need for treatment or rehabilitation.

Mr. A's behavioral functioning is generally consistent with acute psychosis. Milieu-based observational data indicate that he does not independently perform basic daily self-care activities, does not attend scheduled occupational or recreational activities, remains reclusive and socially isolated, maintains a belligerent, irritable demeanor, and demonstrates a moderate degree of odd posturing and talking to himself in the ambient environment.

Mr. A's social history indicates a lack of role performance in the domains of independent living, occupational functioning, and leisure/recreational activities. The role of episodic psychosis in his performance of independent living skills is unclear, as it appears there is usually a significant decrease in functioning associated with the onset of episodes. Occupational and leisure/recreational functioning appears to be relatively independent of episodic psychosis, as he has been unable to maintain employment even during periods of otherwise stable functioning, and a lack of leisure/recreational interests appears to predate onset of his disorder. The history of repeated treatment nonadherence and relapse also suggests insufficient skill performance in the domain of disorder management, although is it unclear how much his baseline skill performance is periodically compromised by acute psychosis.

Mr. A's parents and one sibling live in this area. All three report interest in being involved in rehabilitation. However, Mr. A is adamantly opposed to their involvement. The team will invite the family to attend the Mental Health Center Family Education Program, and will work with Mr. A to reach an accommodation
regarding their involvement in his rehabilitation and recovery.

The initial focus of this rehabilitation plan is further resolution of the acute
psychosis. This is addressed by problem 1, episodic CNS dysregulation. Interventions include continued psychopharmacotherapy and provision of a stable, consistent daily schedule of self-care, low-demand occupational activities, and recreational activities. A behavior management program will be used to enhance
adherence to the daily schedule. A second behavior management program will be
used to monitor aggressive behavior and control it with a time-out-from-reinforcement procedure, with the expectation that it will not be needed after further resolution of the acute psychosis. However, social and self-regulation skills deficits may
also be implicated in Mr. A's aggression, and these will be assessed as resolution of
the psychosis proceeds. At this time, there are no known factors to preempt Mr. A's
response to these interventions.

Preliminary interventions will be started to address deficits in Mr. A's disorder
management, occupational, and leisure skills (problems 2–4). These interventions
will provide additional data on resolution of the acute psychosis and the role of residual skills deficits, but optimal response in these domains is expected to be contingent on further resolution of the acute psychosis. Mr. A's substance abuse (problem
5) and unstable living conditions (problem 6) will have to be addressed before he
can move to a less restrictive rehabilitation setting, but at this time the acute psychosis prevents meaningful progress in these domains.

## MONTHLY PROGRESS REVIEW (7/01/02)

Rehabilitation client: Joe A
Date of this progress review: July 1, 2002
Date of next progress review: August 1, 2002

**Problem 1**

*Problem Title*: Episodic CNS dysregulation
*Priority Level*: 1

| Intervention | Start date | Implementation comments |
|---|---|---|
| Psychopharmacotherapy (psychiatrist) | 6/01/02 | Implemented as planned |

| Behavior management program—TOFR for aggression | 6/01/02 | Implemented as planned |
| Behavior management program—adherence to schedule | 6/04/02 | Implemented upon schedule construction |

*Summary of key indicator activity*: Psychiatrist reports subjective reduction in auditory hallucinations, objective reductions in manifest agitation; BPRS shows Disorganization and Excitement decreased from "moderate" (4–5) to "mild" (1–4), Paranoia remains high (6–7); NOSIE shows decrease in PSY and IRR in first 2 weeks, less change over second 2 weeks. BMPs show reduction of aggression requiring TOFR, from initial 5/week to 2/week, after small initial increase in second week. Performance of scheduled activities shows increase from initial 20% to 80%.

*Rating of progress toward long-term goal*: +1 (minimal to less than expected)
*Rating of progress toward short-term goals*: +1 (minimal to less than expected)
*Comments on progress ratings*: Initial medication response appears to be leveling off at a greatly reduced but still elevated level; paranoia responding slowly, if at all. Disorganization is still sufficient to interfere with rehabilitation and recovery.

**Problem 2**

*Problem Title*: Disorder management deficit
*Priority Level*: 2

| *Intervention* | *Start date* | *Implementation comments* |
| --- | --- | --- |
| Medication counseling (psychiatrist) | 6/01/02 | Implemented as planned |
| Rehabilitation counseling (team coordinator) | 6/01/02 | Implemented as planned |

*Summary of key indicator activity*: Psychiatrist reports no change in awareness that hallucinations are symptoms of mental illness; remains compliant but disagrees that medication is beneficial; treatment coordinator reports no change in understanding of reasons for hospitalization or need for treatment or rehabilitation; both report Mr. A has been cooperative with meetings and his demands for immediate release from hospital have decreased to zero in the past week, but he still appears unable to formulate specific actions to gain release.

*Rating of progress toward long-term goal*: +1 (minimal to less than expected)
*Rating of progress toward short-term goals*: +1 (minimal to less than expected)
*Comments on progress ratings*: Continuing indications of acute psychosis sug-

gest that the psychosis and/or post-acute impairments are interfering with progress on this problem.

## Problem 3

Problem Title: Occupational skills deficit
Priority Level: 2

| Intervention | Start date | Implementation comments |
| --- | --- | --- |
| Rehabilitation counseling (occupational therapist) | 6/01/02 | Implemented as planned |
| Daily occupational schedule | 6/04/02 | Implemented as planned |

Summary of key indicator activity: Occupational therapist reports improved ability to identify and select activities from program menu; interest in activities is moderate; behavior management program shows that adherence to selected schedule has increased from 50% to 80%; therapy/activity/class data show that participation is low to moderate, with slight increase; rating of inappropriate behavior during activities has decreased from "often" to "occasional"; Mr. A becomes interested and engaged in activities while actually performing them but expresses no interest in identifying and selecting activities ahead of time or following a personal schedule. He attributes his adherence to his schedule as due solely to the behavior management program.

Rating of progress toward long-term goal: +1 (minimal to less than expected)
Rating of progress toward short-term goals: +2 (expected progress)
Comments on progress ratings: Has engaged in the occupational resources in the milieu and is accessing them. Is progressing less rapidly in developing the understanding necessary to support a major occupational role in a less structured environment.

## Problem 4

Problem Title: Leisure/recreational skills deficit
Priority Level: 2

| Intervention | Start date | Implementation comments |
| --- | --- | --- |
| Rehabilitation counseling (recreational therapist) | 6/02/02 | Implemented as planned |
| Leisure/recreational schedule | 6/04/02 | Implemented as planned |

Summary of key indicator activity: Recreational therapist reports ability to identify and select activities from program menu; interest in activities is moderate; participates in activities but remains aloof and interacts minimally; behavior management program shows that adherence to selected schedule has been high throughout, 80%–90%. Therapy/activity/class data show participation is low to moderate, with slight increase; rating of inappropriate behavior during activities has remained at "sometimes"; rating of socialization during activities has remained at "seldom or never."

*Rating of progress toward long-term goal*: +1 (minimal to less than expected)
*Rating of progress toward short-term goals*: +2 (expected progress)
*Comments on progress ratings*: Has engaged in the recreational resources in the milieu, is accessing them, but has not developed the understanding necessary to support leisure/recreational pursuits in a less structured environment.

## Problem 5

*Problem Title*: Substance abuse
*Priority Level*: 3

*Intervention*            *Start date*   *Implementation comments*
No interventions scheduled

*Summary of key indicator activity*: Program log data show no attempt to obtain substances or alcohol.

*Rating of progress toward long-term goal*: +0 (no change)
*Rating of progress toward short-term goals*: +2 (expected progress)
*Comments on progress ratings*: Abstinence is attributable to unavailability in milieu; Mr. A does not view himself as having a substance abuse problem.

## Problem 6

*Problem Title*: Unstable living conditions
*Priority Level*: 3

*Intervention*            *Start date*   *Implementation comments*
No interventions scheduled

*Summary of key indicator activity*: Social worker reports that Mr. A is probably eligible for disability pension and subsidized housing; can further assess when acute psychosis is resolved; at present, he refuses to discuss housing or related discharge considerations.

*Rating of progress toward long-term goal*: +0 (no change)

*Rating of progress toward short-term goals*: +2 (expected progress)

*Comments on progress ratings*: Continuing indications of acute psychosis suggest that the psychosis and/or post-acute impairments are interfering with progress on this problem.


## NARRATIVE SUMMARY OF PROGRESS REVIEW (7/01/02)

Mr. A's recovery and rehabilitation have progressed generally as expected, although with a slower than expected rate in some areas. The acute psychosis has diminished in severity and appears to have reached a plateau. Further improvements are expected over the next several weeks as recovery from the acute episode proceeds, but at a slower rate. The trajectory of recovery is considered acceptable, and there appear to be no side effects sufficient to cause distress or compromise functioning, so no further adjustments in the medication regimen are contemplated at this time. Remaining indications of psychosis, especially disorganization and cognitive difficulties in all psychosocial interventions, are now thought to reflect residual impairments that may respond to neurocognitive intervention. Neuropsychological assessment also indicates the presence of persistent, substantial, and pervasive neurocognitive impairment, although at reduced levels. The revised rehabilitation plan will include a new problem to address this area.

Mr. A's aggressive behavior has responded well to combined psychopharmacotherapy and behavior management. The behavior management component has eliminated the need for restraint and seclusion that occurred during previous hospitalizations. The intensity and dangerousness of aggressive episodes have diminished (e.g., from physical to verbal) to levels manageable in a less secure environment, although the risk management protocol requires further time to establish the stability of current intensity levels and further reduce frequency of incidents.

The family report that they attended the Mental Health Center Family Education Program and are interested in helping as much as possible. Mr. A continues to oppose their involvement in his rehabilitation. Negotiations in this regard will continue.

Mr. A's engagement in the rehabilitation program is approaching a level that would permit a less restrictive environment. However, his view of the causes of his commitment and hospitalization continues to represent a significant risk factor for relapse and reactivation of dangerous behavior. In addition, substance abuse leading to relapse and dangerous behavior would likely continue if substances were available in the milieu. Continued behavior management programming is necessary to sustain performance of self-care and daily living activities, and to prevent aggression. The Community Transition Program (CTP) is optimally able to accommodate Mr. A's slightly reduced needs for a secure environment. It is expected that at the current rate of progress, Mr. A will be qualify for placement in the CTP within 4 to 6 weeks. Transfer planning will begin now in anticipation of continued progress.

The following problem was added to the rehabilitation plan after the 7/01/02 review.

## Problem 7

*Problem Title*: Post-acute neurocognitive impairment
*Priority Level*: 1
*Problem Description*: Neurocognitive impairment expressed as behavioral disorganization, neglect of daily living and self-care activities without environmental support, severely limited response to psychosocial rehabilitation activities, and abnormal neuropsychological test data, persisting after partial resolution of acute psychotic episodes.
*Long-Term Goal*: Elimination of neurocognitive impairment and its impact on personal and social functioning.
*Short-Term Goal (1)*: Reduce behavioral disorganization to minimal levels.
*Short-Term Goal (2)*: Increase performance of daily personal schedule to 100%.
*Short-Term Goal (3)*: Reduce impairment on neuropsychological tests to minimal levels.
*Short-Term Goal (4)*: Increase rate of progress in interventions for disorder management deficit, occupational skills deficit, and leisure/recreational skills deficit.
*Interventions*: Neurcognitive recovery group, behavior management program.

1. *Neurcognitive recovery group (NRG), intervention parameters*: Scheduled group, Monday–Friday, 9:00–10:00 A.M.
2. *Behavior management program, intervention parameters*: Contingency management program to provide immediate, salient reinforcement for adherence to personal daily schedule, with minimum necessary staff prompts.

*Key Indicators*:

1. Weekly progress note from neurocognitive recovery group therapist, reporting on response to the groups's procedures.
2. Behavior management program data: Records adherence to personal daily schedule with minimum staff prompts.
3. Therapy/activity/class data system: Records attendance, participation, appropriate/inappropriate behavior, and social interaction during the neurocognitive recovery group meetings, occupational therapy skills, and recreational skills.

Mr. A was transferred to the Community Transition Program, as planned. The CTP is an intensive biopsychosocial rehabilitation program that accepts referrals from the short-term inpatient unit. People are referred to the CTP when, after 2 months, recovery has been insufficient to allow return to a community setting with the expectation of safe and stable functioning and a decent quality of life. The next document provides a summary of his progress review following the transfer.

## NARRATIVE SUMMARY OF PROGRESS REVIEW (9/01/02)

Mr. A has made mixed progress toward his long- and short-term goals during this review period. The acute psychosis that was the primary focus of earlier intervention is now thought to be resolved, and the CNS dysregulation is thought to be in a stable state. However, resolution of the psychotic state has not resolved some problems previously thought to result directly from CNS dysregulation. Mr. A's confusion, agitation, and disorganization have reached a very mild plateau. He no longer describes bizarre conspiratorial delusions, although if directly asked, he does state that he was illegally hospitalized by "authorities" who wish him ill. His interpersonal functioning is still marked by belligerence and irritability. Although his aggressive behavior has reached a low level of frequency and intensity, it remains at socially unacceptable levels. The aggression occurs with staff, in response to prompts to adhere to scheduled activities and/or their implementation of behavior management consequences, and also with other patients, in response to interpersonal conflicts. It has been observed that Mr. A is frequently unassertive with other patients, and his aggression tends to erupt after he has acceded to inappropriate requests (e.g., bumming cigarettes). There has been a slight increase in aggression over the last 3 weeks, which is thought to reflect increasing demands for adherence to a personal schedule, and increased interpersonal interaction associated with more hours spent in occupational and recreational activities.

Mr. A has made further progress in the neurocognitive domain. He has had significant difficulty participating in the neurocognitive rehabilitation group, which supports the hypothesis of post-acute impairment. His progress has been slow but steady. As Mr. A becomes increasingly involved in occupational and recreational activities, his neurocognitive impairments have become more evident in behavioral performance, but he is making acceptable progress. At the current rate, Mr. A is expected to be performing at a level consistent with entry-level employment within 2 to 3 months. In addition, Mr. A's neurocognitive functioning is now thought sufficient to allow an expected response to more structured skills training modalities, although intervention at the neurocognitive level will continue.

Mr. A remains skeptical that he has a mental illness, but he does recognize that he has symptoms that respond to treatment. He attributes his reduced agitation, confusion, and auditory hallucinations to medication and "being in a quiet place" (i.e., the Community Transition Program), but he also insists that "everyone hears those voices, they just don't admit it." He has been adherent to all aspects of his rehabilitation regimen, although he states that he does it only for the consequences of the behavior management programs.

In response to the areas of differential progress, the team will add two new problems to the rehabilitation plan: psychophysiological self-regulation deficit (associated with anger and aggression) and social skills deficit. The former will focus on teaching him how to inhibit aggression and reduce his anger, thereby improving his stress management skills. The latter will focus on teaching him how to resolve immediate interpersonal conflicts, toward a long-term goal of establishing and maintaining stable work relationships and friendships. The episodic CNS dysregulation problem is changed to priority level 4, indicating that the current regimen is at maintenance level and at further improvement is expected in response to neurophysiological interventions. The occupational and recreational skills problems remain at priority level 2, because the residual levels of aggression continue to compromise progress in these areas. Disorder management, psychophysiological self-regulation, social skills, substance abuse, and living conditions problems are all changed to priority level 1, indicating the removal of neurophysiological and neurocognitive barriers and in anticipation of increased intervention via skills training groups and individual counseling. In addition to the respective skills training interventions, Mr. A will begin weekly meetings with the team social worker (as an intervention under problem 6) to formulate plans for a future living situation and economic support.

The following problems were added to the rehabilitation plan after the 9/01/02 review.

## Problem 8

*Problem Title*: Psychophysiological self-regulation deficit

*Priority Level*: 1

*Problem Description*: Episodes of rapid psychophysiological and behavioral escalation, in response to frustration and/or interpersonal conflict, progressing from an angry, belligerent demeanor to physical intimidation to verbal aggression to physical aggression; data indicate that physical aggression is effectively suppressed by a time-out for reinforcement intervention (TOFR) but frequency and intensity of escalations are still at socially unacceptable levels and would likely proceed to physical aggression in a less supportive environment.

*Long-Term Goal*: Elimination of verbal and physical aggression, moderation of anger to normal frequency and intensity, reliable use of socially appropriate assertiveness and interpersonal problem solving in conflict situations.

*Short-Term Goal (1)*: Reduce need for TOFR intervention to zero.

*Short-Term Goal (2)*: Establish psychophysiological relaxation response of sufficient strength to reliably inhibit anger-related escalation.

*Short-Term Goal (3)*: Acquire and use daily stress management skills, including regular stress reduction activities.

*Short-Term Goal (4)*: Acquire and use social skills sufficient to resolve interpersonal conflicts and avoid aggression.

*Interventions*: Relaxation and stress management group, behavior management program, social skills training group, rehabilitation counseling.

1. *Relaxation and stress management group (RSM), intervention parameters*: Scheduled group, Tuesday and Thursday, 10:00–11:00 A.M.
2. *Behavior management program, intervention parameters*: Contingency management program to prompt (1) use of TOFRs, (2) differentially reinforce compliance with TOFR prompts, (3) adhere to relaxation/stress management regimen, (4) avoid aggression, and (5) use socially appropriate means of conflict resolution.
3. *Social skills training group (SST), intervention parameters*: Scheduled group, Mondays, Wednesdays, Fridays, 10:00–11:00 A.M.
4. *Rehabilitation counseling, intervention parameters*: Weekly meeting with treatment coordinator to include (1) discussion of need for self-regulation, (2) discussion of importance of avoiding aggression, (3) review and analysis of recent instances of aggression, and (4) monitor use of relaxation, stress management, and social skills.

*Key Indicators*:

1. Weekly progress note from relaxation and stress management group therapist, reporting on response to group's procedures.
2. Weekly progress note from social skills training group therapist, reporting on response to group's procedure.
3. Monthly note from treatment coordinator, reporting on current understanding of need for self-regulation and suppression of aggression.
4. Behavior management program data: Records adherence to stress management schedule with minimum staff prompts and need for TOFRs.
5. Therapy/activity/class data system: Records attendance, participation, appropriate/inappropriate behavior in the two groups.

## Problem 9

*Problem Title*: Social skills deficit
*Priority Level*: 1
*Problem Description*: History of social isolation; lack of supportive social network. Current observations indicate low levels of ambient socialization; does not identify friends or acquaintances, avoids interpersonal activity, does not use appropriate assertiveness. Incidents of aggression are associated with interpersonal conflicts.
*Long-Term Goal*: Maintain normal, productive interpersonal relationships in work settings; enjoy gratifying friendships and a supportive social network.
*Short-Term Goal (1)*: Increase social and interpersonal problem-solving skills to normal levels as measured by clinical/laboratory assessments.

*Short-Term Goal (2):* Increase performance of daily personal schedule to 100%.

*Short-Term Goal (3):* Reduce impairment on neuropsychological tests to minimal levels.

*Short-Term Goal (4):* Increase rate of progress in interventions for disorder management deficit, occupational skills deficit, and leisure/recreational skills deficit.

*Interventions:* Social skills training, rehabilitation counseling.

1. *Social skills training group (SST), intervention parameters:* Scheduled group, Mondays, Wednesdays, Fridays, 10:00–11:00 A.M.
2. *Rehabilitation counseling, intervention parameters:* Weekly scheduled meeting with treatment coordinator, to include discussion of interpersonal relationships at work (OT work activities) and friendships.

*Key Indicators:*

1. Weekly progress note from social skills training therapist, reporting on response to group's procedures.
2. Monthly progress note from treatment coordinator, reporting on development of work relationships and friendships.
3. Therapy/activity/class data system: Records social interaction in occupational therapy and recreational activities.

## NARRATIVE SUMMARY OF PROGRESS REVIEW (1/02/03)

After 3 months (9/02–12/02) of steady, expected progress, Mr. A experienced a setback during this review period. Progress had been demonstrated on all problems identified on the rehabilitation plan. Mr. A's CNS dysregulation was assessed to be stable and optimally medicated. His neurocognitive functioning, measured by progress in the neurocognitive rehabilitation group, steadily improved, as did his performance and acquisition in his other skills training groups. By the end of November, neuropsychological testing showed that his residual impairments had reduced, although they are still sufficient to retard rehabilitation progress and interfere with personal and social functioning. Mr. A's self-regulation of aggression also improved. His response to the relaxation and stress management group was observed to be good, and his need for TOFRs has reduced to zero. His angry, belligerent demeanor has diminished, and his interactions with staff and others are generally appropriate. He has shown appropriate assertiveness on several occasions. He reports considerable reduction in subjective distress, which he associates with performance of his daily relaxation and stress management regimen. Although he does not characterize anybody as "a friend," his level of ambient social interaction has increased in occupational therapy and recreational activities. He was reported to be progressing, as expected, in social skills training, rehabilitation counseling, and planning for his future living situation and economic support. He was adherent to his personal daily schedule and rehabilitation regimen; behavior management contingencies had been steadily reduced in anticipation of conditions in the aftercare environment. A preliminary target date of February 1 had been identified for discharge from the Community Transition Program to the Supported Community Living Program, with a plan to (1) continue in the occupational therapy workshop program, (2) join the Community Social and Recreational Program, (3) receive disability (financial) support, (4) live in a subsidized housing program apartment, and (5) continue rehabilitation in consultation with a Mental Health Center case manager.

In mid-December, Mr. A's mood state evidenced sadness, a mild resurgence of anger (but without aggression), and lethargy. His attendance and performance at the occupational therapy work program dropped from a previously high level. He reported feelings of frustration, a sense of demoralization, an increase in the intensity of auditory hallucinations (which previously had been quite subdued), and "feelings" about being persecuted that he recognized as characteristic of his previous acute psychosis. He had been making considerable progress in acquiring disorder management skills and had graduated from the disorder management group, although he continued to be skeptical that the information from that group actually applied to him. He was having considerable difficulty constructing his relapse prevention plan, because the need for continuing medication and other rehabilitation seemed inconsistent with his desire for complete independence. Similarly, after making excellent progress in learning the risks of substance abuse and developing alternative skills, Mr. A reacted markedly to the suggestion that past substance abuse may have been, in part, an attempt to escape from the realities of having a mental illness. By the end of December, he was reporting suicidal feelings and had been placed on special precautions on two occasions.

All data available to the team indicate that this turn of events is a response to the resulting demoralization of Mr. A's increasing awareness that he has a serious disability, possibly exacerbated by the stress and self-examination that often accompany the holidays. The team considered adding a new problem to reflect either (1) a tonic CNS dysregulation of the type associated with depression, (2) an affect-linked attribution problem, and/or (3) a second psychophysiological problem (the current one addresses aggression). The second alternative was chosen, reflecting a hypothesis that the current depression was precipitated mostly by Mr. A's confrontation with personal desires, values, and expectations that are unrealistic. The history does not suggest a neurophysiological or psychophysiological vulnerability to depression. It is expected that continued progress in the most functional aspects of rehabilitation, especially in work and independent living, combined with careful attention to relevant affective and attributional issues in rehabilitation counseling, will be sufficient to overcome the demoralization. To amplify the role of rehabilitation counseling in addressing this problem, a course of individual therapy will be added to the rehabilitation plan, under the new affect-linked attribution problem.

During the previous review period, concerns were raised about Mr. A's independent living skills. Although he has regained an ability to perform routine activities of self-care and housekeeping with minimal environmental support, his ability to manage personal finances remains in doubt. Subsequent assessments confirm that his financial knowledge and management skills are quite limited. His own concerns about this, in the face of the anticipated discharge, may be contributing to his current depression. An independent living skills problem, addressing personal financial management, will be added to the rehabilitation plan.

Mr. A's antipsychotic medication has been titrated downward to a maintenance dose. The reappearance of psychotic symptoms suggests that the current dose may be too low to protect against stress-related recurrences. Therefore, the CNS dysregulation problem will be returned to priority level 1, and the dosage will be titrated upward.

To allow for addressing the new attributional and living skills problems, and to ensure a smooth transition to a less supportive environment, the target date for discharge to the Mental Health Center case management and supported living programs is moved to April 15, 2003. Preliminary plans for this move are nearing completion. By that time, Mr. A's work schedule needs to reflect a post-discharge level, his behavior management programs need to reflect post-discharge conditions, the relapse prevention plan needs to be completed, and Mr. A needs to have demonstrated reliable adherence to the relapse prevention plan and his anticipated post-discharge schedule.

Mr. A has signed a release of information to his three local family members, and he has agreed to engage in a preliminary discussion about their possible role in his life. The team social worker will meet with the family and Mr. A for this purpose (as an assessment, not an intervention).

In response to the progress review, the following problems were added to the rehabilitation plan.

## Problem 9

*Problem Title*: Affect-linked attribution deficit

*Priority Level*: 1

*Problem Description*: Dysphoria, distress, sadness, demoralization, frustration, and suicidal feelings, resulting from incompatible desires, values, and beliefs; a belief that one cannot have a decent and meaningful life and also have a disabling mental illness.

*Long-Term Goal*: Establish and maintain an understanding of mental illness as comprised of disabilities to be overcome, accept personal limitations as a challenge, and pursue a meaningful and gratifying lifestyle within those limitations, free from protracted demoralization and suicidal feelings.

*Short-Term Goal (1)*: Complete a realistic appraisal of personal limitations, including but not limited to those associated with mental illness, and identify short- and long-term consequences of those limitations.

*Short-Term Goal (2)*: Complete a realistic plan for achieving the best possible personal and social functioning, including maximum personal gratification, dignity, and self-respect.

*Short-Term Goal (3)*: Incorporate plans for meeting personal goals and desires into the master rehabilitation plan and the relapse prevention plan.

*Short-Term Goal (4)*: Adhere to all provisions of the master rehabilitation plan and the relapse prevention plan.

*Interventions*: Social skills training, CBT.

1. *Social skills training group (SST), intervention parameters*: Scheduled group, Mondays, Wednesdays, Fridays, 10:00–11:00 A.M.
2. *Individual cognitive-behavioral psychotherapy (CBT), intervention parameters*: Weekly scheduled meeting with psychotherapist to address personal beliefs regarding achievement, autonomy, and other values, and to identify how these values can be realized despite limitations imposed by mental illness; 12 sessions planned at this time.

*Key Indicators*:

1. Weekly progress note from CBT therapist, reporting on response to CBT procedures.
2. Monthly progress note from treatment coordinator, reporting on adherence to and understanding of rehabilitation plan and relapse prevention plan, and feelings of demoralization and suicide.
3. Clinical/lab measures of affective state, including depression and hopelessness.
4. Program log reporting incidents of suicidal feelings, precautionary responses.
5. Therapy/activity/class data system: Records demeanor and social interactions in occupational therapy and recreational activities.

## Problem 10

*Problem Title*: Independent living deficit

*Priority Level*: 1

*Problem Description*: Recent history of financial problems, not paying rent and bills; has not had a checking account for several years; unable to demonstrate basic personal finance skills, including bookkeeping and budgeting.

*Long-Term Goal*: Reliably manage personal finances, pay bills on time, conform consumer choices to financial resources, maintain a bank account and savings.

*Short-Term Goal (1)*: Construct a personal budget showing expected income and expenditures as they currently exist, and follow the budget.

*Short-Term Goal (2)*: Construct a personal budget showing expected income and expenditures as they will exist in the aftercare environment.

*Short-Term Goal (3)*: Incorporate plans for meeting personal goals and desires into the master rehabilitation plan and the relapse prevention plan.

*Short-Term Goal (4)*: Adhere to all provisions of the master rehabilitation plan and the relapse prevention plan.

*Interventions:* Personal finances group, budgeting coach, discharge planning.

1. *Personal finances group (PFG), intervention parameters*: Scheduled group, Tuesdays and Thursdays, 3:00–4:00 P.M..
2. *Personal budgeting coach, intervention parameters*: Weekly scheduled meeting with personal budgeting coach to apply information learned in personal finances group, identify income sources and expenditures, construct a personal budget, follow it, and keep the books.
3. *Discharge planning, intervention parameters*: Semiweekly meeting with social worker to include planning for personal finances in aftercare setting (i.e., obtaining disability income, opening a bank account, and paying rent and other bills.

*Key Indicators:*

1. Weekly progress note from personal finances group therapist, reporting on responses to the group's procedures.
2. Weekly progress note from the budgeting coach, reporting on progress in constructing and following budget.
3. Monthly progress note from social worker, reporting on setting up aftercare finances.

The last document, the narrative summary from the last monthly progress review, summarizes Mr. A's progress prior to his discharge to a supported living apartment, case management, and aftercare rehabilitation.

## NARRATIVE SUMMARY OF PROGRESS REVIEW (4/01/03)

Mr. A has made expected progress in his rehabilitation and recovery. He is expected to be discharged from the Community Transition Program later this month, pending completion of arrangements for his aftercare services and living situation. He will live in an apartment in the Mental Health Center subsidized housing program, will work in the occupational therapy workshop, attend the center's socialization and recreational program two to three times per week, and will attend selected mo-

dalities in the center's outpatient rehabilitation program. A letter of notification will
be sent to the Mental Health Board upon completion of arrangements for this plan.

Mr. A has now been on the current dose of antipsychotic medication for 3
months. He reports that the symptoms that reappeared in December had subsided
by mid-January. There is no evidence of side effects, and the history suggests that
the current dose is necessary to prevent breakthrough symptoms. No further change
is expected, and the CNS dysregulation problem has been put at priority level 4.

Mr. A's neurocognitive functioning showed a slow but steady improvement
over the 6 months following its inclusion in the rehabilitation plan. Temporary increases in impairments were associated with December's depression and breakthrough symptoms. There has been no evidence of further change for about 3
months. On neuropsychological testing, Mr. A continues to show mild impairment
in memory and executive functions. These are now thought to be residual, rather
than post-acute, impairments, and are too mild to be significant factors in rehabilitation and recovery. This problem has been put at priority level 4. It is not considered fully resolved, because it could recur with subsequent psychotic episodes.

This week Mr. A will complete a 12-session course of cognitive-behavioral
therapy, addressing affect-linked attribution problems. The therapist reports that he
has responded well, which is corroborated by reports from the treatment coordinator, occupational and recreational therapists, and by lab measures of his mood
states. He now expresses an adaptive attitude about his mental illness and disabilities, as well as determination to achieve the best possible life despite these
challenges. Although he remains skeptical of the concept of mental illness, and especially of psychiatric diagnoses, he fully acknowledges the importance and benefits
of following his comprehensive relapse prevention plan, and of continuing to build
on his occupational and social skills. The affect-linked attribution problem and the
disorder management problem are thought to be resolved, at least in the current
context. They will be kept on the outpatient rehabilitation plan, but at a priority
level 4, until sustained performance in the aftercare setting indicates they can be removed. The case manager will review the relapse prevention plan with Mr. A during
their monthly sessions.

Mr. A has been working on his personal budgeting skills for 3 months. During
this review period he constructed the budget he will follow after discharge. The personal finances group therapist, budgeting coach, and social worker all report good
progress and achievement of short-term goals. Although his skills are much improved, it is expected he will continue to need some assistance after discharge, especially as his income fluctuates with changes in his occupational functioning. This
problem will be included on the outpatient rehabilitation plan at a priority level of
1. It is expected that the outpatient case manager will provide budget coaching pur-
suant to this need.

The team social worker met with Mr. A and members of his family. They
agreed to plan one or two family activities per month, such as going out to dinner,
attending sporting events, or observing holidays. Mr. A reports comfort with this

plan and no longer fears that his family will attempt to change him or impose unreasonable expectations. The family report that their experience in the family education program should help them avoid problems they encountered in the past. No further action appears necessary in this domain. The case manager will be available to the family in case of future concerns.

Mr. A has not demonstrated aggressive behavior for almost 5 months. Based on the history, this appears to be the longest period free of aggression he has experienced since the onset of the illness. He regularly performs his relaxation and stress management exercises and consistently uses appropriate assertive skills, when needed. He has successfully resolved routine interpersonal conflicts in the work environment. His self-regulation skills are now such that the psychophysiological self-regulation problem is considered resolved and will be removed from the rehabilitation plan.

Mr. A plans to progress from the occupational therapy workshop to the center's transitional employment program after he has adapted to the discharge itself. Adaptation is expected to take 2–3 months. The occupational skill problem will remain on the outpatient rehabilitation plan at a priority level 1. The case manager will oversee the transition between programs.

Mr. A expresses satisfaction with his current repertoire of leisure/recreational skills. There is some concern that he relies too much on solitary activities, leaving him vulnerable to social isolation. This tendency toward isolation will be addressed as part of the social skills problem, which will be kept on the outpatient rehabilitation plan. The aftercare regimen will include socially oriented recreational activities, and Mr. A's interpersonal functioning can be monitored in this context; Mr. A also expresses interest in further developing his social skills. The recreational skills problem is considered resolved and will be removed from the plan.

Mr. A continues to report discomfort with attending Alcoholics Anonymous meetings, so this venue does not appear to be a feasible source of support for his continued abstinence. Realistically, street drugs will be available in the aftercare environment. Mr. A expresses determination to remain abstinent but acknowledges the risk for relapse. He has agreed to undergo random drug screens as a condition for participating in the supported housing and work programs. Abstinence is part of his relapse prevention plan, to be monitored by the case manager. Considering that he has graduated from all the substance abuse skills training groups offered by the center, and that virtually all his socialization will be in the context of the center's work and recreation activities, the center's influence and containment is judged to be sufficient as an anti-substance abuse plan at this time. This problem will be kept on the outpatient plan at a priority level of 1.

The final problem, unstable living conditions, will be resolved upon completion of housing and financial arrangements, at which time it will be considered resolved and removed from the plan.

# Appendix 3

# An Algorithm for Treatment and Rehabilitation of Schizophrenia[1]

*Preliminary differential diagnosis*: Rule out presence of other conditions as possible causes of psychotic behavior:

Acute neuropathy
Bipolar disorder
Factitious report of symptoms
Febrile delerium
Intoxication
Known chronic or progressive neurological conditions
Malingering
Psychotic depression
Psychotic-like behavior associated with cultural or sociological circumstances (e.g., spiritual, religious, or political beliefs, associated with identifiable groups or ideologies, that appear bizarre to other groups)
Transient periods of psychotic-like behavior associated with extreme stress, anxiety, depression, or severe personality disorder

*Proceed with algorithm if*, after ruling out or resolving these causes, a clinical picture of schizophrenia or other severe, adult-onset psychiatric condition persists, including continuous or episodic psychotic symptoms that, when untreated, result in significant compromise of personal and social functioning (the functional deficits need not be attributable to the psychotic symptoms).

1. Begin functional assessment and rehabilitation counseling to identify problems and treatment goals.
2. Does historical or current behavioral–observational data indicate prob-

---

[1]From Spaulding, Johnson, and Coursey (2001). Copyright ©2001 by the American Psychological Association. Adapted with permission.

lems in adherence to treatment and rehabilitation regimens and/or inability to give informed consent to treatment? *If yes,* assess thoroughly and take action, as indicated, to protect those at risk and engage treatment (these actions must be reevaluated repeatedly, as recovery permits greater participation and less restriction, and restores legal competence):

- Establish means of appropriate substitute decision-making (e.g., appointment of guardian, civil commitment, judicial supervision of treatment, etc.), when necessary.
- Provide environmental structure sufficient to ensure safety at lowest possible level of restriction (e.g., hospitalization, crisis respite, supervised residential services, etc.).
- Negotiate contingency management programs sufficient to establish engagement in treatment and rehabilitation at the lowest possible level of restriction.

3. (*Under most circumstances, this step is conducted simultaneously with the previous step.*) Does history and presentation suggest that the affected individual is currently experiencing an acute psychotic episode? *If yes,* take action to resolve acute episode:

- Provide crisis intervention, as circumstances demand.
- Initiate clinical trial of antipsychotic medication, beginning with first recourse selection; titrate dose upward or select alternative, as indicated by treatment response.
- Administer adjunctive medication to control side effects, as necessary.
- Provide psychosocial interventions to enhance resolution of acute psychosis (e.g., specialized CBT) and suppress dangerous or unacceptable behaviors (e.g., TOFR contingency management programs).

4. (*When the antipsychotic used in resolving acute psychosis is a neuroleptic:*) Is there evidence of residual negative symptoms, deficit states, side effects, or psychophysiological or affective dysregulation, for which an atypical antipsychotic would be more beneficial? *If yes,* begin controlled trial of an atypical antipsychotic (under most circumstances, the switch should be gradual and staggered).

   *Proceed to next step* when data indicate that acute episode is stabilized as much as possible; that is, psychotic symptoms, related behaviors, and acute cognitive impairments are not expected to respond to further adjustments in medication and/or more time in the therapeutic milieu.

5. Is there evidence of residual negative symptoms, deficit states, or psychophysiological or affective dysregulation for which adjunctive pharmacotherapy may be beneficial? *If yes,* begin controlled trial of adjunctive pharmacotherapy targeting specific residual problems (e.g., antidepressant

medication if residual state is suspected to be depression-related; anti-convulsant for agitation or aggression).

6. Does assessment reveal residual neurocognitive impairments sufficient to compromise personal or social functioning or response to rehabilitation? *If yes,* provide neuropsychological intervention:

   • Begin trial of cognitive–rehabilitative intervention (e.g., IPT, CET).
   • Provide supportive and prosthetic environmental conditions for residual impairments that limit functioning and are not eliminated by treatment.

7. Is there evidence of residual symptoms, affective dysregulation, or other persistent condition for which psychosocial treatment may be effective? *If yes,* begin trial of psychosocial treatment targeting specific problem (e.g., CBT for symptom control or depression; relapse prevention for substance abuse).

8. (*This step is usually conducted simultaneously with the previous step*) Does functional assessment reveal deficits in skills-related areas needed for the recovering person to achieve full potential, live in the least restrictive environment possible, and enjoy a satisfactory quality of life? *If yes,* begin psychosocial rehabilitation targeting specific skill deficits.

9. Does progress in rehabilitation allow (a) titration of antipsychotic dose to maintenance level, (b) discontinuation of adjunctive pharmacotherapy, (c) reduction or discontinuation of restrictive environmental supports, or (d) contingency management programs? *If yes,* adjust regimen accordingly.

10. Is recovery proceeding as expected, toward measurable goals identified by the entire treatment team (including identified patient and relevant family)? *If no,* identify barriers to progress, reformulate the treatment and rehabilitation plan, and repeat the entire algorithm.

# References

Abrams, M., & Reber, A. S. (1988). Implicit learning: Robustness in the face of psychiatric disorders. *Journal of Psycholinguistic Research, 17,* 425–439.

Addington, J., & Addington, D. (1999). Neurocognitive and social functioning in schizophrenia. *Schizophrenia Bulletin, 25*(1), 173–182.

Alford, B., & Correia, C. (1994). Cognitive therapy of schizophrenia: Theory and empirical status. *Behavior Therapy, 25,* 17–33.

Alford, H., Fleece, L., & Rothblum, E. (1982). Hallucinatory-delusional verbalizations: Modification in a chronic schizophrenic by self-control and cognitive restructuring. *Behavior Modification, 6,* 412–435.

Allen, D., Aldarondo, F., Goldstein, G., Huegel, S., Gilbertson, M., & van Kammen, D. (1998). Construct validity of neuropsychological tests in schizophrenia. *Assessment, 5,* 365–374.

Allness, D., & Knoedler, W. (1998). *The PACT model of community-based treatment for persons with severe and persistent mental illnesses: A manual for PACT start-up.* Arlington, VA: National Alliance for the Mentally Ill.

Amador, X., Flaum, M., Andreasen, N., Strauss, D., Yale, S., Clark, S., & Gorman, J. (1994). Awareness of illness in schizophrenia and schizoaffective and mood disorders. *Archives of General Psychiatry, 51,* 826–836.

Amador, X., & Johanson, A. (2000). *I am not sick I don't need help: Helping the seriously mentally ill accept treatment.* Peconic, NY: VidaPress.

American Psychiatric Association. (1994). *Diagnostic and statistical manual of mental disorders* (4th ed.). Washington, DC: Author.

Andreae, D. (1996). Systems theory and social work treatment. In F. Turner (Ed.), *Social work treatment: Interlocking theoretical approaches* (4th. ed., pp. 601–616). New York: Free Press.

Andreasen, N. (1986). Scale for the assessment of thought, language and communication (TLC). *Schizophrenia Bulletin, 12,* 473–482.

Anthony, W. A. (1979). *Principles of psychiatric rehabilitation.* Baltimore: University Park Press.

Anthony, W. A., Cohen, M., & Nemec, P. (1986). Assessment in psychiatric rehabilitation. In B. Bolton (Ed.), *Handbook of measurement and evaluation in rehabilitation* (2nd ed.). Baltimore: Brookes.

Anthony, W. A., & Liberman, R. P. (1986). The practice of psychiatric rehabilitation:

Historical, conceptual, and research base. *Schizophrenia Bulletin, 12*(4), 542–559.

Antony, M., & Swinson, R. (2001). Comparative and combined treatments for obsessive–compulsive disorder. In M. T. Sammons & N. B. Schmidt (Eds.), *Combined treatments for mental disorders: A guide to psychological and pharmacological interventions.* Washington, DC: American Psychological Association.

Arango, C., Kirkpatrick, B., & Koenig, J. (2001). At issue: Stress, hippocampal neuronal turnover, and neuropsychiatric disorders. *Schizophrenia Bulletin, 27,* 477–480.

Ashcraft, M., Fries, B., Nerenz, D., & Falcon, S. (1989). A psychiatric patient classification system: An alternative to diagnosis-related groups. *Medical Care, 27,* 543–557.

Ashe, P., Berry, M., & Boulton, A. (2001). Schizophrenia, a neurodegenerative disorder with neurodevelopmental antecedents. *Progress in Neuro-Psychopharmacology and Biological Psychiatry, 25,* 691–707.

Austin, N., Liberman, R., King, L., & DeRisi, W. (1976). A comparative evaluation of two day hospitals: Goal attainment scaling of behavior therapy vs. milieu therapy. *Journal of Nervous and Mental Disease, 163,* 253–262.

Ayllon, T., & Azrin, N. H. (1968). *The token economy.* New York: Appleton-Century-Crofts.

Aylward, A., Schloss, P., Alper, S., & Green, C. (1996). Improving direct-care staff consistency in a residential treatment program through the use of self-recording and feedback. *International Journal of Disability, Development and Education, 43,* 43–53.

Baars, B. J. (1986). *The cognitive revolution in psychology.* New York: Guilford Press.

Bachrach, L. (1983). *Desinstitutionalization.* San Francisco: Jossey-Bass.

Bachrach, L. (1994). What do patients say about program planning? Perspectives from the patient-authored literature. In J. Bedell (Ed.), *Psychological assessment and treatment of persons with severe mental disorders* (pp. 75–91). Philadelphia: Taylor & Francis.

Bachrach, L. (1999). The state of the state mental hospital at the turn of the century. In W. Spaulding (Ed.), *The state hospital in the 21st century: New directions for mental health services* (Vol. 84, pp. 7–24). San Francisco: Jossey-Bass.

Baer, L., Rauch, S., Ballantine, T., Martuza, R., Cosgrove, R., Cassem, E., Giriunas, I., Manzo, P., Dimino, C., & Jenike, M. (1995). Cingulotomy for intractable obsessive–compulsive disorder: Prospective long-term follow-up of 18 patients. *Archives of General Psychiatry, 52,* 384–392.

Baldwin, L., Beck, N., Menditto, A., Arms, T., & Corrier, G. (1992). Decreasing excessive water drinking by chronic mentally ill forensic patients. *Hospital and Community Psychiatry, 43,* 507–509.

Banchard, J., Mueser, K., & Bellack, A. (1998). Anhedonia, positive and negative affect, and social functioning in schizophrenia. *Schizophrenia Bulletin, 24,* 413–424.

Bandura, A. (1969). *Behavior modification.* New York: Holt, Rinehart & Winston.

Barkow, J. H., Cosmides, L., & Tooby, J. (Eds.). (1992). *The adapted mind: Evolutionary psychology and the generation of culture.* New York: Oxford University Press.

Barrowclough, C., Haddock, G., Tarrier, N., Lewis, S., Moring, J., O'Brien, R., Schofield, N., & McGovern, J. (2001). Randomized controlled trial of motivational interviewing, cognitive behavior therapy, and family intervention for patients with comorbid schizophrenia and substance use disorders. *American Journal of Psychiatry, 15*, 1706–1713.

Basavaraju, N., & Phillips, S. (1989). Cortisol deficient state: A cause of reversible cognitive impairment and delirium in the elderly. *Journal of the American Geriatric Society, 37*, 49–51.

Bebbington, P., & Kuipers, L. (1988). Social influences on schizophrenia. In P. Bebbington & P. McGuffin (Eds.), *Schizophrenia: The major issues* (pp. 201–225). Oxford, England: Heinemann.

Beck, A. T., Rush, A. J., Shaw, B. F., & Emery, G. (1979). *Cognitive therapy of depression*. New York: Guilford Press.

Beidel, D. (1983). Using the goal attainment scale to measure treatment outcome in schizophrenia. *International Journal of Partial Hospitalization, 21*, 33–41.

Belenko, S. (2002). Drug courts. In F. Tims (Ed.), *Treatment of drug offenders: Policies and issues* (pp. 301–318). New York: Springer.

Bell, M. (2001). Object-relations and reality-testing deficits in schizophrenia. In P. Corrigan & D. Penn (Eds.), *Social cognition and schizophrenia* (pp. 285–311). Washington, DC: American Psychological Association.

Bell, M., Bryson, G., Greig, T., Corcoran, C., & Wexler, B. (2001). Neurocognitive enhancement therapy with work therapy: Effects on neurocognitive test performance. *Archives of General Psychiatry, 58*, 763–768.

Bellak, A., Morrison, R., & Mueser, K. (1989). Social problem solving in schizophrenia. *Schizophrenia Bulletin, 15*, 101–116.

Benedict, R., Harris, A., Markow, T., McCormick, J., Neuchterlein, K., & Asarnow, R. (1996). Effects of training on information processing in schizophrenia. *Schizophrenia Bulletin, 20*, 537–546.

Benes, F. (1989). Myelination of cortical–hippocampal relays during late adolescence. *Schizophrenia Bulletin, 15*(4), 585–593.

Benes, F. (1997). The role of stress and dopamine–GABA interactions in the vulnerability for schizophrenia. *Journal of Psychiatry Research, 31*, 257–275.

Bennett, M., Bellack, A., & Gearon, J. (2001). Treating substances abuse in schizophrenia: An initial report. *Journal of Substance Abuse Treatment, 20*, 163–175.

Bentall, R. (2001). Social cognition and delusional beliefs. In P. Corrigan & D. Penn (Eds.), *Social cognition and schizophrenia* (pp. 123–148). Washington, DC: American Psychological Association.

Bentall, R., & Kinderman, P. (1998). Psychological processes and delusional beliefs: Implications for the treatment of paranoid states. In T. Wykes, N. Tarrier, & S. Lewis (Eds.), *Outcome and innovation in psychological treatment of schizophrenia* (pp. 117–144). London: Wiley.

Benton, M., & Schroeder, H. (1990). Social skills training with schizophrenics: A meta-analytic evaluation. *Journal of Consulting and Clinical Psychology, 58*(6), 741–747.

Ben-Yishay, Y., Rattok, J., Lakin, P., Piasetsky, E., Ross, B., Silver, S., Zide, E., & Ezrachi, O. (1985). Neuropsychological rehabilitation: Quest for a holistic approach. *Seminars in Neurology 5*, 252–299.

Birchwood, M. (1995). Early intervention in psychotic relapse: Cognitive approaches to detection and management. *Behaviour Change, 12*(1), 2–19.

Birchwood, M., & Cochrane, R. (1992). Specific and non-specific effects of educational intervention for families living with schizophrenia. *British Journal of Psychiatry, 160,* 806–814.

Bisiach, E., Meregalli, S., & Berti, A. (1985). *Mechanisms of production-control and belief-fixation in human visuospatial processing: Clinical evidence from hemispatial neglect.* Paper presented at the Eighth Symposium on Quantitative Analyses of Behavior, Harvard University, Cambridge, MA.

Bleuler, E. (1950). Dementia praecox or the group of schizophrenias. In G. Aschaffenburg (Ed.), *Handbook of mental illness.* (G. Zinkin, Trans.). New York: International Universities Press. (Original work published 1911)

Bond, G., Dincin, J., Setze, P., & Witheridge, T. (1984). The effectiveness of psychiatric rehabilitation: A summary of research at Thresholds. *Psychosocial Rehabilitation Journal, 7,* 6–22.

Bowden, C. (1998). Treatment of bipolar disorder. In A. F. Schatzberg & C. B. Nemeroff (Eds.), *Textbook of psychopharmacology* (2nd ed., pp. 733–746). Washington, DC: American Psychiatric Press.

Bowen, L., Glynn, S., Marshall, B., Kurth, C., & Hayden, J. (1990). Successful behavioral treatment of polydipsia in a schizophrenic patient. *Journal of Behavior Therapy and Experimental Psychiatry, 21,* 53–61.

Bowen, L., Wallace, C., Glynn, S., Neuchterlein, K., Lutzger, J., & Kuehnel, T. (1994). Schizophenics' cognitive functioning and performance in interpersonal interactions and skills training procedures. *Journal of Psychiatry Research, 28*(3), 289–301.

Bradshaw, J., & Sheppard, D. (2000). The neurodevelopmental frontostriatal disorders: Evolutionary adaptiveness and anomalous lateralization. *Brain and Language, 73,* 297–320.

Braginsky, B. M., Braginsky, D. D., & Ring, K. (1969). *Methods of madness: The mental hospital as last resort.* New York: Holt, Rhinehart & Winston.

Brandt, E., & Pope, A. (1997). *Enabling America: Assessing the role of rehabilitation science and engineering.* Washington, DC: National Academy Press.

Breggin, P. R. (1991). *Toxic psychiatry: Why therapy, empathy, and love must replace the drugs, electroshock, and biochemical theories of the "new psychiatry."* New York: St. Martin's Press.

Brenner, H. (1987). On the importance of cognitive disorders in treatment and rehabilitation. In J. Strauss, W. Baker, & H. Brenner (Eds.), *Psychosocial treatment of schizophrenia.* Toronto: Huber.

Brenner, H., Roder, V., Hodel, B., Kienzle, N., Reed, D., & Liberman, R. (1994). *Integrated psychological therapy for schizophrenic patients.* Toronto: Hogrefe & Huber.

Bressi, S., Miele, L., Bressi, C., Vita, A., Astori, S., Gimosti, E., Linciano, A., Sessini, M., Sferlazza, A., & Zirulia, G. (1998). Sequence skill learning and semantic priming in schizophrenia. Evidence for a differential impairment of the implicit memory system. *New Trends in Experimental and Clinical Psychiatry, 14,* 179–188.

Broen, W., & Storms, L. (1966). Lawful disorganization: The process underlying a schizophrenic syndrome. *Psychological Review, 73,* 265–279.

Brown, C., Harwood, K., Hays, C., Heckman, J., & Short, J. (2000). Effectiveness of cognitive rehabilitation for improving attention in patients with schizophrenia. *Occupational Therapy Journal of Research, 13,* 71–86.

Bruch, M. (1998). Cognitive behavioral case formulation. In E. Sanavio (Ed.), *Behavior and cognitive therapy today: Essays in honor of Hans J. Eysenck* (pp. 31–48). Oxford, England: Elsevier Science.

Buchanan, R. (1995). Clozapine: Efficacy and safety. *Schizophrenia Bulletin, 21*(4), 579–591.

Buckley, W. (1967). *Modern systems research for the behavioral scientist.* Chicago: Aldine.

Buican, B., Spaulding, W., Gordon, B., & Hindman, T. (1999). Clinical decision support systems in state hospitals. In W. Spaulding (Ed.), *The role of the state hospital in the 21st century* (Vol. 84, pp. 99–112). San Francisco: Jossey-Bass.

Burns, B., & Santos, A. (1995). Assertive Community Treatment: An update of randomized trials. *Psychiatric Services, 46,* 669–675.

Burns, D. (1995). *Therapist's tool kit: Comprehensive assessment and treatment tools for the mental health professional.* Gladwyne, PA: Author.

Bynum, W., Porter, R., & Shepherd, M. (Eds.). (1988). *The asylum and its psychiatry* (Vol. 3). London: Routledge.

Calsyn, R., & Davidson, W. (1978). Do we really want a program evaluation strategy based solely on individualized goals? A critique of goal attainment scaling. *Community Mental Health Journal, 14,* 300–308.

Carter, M., & Flesher, S. (1995). The neuropsychology of schizophrenia: Vulnerability and functional disability. *Psychiatry, Interpersonal and Biological Processes, 58,* 209–224.

Casey, B., Giedd, J., & Thomas, K. (2000). Structural and functional brain development and its relations to cognitive development. *Biological Psychology, 54,* 241–257.

Cesare-Murphy, M., McMahill, C., & Schyve, P. (1997). Joint commission evaluation of behavioral health care organizations. *Evaluation Review, 21,* 322–329.

Chadwick, P., Birchwood, M., & Trower, P. (1996). *Cognitive therapy for delusions, voices and paranoia.* New York: Wiley.

Chapman, L. J., & Chapman, J. P. (1978). The measurement of differential deficit. *Journal of Psychiatric Research, 14,* 303–311.

Cheng, P. W., & Novick, L. R. (1992). Covariation in natural causal induction. *Psychological Review, 99,* 365–382.

Choca, J., Peterson, C., & Shanley, L. (1987). DRGs: Forests and trees. *American Psychologist, 42,* 189–191.

Claridge, G. (1990). Can a disease model of schizophrenia survive? In R. Bentall (Ed.), *Reconstructing schizophrenia* (pp. 157–183). London: Routledge.

Cline, D., Rouzer, D., & Bransford, D. (1973). Goal attainment scaling as a method for evaluating mental health programs. *American Journal of Psychiatry, 130,* 105–108.

Corcoran, R. (2001). Theory of mind and schizophrenia. In P. Corrigan & D. Penn (Eds.), *Social cognition and schizophrenia* (pp. 149–174). Washington, DC: American Psychological Association.

Corrigan, P., Hirschbeck, J., & Wolfe, M. (1995). Memory and vigilance training to improve social perception in schizophrenia. *Schizophrenia Research, 17,* 257–265.

354 References

Corrigan, P., Holmes, E., Luchns, D., & Basit, A. (1995). The effects of interactive staff training on staff programing and patient aggression in a psychiatric inpatient ward. *Behavioral Interventions, 10*, 17–32.

Corrigan, P., & Liberman, R. (1994). *Behavior therapy in psychiatric hospitals.* New York: Springer.

Corrigan, P., Liberman, R., & Wong, S. (1993). Recreational therapy and behavior management on inpatient units: Is recreational therapy therapeutic? *Journal of Nervous and Mental Disease, 181*(10), 644–646.

Corrigan, P., & McCracken, S. (1997a). *Interactive staff training: Rehabilitation teams that work.* New York: Plenum Press.

Corrigan, P., & McCracken, S. (1997b). Intervention research: Integrating practice guidelines with dissemination strategies—a rejoinder. *Applied and Preventative Psychology, 6*, 205–209.

Corrigan, P., & Nelson, D. (1998). Factors that affect social cue recognition in schizophrenia. *Psychiatry Research, 78*, 189–196.

Corrigan, P., & Penn, D. (1995). The effects of antipsychotic and antiparkinsonian medication on psychosocial skill learning. *Clinical Psychology: Science and Practice, 2*(3), 251–262.

Corrigan, P., & Penn, D. (1999). Lessons from social psychology on discrediting psychiatric stigma. *American Psychologist, 54*(9), 765–776.

Corrigan, P., & Penn, D. (Eds.). (2001). *Social cognition and schizophrenia.* Washington, DC: American Psychological Association.

Corrigan, P., & Storzbach, D. (1993). The ecological validity of cognitive rehabilitation for schizophrenia. *Journal of Cognitive Rehabilitation, 11*, 14–21.

Cosoff, S., & Hafner, R. (1998). The prevalence of comorbid anxiety in schizophrenia, schizoaffective disorder and bipolar disorder. *Australian and New Zealand Journal of Psychiatry, 32*, 67–72.

Cromwell, R. L. (1975). Assessment of schizophrenia. *Annual Review of Psychology, 26*, 593–619.

Cromwell, R. L. (1984). Preemptive thinking and schizophrenia research. In W. D. Spaulding & J. K. Cole (Eds.), *Theories of schizophrenia and psychosis* (pp. 1–46). Lincoln: University of Nebraska Press.

Cromwell, R. L., Elkins, I., McCarthy, M., & O'Neil, T. (1994). Searching for the phenotypes of schizophrenia. *Acta Psychiatrica Scandinavica, 90*(384, Suppl.), 34–39.

Cromwell, R. L., & Spaulding, W. (1978). How schizophrenics handle information. In W. E. Fann, I. Karacan, A. D. Pokorny, & R. L. Williams (Eds.), *The phenomenology and treatment of schizophrenia* (pp. 127–162). New York: Spectrum.

Crow, T. (1985). The two-syndrome concept: Origins and current status. *Schizophrenia Bulletin, 11*, 471–486.

Cytrynbaum, S., Ginath, Y., Birdwell, J., & Brandt, L. (1979). Goal attainment scaling: A critical review. *Evaluation Quarterly, 3*, 5–40.

Danion, J., Meulemans, T., Kauffmann-Muller, F., & Vermaat, H. (2001). Intact implicit learning in schizophrenia. *American Journal of Psychiatry, 158*, 944–948.

David, A., & Cutting, J. (Eds.). (1994). *The neuropsychology of schizophrenia.* Hillsdale, NJ: Erlbaum.

Davis, S. (2001). What gene activation can tell us about synaptic plasticity and the mechanisms underlying the encoding of the memory trace. In C. Hoelscher (Ed.), *Neuronal mechanisms of memory formation: Concepts of long-term potentiation and beyond* (pp. 450–475). New York: Cambridge University Press.

Davis, A., Davis, S., Moss, N., Marks, J., et al. (1993). First steps towards an interdisciplinary approach to rehabilitation. *Clinical Rehabilitation, 6*, 237–244.

Davis, P., & Blankenship, C. (1996). Group-oriented contingencies: Applications for community rehabilitation programs. *Vocational Evaluation and Work Adjustment Bulletin, 29*, 114–118.

Dawson, M. E., & Neuchterlein, K. H. (1984). Psychophysiological dysfunctions in the developmental course of schizophrenic disorders. *Schizophrenia Bulletin, 10*, 204–232.

de Haan, L. van der Gaag, M., & Wolthaus, J. (2000). Duration of untreated psychosis and the long-term course of schizophrenia. *European Psychiatry, 15*, 264–267.

de Jesus-Marie, J., & Streiner, D. (1994). An overview of family interventions and relapse on schizophrenia: Meta-analysis of research findings. *Psychological Medicine, 24*(3), 565–578.

DeLeon, P., Howell, W., Newman, R., Brown, A., Keita, G., & Sexton, J. (1996). Expanding roles in the twenty-first century. In R. Resnick & R. Rozensky (Eds.), *Health psychology through the life span: Practice and research opportunities* (pp. 427–453). Washington, DC: American Psychological Association.

Dennis, D., & Monahan, J. (Eds.). (1996). *Coercion and aggressive community treatment*. New York: Plenum Press.

Dickens, P. (1994). *Quality and excellence in human services*. New York: Wiley.

Dienstbier, R. (1991). Behavioral correlates of sympathoadrenal reactivity: The toughness model. *Medicine and Science in Sports and Exercise, 23*, 846–852.

Dixon, L. (1999). Dual diagnosis of substance abuse in schizophrenia: Prevalence and impact on outcomes. *Schizophrenia Research, 35*(Suppl.), S93–S100.

Donahoe, C. P. *Assessment instrument for problem-solving skills*. Unpublished manuscript.

Donahoe, C. P., Carter, M., Bloem, W., Hirsch, G., Lassi, N., & Wallace, C. (1990). Assessment of interpersonal problem solving skills. *Psychiatry, 53*(4), 329–339.

Drury, V., Birchwood, M., Cochrane, R., & MacMillan, F. (1996a). Cognitive therapy and recovery from acute psychosis: A controlled trial: I. Impact on psychotic symptoms. *British Journal of Psychiatry, 169*, 593–601.

Drury, V., Birchwood, M., Cochrane, R., & MacMillan, R. (1996b). Cognitive therapy and recovery from acute psychosis: A controlled trial: II. Impact on recovery time. *British Journal of Psychiatry, 169*, 602–607.

Duncan, C. C. (1988). Event-related brain potentials: A window on information processing in schizophrenia. *Schizophrenia Bulletin, 14*, 199–203.

Durham, T. (1997). Work-related activity for people with long-term schizophrenia: A review of the literature. *British Journal of Occupational Therapy, 60*(6), 248–252.

D'Zurilla, T. J. (1986). *Problem-solving therapy: A social competence approach to clinical intervention*. New York: Springer.

D'Zurilla, T. J. (1988). Problem-solving therapies. In K. S. Dobson (Ed.), *Handbook of cognitive-behavioral therapies* (pp. 85–135). New York: Guilford Press.

D'Zurrila, T. J., & Goldfried, M. R. (1971). Problem-solving and behavior modification. *Journal of Abnormal Psychology, 78*, 107–126.

D'Zurilla, T. J., & Maydeu-Olivares, A. (1995). Conceptual and methodological issues in social problem-solving assessment. *Behavior Therapy, 26*(3), 409–432.

D'Zurilla, T. J., & Nezu, A. (1982). Social problem solving in adults. In P. C. Kendall (Ed.), *Advances in cognitive-behavioral research and therapy* (Vol. I, pp. 202–274). New York: Academic Press.

Eckman, T. A., Liberman, R. P., Phipps, C. C., & Blair, K. E. (1990). Teaching medication management skills to schizophrenic patients. *Journal of Clinical Psychopharmacology, 10*, 33–38.

Eells, T. D. (Ed.). (1997). *Handbook of psychotherapy case formulation*. New York: Guilford Press.

Elbogen, E., & Tomkins, A. (1999). The psychiatric hospital and therapeutic jurisprudence: Applying the law to promote mental health. In W. Spaulding (Ed.), *The state hospital in the 21st century: New directions for mental health services* (Vol. 84, pp. 71–84). San Francisco: Jossey-Bass.

Ellis, H., & dePauw, D. (1994). The cognitive neuropsychiatric origins of the Capgras delusion. In A. David & J. Cutting (Eds.), *The neuropsychology of schizophrenia* (pp. 317–335). Hillsdale, NJ: Erlbaum.

English, J. (1986). Diagnosis-related groups and general hospital psychiatry: The APA study. *American Journal of Psychiatry, 143*, 131–139.

Erickson, R. (1994). Neuropsychological assessment and consultation in psychiatric rehabilitation, in W. Spaulding (Ed.), *Cognitive technology in psychiatric rehabilitation* (pp. 27–48). Lincoln: University of Nebraska Press.

Fadden, G. (1997). Implementation of family interventions in routine clinical practice following staff training programs: A major cause for concern. *Journal of Mental Health, 6*, 599–612.

Fairweather, G., Sanders, D., Maynard, H., & Cressler, D. (1969). *Community life for the mentally ill: An alternative to institutional care*. Chicago: Aldine.

Falloon, I. R. H. (1990). Family management of schizophrenia. In M. Weller (Ed.), *International perspectives in schizophrenia: Biological, social and epidemiological findings* (pp. 293–305). London: Libbey.

Falloon, I. R. H., Boyd, J. L., & McGill, C. W. (1984). *Family care of schizophrenia: A problem-solving approach to the treatment of mental illness*. New York: Guilford Press.

Falloon, I. R. H., Laporta, M., Fadden, G., & Graham-Hole, V. (1993). *Managing stress in families: Cognitive and behavioural strategies for enhancing coping skills*. London: Routledge.

Faulkner, L. (1986). Small group work therapy for the chronic mentally ill. *Hospital and Community Psychiatry, 37*, 273–279.

Fauman, M. (1990). Quality assurance monitoring in psychiatry. *American Journal of Psychiatry, 146*, 1112–1130.

Fennell, M. (1998). Low self-esteem. In N. Tarrier, A. Wells, & G. Haddock (Eds.), *Treating complex cases: The cognitive behavioral therapy approach* (pp. 217–240). Chichester, England: Wiley.

Fischer, J., & Corcoran, K. (1994). *Measures for clinical practice: A sourcebook* (2nd ed.). New York: Free Press.

Flannery, R., Penk, W., & Addo, L. (1996). Resolving learned helplessness in the seriously and persistently mentally ill. In S. Soreff (Ed.), *Handbook for the treatment of the seriously mentally ill* (pp. 239–256). Kirkland, WA: Hogrefe & Huber.

Fodor, J. (1983). *The modularity of mind.* Boston: MIT Press.

Fodor, J. (2000). *The mind doesn't work that way.* Boston: MIT Press.

Ford, L. (1995). *Providing employment support for people with long-term mental illness: Choices, resources and practical strategies.* Baltimore: Brookes.

Fordyce, W. (1982). Interdisciplinary processes: Implications for rehabilitation psychology. *Rehabilitation Psychology, 27,* 5–11.

Foster, K. (1988). The role of behavior management programs in the rehabilitation process. *Cognitive Rehabilitation, 6,* 16–19.

Frank, J. D., & Frank, J. B. (1991). *Persuasion and healing: A comparative study of psychotherapy* (3rd ed.). Baltimore: Johns Hopkins University Press.

Gabrielli, J. (1995). Contribution of the basal ganglia to skill learning and working memory in humans. In J. Houk & J. Davis & D. Beiser (Eds.), *Models of information processing in the basal ganglia* (pp. 277–294). Cambridge, MA: MIT Press.

Gambrill, E. (1990). *Critical thinking in clinical practice.* San Francisco: Jossey-Bass.

Gardner, H. (1987). *The mind's new science: A history of the cognitive revolution.* New York: Basic Books.

Gay, E., Kronenfeld, J., Baker, S., & Amidon, R. (1989). An appraisal of organizational response to fiscally constraining regulation: The case of hospitals and DRGs. *Journal of Health and Social Behavior, 30,* 41–55.

Geist, P., & Hardesty, M. (1992). *Negotiating the crisis: DRGs and the transformation of hospitals.* Hillsdale, NJ: Elrbaum.

Gelfand, D., Gelfand, S., & Dobson, W. (1967). Unprogrammed reinforcement of patients' behavior in a mental hospital. *Behavior Research and Therapy, 5,* 201–207.

Gershater, R., Lutzker, J., & Kuehnel, T. (1997). Activity scheduling to increase staff–patient interactions. *Clinical Supervisor, 15,* 115–128.

Gervey, R., & Bedell, J. (1994). Supported employment in vocational rehabilitation. In J. Bedell (Ed.), *Psychological assessment and treatment of persons with severe mental disorders* (pp. 31–56). Philadelphia: Taylor & Francis.

Glasscote, R. M. (1971). *Rehabilitating the mentally ill in the community.* Washington, DC: Joint Information Service of the American Psychiatric Association.

Glynn, S. (1990). The token economy: Progress and pitfalls over 25 years. *Behavior Modification, 14,* 383–407.

Goffman, E. A. (1961). *Asylums.* Garden City, NY: Anchor Books.

Goldberg, J. (1994). Cognitive retraining in a community psychiatric rehabilitation program. In W. Spaulding (Ed.), *Cognitive technology in psychiatric rehabilitation* (pp. 67–86). Lincoln: University of Nebraska Press.

Goldberg, S. C., Schooler, N. R., Hogarty, G. E., & Roper, M. (1977). Prediction of relapse in schizophrenia outpatients treated by drug and sociotherapy. *Archives of General Psychiatry, 34,* 171–184.

Goldstein, G. (1978). Cognitive and perceptual differences between schizophrenics and organics. *Schizophrenia Bulletin, 4,* 160–185.

Goldstein, G. (1986). The neuropsychology of schizophrenia. In I. Grant & K. Adams

(Eds.), *Neuropsychological assessment of neuropsychiatric disorders*. New York: Oxford University Press.

Goldstein, G. (1990). Neuropsychological heterogeneity in schizophrenia: A consideration of abstraction and problem-solving abilities. *Archives of Clinical Neuropsychology, 5*, 251–264.

Goldstein, G. (1991). Comprehensive neuropsychological test batteries and research in schizophrenia. In S. R. Steinhauer, J. H. Gruzelier, & J. Zubin (Eds.), *Handbook of schizophrenia. Vol. 5: Neuropsychology, psychopathology and information processing* (pp. 525–551). Amsterdam: Elsevier Science.

Goldstein, G., & Halperin, K. M. (1977). Neuropsychological differences among subtypes of schizophrenia. *Journal of Abnormal Psychology, 86*, 34–40.

Goldstein, G., & Shemansky, W. (1995). Influences on cognitive heterogeneity in schizophrenia. *Schizophrenia Research, 18*, 59–69.

Goldstein, M. (1991). Schizophrenia and family therapy. In B. Beitman & G. Klerman (Eds.), *Integrating pharmacotherapy and psychotherapy*. Washington, DC: American Psychiatric Press.

Gottesman, I. I., Shield, J., & Hanson, D. R. (1982). *Schizophrenia: The epigenetic puzzle*. Cambridge, England: Cambridge University Press.

Gray, J., Buhusi, C., & Schmajuk, N. (1997). The transition from automatic to controlled processing. *Neural Networks, 10*, 1257–1268.

Green, M. (1998). *Schizophrenia as a neurocognitive disorder*. Boston: Allyn & Bacon.

Green, M. (2001). *Schizophrenia revealed: From neurons to social interactions*. New York: Norton.

Green, M., Kern, R., Williams, O., McGurk, S., & Kee, D. (1997). Procedural learning in schizophrenia: Evidence from serial reaction time. *Cognitive Neuropsychiatry, 2*, 123–134.

Green, M., & Neuchterlein, K. (1999). Should schizophrenia be treated as a neurocognitive disorder? *Schizophrenia Bulletin, 25*, 309–319.

Greene, B. (1999). *The elegant universe*. New York: Norton.

Griffith, R. (1980). An administrative perspective on guidelines for behavior modification: The creation of a legally safe environment. *Behavior Therapist, 3*, 5–7.

Grob, G. (1973). *Mental institutions in America: Social policy to 1875*. New York: Free Press.

Grob, G. (1983). *Mental illness and American society, 1875–1940*. Princeton, NJ: Princeton University Press.

Gruzelier, J. H. (1991). Hemispheric imbalance: Syndromes of schizophrenia, premorbid personality, and neurodevelopmental influences. In S. R. Steinhauer, J. H. Gruzelier, & J. Zubin (Eds.), *Handbook of schizophrenia. Vol. 5: Neuropsychology, psychopathology and information processing* (pp. 599–650). Amsterdam: Elsevier Science.

Gruzelier, J. H., Wilson, L., & Richardson, A. (1999). Cognitive asymmetry patterns in schizophrenia: Retest reliability and modification with recovery. *International Journal of Psychophysiology, 34*, 323–331.

Gur, R. E., & Chin, S. (1999). Laterality in functional brain imaging studies of schizophrenia. *Schizophrenia Bulletin, 25*, 141–156.

Gur, R. E., & Gur, R. C. (1991). Laterality in schizophrenia: Positron-emission tomography studies. In N. D. Volkow & A. P. Wolf (Eds.), *Positron-emission tomography in schizophrenia research* (pp. 47–58). Washington, DC: American Psychiatric Press.

Haddock, G., & Tarrier, N. (1998). Assessment and formulation in the cognitive behavioral treatment of psychosis. In G. Haddock (Ed.), *Treating complex cases: The cognitive behavioral therapy approach.* Chichester, England: Wiley.

Haddock, G., Tarrier, N., Spaulding, W., Yusupoff, L., Kinney, C., & McCarthy, E. (1998). Individual cognitive-behavior therapy in the treatment of hallucinations and delusions: A review. *Clinical Psychology Review, 18*(7), 821–838.

Haley, J. (1986). *The power tactics of Jesus Christ and other essays.* Rockville, MD: Triangle Press.

Halperin, S., Nathan, P., Drummond, P., & Castle, D. (2000). A cognitive-behavioral, group-based intervention for social anxiety in schizophrenia. *Australian and New Zealand Journal of Psychiatry, 34,* 809–813.

Harmon-Jones, E., & Mills, J. (Eds.). (1999). *Cognitive dissonance: Progress on a pivotal theory in social psychology.* Washington, DC: American Psychological Association.

Heaton, R. (1981). *Wisconsin card sorting test manual.* Odessa, FL: Psychological Assessment Resources.

Heavlin, W., Lee-Merrow, S., & Lewis, V. (1982). The psychometric foundations of goal attainment scaling. *Community Mental Health Journal, 18,* 230–241.

Heinssen, R. (1996). The cognitive exoskeleton: Environmental interventions in cognitive rehabilitation. In P. Corrigan & S. Yudofsky (Eds.), *Cognitive rehabilitation of neuropsychiatric disorders.* Washington, DC: American Psychiatric Press.

Heinssen, R., Levendusky, P., & Hunter, R. (1995). Client as colleague: Therapeutic contracting with the seriously mentally ill. *American Psychologist, 50*(7), 522–532.

Heinssen, R., & Victor, B. (1994). Cognitive-behavioral treatments for schizophrenia: Evolving rehabilitation techniques. In W. Spaulding (Ed.), *Cognitive technology in psychiatric rehabilitation* (pp. 159–182). Lincoln: University of Nebraska Press.

Hermanutz, M., & Gestrich, J. (1991). Computer-assisted attention training in schizophrenics. *European Archives of Psychiatry and Clinical Neuroscience, 24,* 282–287.

Hersen, M., Bellak, A., & Harris, F. (1993). Staff training and consultation. In A. Bellak & M. Hersen (Eds.), *Handbook of behavior therapy in the psychiatric setting: Critical issues in psychiatry* (pp. 143–164). New York: Plenum Press.

Herz, M. (1986). Toward an integrated approach to the treatment of schizophrenia. *Psychotherapy and Psychodynamics, 46,* 45–57.

Herz, M. I., Lamberti, S., Mintz, J., Scott, R., O'Dell, S., McCartan, L., & Nix, G. (2000). A program for relapse prevention in schizophrenia: A controlled study. *Archives of General Psychiatry, 57,* 277–283.

Herz, M. I., & Melville, C. (1980). Relapse in schizophrenia. *American Journal of Psychiatry, 137,* 801–805.

Higgins, E., & Bargh, J. (1987). Social cognition and social perception. *Annual Review of Psychology, 38,* 369–425.

Himadi, B., & Kaiser, A. (1992). The modification of delusional beliefs: A single subject evaluation. *Behavioral Residential Treatment, 7*(1), 1–14.

Hodel, B., & Brenner, H. D. (1997). A new development in integrated psychological therapy for schizophrenic patients (PS): First results of emotional management training. In H. D. Brenner & W. Boeker (Eds.), *Towards a comprehensive therapy for schizophrenia* (pp. 118–134). Kirkland, WA: Hogrefe & Huber.

Hodel, B., Brenner, H. D., Merlo, M., & Teuber, J. (1998). Emotional management therapy in early psychosis. *British Journal of Psychiatry, 172*(33, Suppl.), 128–133.

Hoffman, H., & Kupper, Z., (1996). Patient dynamics in early stages of vocational rehabilitation: A pilot study. *Comprehensive Psychiatry, 37*, 216–221.

Hogarty, G. (1977). Treatment and the course of schizophrenia. *Schizophrenia Bulletin, 3*(4), 587–599.

Hogarty, G., Anderson, C., Reiss, D., Kornblith, S., Greenewald, D., Javno, C., & Madonia, M. (1986). Family psycho-education, social skills training and maintenance chemotherapy: I. One-year effects of a controlled study on relapse and expressed emotion. *Archives of General Psychiatry, 43*, 633–642.

Hogarty, G., & Flesher, S. (1999a). A developmental theory for cognitive enhancement therapy of schizophrenia. *Schizophrenia Bulletin, 25*(4), 677–692.

Hogarty, G., & Flesher, S. (1999b). Practice principles of cognitive enhancement therapy for schizophrenia. *Schizophrenia Bulletin, 25*(4), 693–708.

Holcomb, W., & Thompson, W. (1988). Medicare prospective reimbursement for mental health services: A literature review. *Administration in Mental Health, 15*, 127–138.

Honigfeld, G., Gillis, R., & Klett, J. (1966). NOSIE-30: A treatment-sensitive ward behavior scale. *Psychological Reports, 19*(1), 180–182.

Hooley, J. M. (1985). Expressed emotion: A review of the critical literature. *Clinical Psychology Review, 5*, 119–139.

Horn, S., Chambers, A., Sharkey, P., & Horn, R. (1989). Psychiatric severity of illness: A case mix study. *Medical Care, 27*, 69–83.

Horowitz, M. (1999). Thinking through psychotherapy: Configurational analysis method of case formulation. In D. Spiegel (Ed.), *Efficacy and cost-effectiveness of psychotherapy* (pp. 1–20). Washington, DC: American Psychiatric Press.

Houk, J. (1995). Information processing in modular circuits linking basal ganglia and cerebral cortex. In J. Hauk & J. Davis & D. Bieser (Eds.), *Models of information processing in the basal ganglia* (pp. 3–9). Cambridge, MA: MIT Press.

Houk, J., & Wise, S. (1993). Outline for a theory of motor behavior. In P. Rudomin, M. Arbib, & F. Cervantes-Perez (Eds.), *From neural networks to artificial intelligence* (pp. 452–470). Heidelberg, Germany: Springer-Verlag.

House, R., & Scott, J. (1996). Problems in measuring problem-solving: the suitability of the means-ends problem-solving (MEPS) procedure. *International Journal of Methods in Psychiatric Research, 6*, 243–251.

Howells, K. (1998). Cognitive behavioral interventions for anger, aggression and violence. In N. Tarrier, A. Wells, & G. Haddock (Eds.), *Treating complex cases: The cognitive behavioral therapy approach* (pp. 295–318). Chichester, England: Wiley.

Huberman, W., & O'Brien, R. (1999). Improving therapist and patient performance in chronic psychiatric group homes through goal-setting, feedback and positive reinforcement. *Journal of Organizational Behavior Management, 19*, 13–36.

Hunter, R. (1999). Public policy and state hospitals. In W. Spaulding (Ed.), *The role of the state hospital in the 21st century* (Vol. 84, pp. 25–35). San Francisco: Jossey-Bass.

Hunter, R. (2000). Treatment, management and control: Improving outcomes through more treatment and less control. In F. Frese (Ed.), *The role of organized psychology in treatment of the seriously mentally ill* (Vol. 88, pp. 5–15). San Francisco: Jossey-Bass.

Hurley, R., & Draper, D. (1998). Medicaid managed care for special needs populations: Behavioral health as "tracer condition." In D. Mechanic (Ed.), *Managed behavioral health care: Current realities and future potential* (Vol. 78). San Francisco: Jossey-Bass.

Ito, M. (1990). Neural control as a major aspect of high-order brain function. In J. C. Eccles & J. Creutzfeldt (Eds.), *The principles of design and operation of the brain* (pp. 281–301). New York: Springer-Verlag.

Iwata, B., Kahng, S., Wallace, M., & Lindberg, J. (2000). The functional analysis model of behavioral assessment. In J. Austin & J. Carr (Eds.), *Handbook of applied behavior analysis* (pp. 61–89). Reno, NV: Context Press.

Jacobs, S., Hoge, M., Sledge, W., & Bunney, B. (1997). Managed care, health care reform and academic psychiatry. *Academic Psychiatry, 21*, 72–85.

Jansen, L., Gispen de Wied, C., Gademan, P., DeJonge, R., van der Linden, J., & Kahn, R. (1998). Blunted cortisol response to a psychosocial stressor in schizophrenia. *Schizophrenia Research, 33*, 87–94.

Jewell, T., Silverstein, S., & Stewart, D. (2001). Development and evaluation of a treatment manual and course for writing behavior contracts for people with severe mental illness. *Psychiatric Rehabilitation Skills, 5*, 255–271.

Jones, E., Kanouse, D., Kelly, H., Nisbett, R., Calins, S., & Weiner, B. (Eds.). (1971). *Attribution: Perceiving the causes of behavior.* Morristown, NJ: General Learning Press.

Jones, M. (1953). *The therapeutic community.* New York: Basic Books.

Karp, B., Garvey, M., Jocabsen, L., Frazier, J., Hamberger, A., Bedwell, J., & Rapoport, J. (2001). Abnormal neurologic maturation in adolescents with early-onset schizophrenia. *American Journal of Psychiatry, 158*, 118–122.

Kasapis, C., Amador, X., Yale, S., Strauss, D., & Gorman, J. (1995). Poor insight in schizophrenia: Neuropsychological and defensive aspects. *Schizophrenia Research, 15*, 123.

Kavanagh, D. J. (1992a). Recent developments in expressed emotion and schizophrenia. *British Journal of Psychiatry, 160*, 601–620.

Kavanagh, D. J. (1992b). Schizophrenia. In P. H. Wilson (Ed.), *Principles and practice of relapse prevention* (pp. 157–190). New York: Guilford Press.

Kay, S., Fizbein, A., & Opler, L. (1987). The positive and negative syndrome scale (PANSS) for schizophrenia. *Schizophrenia Bulletin, 13*, 261–276.

Kazdin, A. (1980). *Research design in clinical psychology.* New York: Harper & Row.

Kazdin, A., & Bootsin, R. (1972). The token economy: An evaluative review. *Journal of Applied Behavior Analysis, 5*, 1–30.

Kellendonk, C., Gass, P., Kretz, O., Schuetz, G., & Tronche, F. (2002). Corticosteroid receptors in the brain: Gene targeting studies. *Brain Research Bulletin, 57*, 73–83.

Kern, R., Green, M., & Goldstein, M. (1995). Modification of performance on the span of apprehension, a putative marker of vulnerability to schizophrenia. *Journal of Abnormal Psychology, 104*(2), 385–389.

Kinderman, P. (2001). Changing causal attributions. In P. Corrigan & D. Penn (Eds.), *Social cognition and schizophrenia* (pp. 195–215). Washington, DC: American Psychological Association.

Kingdon, D. G., & Turkington, D. (1994). *Cognitive-behavioral therapy of schizophrenia.* New York: Guilford Press.

Kiresuk, T., Stelmachers, Z., & Schultz, S. (1982). Quality assurance and goal attainment scaling. *Professional Psychology: Research and Practice, 13*, 145–152.

Kirk, S., & Kutchins, H. (1993). *The selling of the DSM-III: The rhetoric of science of psychiatry.* New York: Aldine.

Klein, D. (1980). Psychosocial treatment of schizophrenia, or psychosocial help for people with schizophrenia? *Schizophrenia Bulletin, 6*, 122.

Klerman, G. (1978). The evolution of a scientific nosology. In J. Shershow (Ed.), *Schizophrenia: Research and practice* (pp. 99–121). Cambridge, MA: Harvard University Press.

Knable, M., Kleinman, J., & Weinberger, D. (1998). Neurobiology of schizophrenia. In A. F. Schatzberg & C. B. Nemeroff (Eds.), *Textbook of psychopharmacology* (2nd ed., pp. 589–608). Washington, DC: American Psychiatric Press.

Knoll, J., Garner, D., Ramberg, J., Kingsbury, S., Croissant, D., & McDermott, B. (1999). Heterogeneity of the psychoses: Is there a neurodegenerative psychosis? *Schizophrenia Bulletin, 24*(3), 365–380.

Kowalski, R., & Leary, M. (Eds.). (1999). *The social psychology of emotional and behavioral problems: Interfaces of social and clinical psychology.* Washington, DC: American Psychological Association.

Kraepelin, E. (1987). Dementia praecox. In M. Shepherd (Ed.), *The clinical roots of the schizophrenia concept* (pp. 426–441). Cambridge, England: Cambridge University Press. (Original work published 1896)

Kremen, W., Seidman, L., Goldstein, G., Faraone, S., & Tsuang, M. (1994). Systematized delusions and neuropsychological function in paranoid and nonparanoid schizophrenia. *Schizophrenia Research, 12*, 223–236.

Kuehnel, T. G., Liberman, R. P., Storzbach, D., & Rose, G. (1990). *Resource book for psychiatric rehabilitation* (2nd ed.). Baltimore: Williams & Wilkins.

Kuhn, T. (1962). *The structure of scientific revolutions.* Chicago: University of Chicago Press.

Kuipers, L., Leff, J., & Lam, D. (1992). *Family work for schizophrenia: A practical guide.* London: Gaskell/Royal College of Psychiatrists.

Kutchins, H., & Kirk, S. (1997). *Making us crazy: The psychiatric bible and the creation of psychiatric disorders.* New York: Free Press.

Laing, R. (1969). *The divided self.* New York, Pantheon.

Lam, D. (1991). Psychosocial family intervention in schizophrenia: A review of empirical studies. *Psychological Medicine, 21*, 423–441.

Lecompte, D., & Pelc, I. (1996). A cognitive-behavioral program to improve compliance with medication in patients with schizophrenia. *International Journal of Mental Health, 25*(1), 51–56.

Lehman, A., Steinwachs, D., Dixon, L., Goldman, H., Osher, F., Postrado, L., Scott, J., Thompson, J., Fahey, M., Fischer, P., Kasper, J., Lyles, A., Skinner, E., Buchanan, R., Carpenter, W., Levine, J., McGlynn, E., Rosenheck, R., & Zito, J. (1998). Translating research into practice: The schizophrenia patient outcomes research team (PORT) treatment recommendations. *Schizophrenia Bulletin, 24*(1), 1–10.

Lehman, A., Steinwachs, D., Dixon, L., Postrado, L., Scott, J., Fahey, M., Fischer, P., Hoch, J., Kasper, J., Lyles, A., Shore, A., & Skinner, E. (1998). Patterns of usual care for schizophrenia: Initial results from the schizophrenia patient outcomes research team (PORT) client survey. *Schizophrenia Bulletin, 24*(1), 11–20.

Leonhard, C., & Corrigan, P. (2001). Social perception in schizophrenia. In P. Corrigan & D. Penn (Eds.), *Social cognition and schizophrenia* (pp. 41–72). Washington, DC: American Psychological Association.

Leven, S. J. (1992). Learned helplessness, memory, and the dynamics of hope. In D. S. Levine & S. J. Leven (Eds.), *Motivation, emotion, and goal direction in neural networks* (pp. 259–299). Hillsdale, NJ: Erlbaum.

Levin, S., Yurgelun-Todd, D., & Craft, S. (1989). Contributions of clinical neuropsychology to the study of schizophrenia. *Journal of Abnormal Psychology, 98,* 341–356.

Lewinsohn, P. M., Sullivan, J. M., & Grosscup, S. J. (1982). Behavior therapy: Clinical applications. In A. J. Rush (Ed.), *Short-term psychotherapies for depression: Behavioral, interpersonal, cognitive, and psychodynamic approaches* (pp. 50–87). New York: Guilford Press.

Lewis, A., Spencer, J., Haas, G., & DiVittis, A. (1987). Goal attainment scaling: Relevance and replicability in follow-up of inpatients. *Journal of Nervous and Mental Disease, 175,* 408–418.

Lewis, J., Lewis, M., & Souflee, F. (1991). *Management of human service programs.* Pacific Grove, CA: Brooks/Cole.

Lezak, M. (1982). The problem of assessing executive functions. *International Journal of Psychology, 17,* 281–297.

Lezak, M. (1994). Domains of behavior from a neuropsychological perspective: The whole story. In W. Spaulding (Ed.), *Nebraska symposium on motivation (Vol. 41): Integrative views of motivation, cognition and emotion* (pp. 23–56). Lincoln: University of Nebraska Press.

Liberman, R. P. (1979). Social and political challenges of the development of behavioral programs in organizations. In P. O. Sjödén, S. Bates, & W. Dockens (Eds.), *Trends in behavior therapy* (pp. 369–398). New York: Academic Press.

Liberman, R. P. (1986). Coping and competence as protective factors in the vulnerability–stress model of schizophrenia. In M. J. Goldstein, I. Hand, & K. Hahlweg (Eds.), *Treatment of schizophrenia: Family assessment and intervention* (pp. 201–216). Berlin: Springer Verlag.

Liberman, R. P. (Ed.). (1992). *Handbook of psychiatric rehabilitation.* New York: Macmillan.

Liberman, R. P., & Marshall, B. (1993). Polydipsia and hyponatremia. *Hospital and Community Psychiatry, 44,* 184.

Liberman, R. P., Mueser, K. T., Wallace, C. J., Jacobs, H. E., Eckman, T., & Massel, H.

K. (1986). Training skills in the psychiatrically disabled: Learning coping and competence. *Schizophrenia Bulletin, 12,* 631–647.

Liberman, R. P., Neuchterlein, K. H., & Wallace, C. J. (1982). Social skills training and the nature of schizophrenia. In J. P. Curran & P. M. Monti (Eds.), *Social skills training: A practical handbook for assessment and treatment* (pp. 5–56). New York: Guilford Press.

Liberman, R. P., Teigen, J., Patterson, R., & Baker, V. (1973). Reducing delusional speech in chronic paranoid schizophrenics. *Journal of Applied Behavior Analysis, 6,* 57–64.

Linehan, M. M. (1993). *Cognitive-behavioral treatment of borderline personality disorder.* New York: Guilford Press.

Lipe, M. G. (1991). Counterfactual reasoning as a framework for attribution theories. *Psychological Bulletin, 109*(3), 456–471.

Magaro, P., Gripp, R., McDowell, D., & Miller, I. (1978). *The mental health industry: A cultural phenomenon.* New York: Wiley.

Maher, B. (1966). *Principles of psychopathology.* New York: McGraw Hill.

Malec, J. (1999). Goal attainment scaling in rehabilitation. *Neuropsychological rehabilitation, 9,* 253–275.

Malle, B. (2001). Folk explanation of intentional action. In B. Malle & L. Moses (Eds.), *Intentions and intentionality: Foundations of social cognition* (pp. 265–286). Cambridge, MA: MIT Press.

Marder, S. (1998). Antipsychotic medications. In A. F. Schatzberg & C. B. Nemeroff (Eds.), *Textbook of psychopharmacology* (2nd ed., pp. 309–321). Washington, DC: American Psychiatric Press.

Marlatt, G. A., & Gordon, J. R. (Eds.). (1985). *Relapse prevention: Maintenance strategies in the treatment of addictive behaviors.* New York: Guilford Press.

Martin, R. (1976). *Legal challenges to behavior modification: Trends in schools, corrections and mental health.* Champaign, IL: Research Press.

Mason, G., & Soreff, S. (1996). Quality improvement and serious mental illness. In S. Soreff (Ed.), *Handbook for the treatment of the seriously mentally ill* (pp. 517–530). Kirkland, WA: Hogrefe & Huber.

Masterpasqua, F., & Perna, P. (Eds.). (1997). *The psychological meaning of chaos: Translating theory into practice.* Washington, DC: American Psychological Association.

Matson, J., & Kazdin, A. (1981). Punishment in behavior modification: Pragmatic, ethical and legal issues. *Clinical Psychology Review, 1,* 197–210.

May, P., Tuma, H., & Dixon, W. (1981). Schizophrenia: A follow-up study of the results of five forms of treatment. *Archives of General Psychiatry, 38,* 776–784.

Mazmanian, P., Kreutzer, J., Devany, C., & Martin, K. (1994). A survey of accredited and other rehabilitation facilities: Education, training and cognitive rehabilitation in brain-injury programs. *Brain Injury, 7,* 319–331.

McClure, R., & Weinberger, D. (2001). The neurodevelopmental hypothesis of schizophrenia: A review of the evidence. In A. Breier & P. Tran (Eds.), *Current issues in the psychopharmacology of schizophrenia.* Philadelphia: Lippincott, Williams & Wilkins.

McEvoy, J., Scheifler, P., & Frances, A. (Eds.). (1999). *Treatment of schizophrenia, 60*(Suppl. 11).

McFarlane, W., & Cunningham, K. (1996). Multiple-family groups and psychoeducation: Creating therapeutic social networks. In J. Vaccaro & G. Clark (Eds.), *Practicing psychiatry in the community: A manual*. Washington, DC: American Psychiatric Press.

McGlashan, T. (1999). Duration of untreated psychosis in first-episode schizophrenia: Marker or determinant of course? *Biological Psychiatry, 44*, 899–907.

McHugh, P. (1992). A structure for psychiatry at the century's turn: The view from Johns Hopkins. *Journal of the Royal Society of Medicine, 85*, 483–487.

McRae, S., & Lutzker, J. (1982). Applied behavior analysis and rehabilitation administration: End of courtship, time for marriage. *Journal of Rehabilitation Administration, 6*, 105–112.

Medalia, A., Aluma, M., Tyron, W., & Merriam, A. (1998). Effectiveness of attention training in schizophrenia. *Schizophrenia Bulletin, 24*(1), 147–152.

Meinecke, D. E. (2001). The developmental etiology of schizophrenia: What is the evidence? *Schizophrenia Bulletin, 27*(3), 335–476.

Meltzer, H., & Fatemi, H. (1998). Treatment of schizophrenia. In C. Nemeroff (Ed.), *Textbook of psychopharmacology* (2nd ed., pp. 747–774). Washington, DC: American Psychiatric Press.

Menditto, A., Beck, N., Stuve, P., Fisher, J., Stacy, M., Logue, M., & Baldwin, L. (1996). Effectiveness of clozapine and a social learning program for severely disabled psychiatric inpatients. *Psychiatric Services, 47*(1), 46–51.

Menditto, A., Wallace, C., Liberman, R., Vander Wal, J., Jones, N., & Stuve, P. (1999). Functional assessment of independent living skills. *Psychiatric Rehabilitation Skills, 3*, 200–219.

Meredith, J., Lambert, M., & Drozd, J. (2001). Clinical outcomes assessment for the practicing clinician. In M. T. Sammons & N. B. Schmidt (Eds.), *Combined treatments for mental disorders: A guide to psychological and pharmacological interventions*. Washington, DC: American Psychological Association.

Meyer, R., & McLaughlin, C. (Eds.). (1998). *Between mind, brain and managed care: The now and future world of academic psychiatry*. Washington, DC: American Psychiatric Press.

Milne, D., Gorenski, O., Westerman, C., Leck, C., & Keegan, D. (2000). What does it take to transfer training? *Psychiatric Rehabilitation Skills, 4*, 259–281.

Milne, D., Keegan, D., Westerman, C., & Dudley, M. (2000). Systematic process and outcome evaluation of brief staff training in psychosocial interventions for severe mental illness. *Journal of Behavioral Therapy and Experimental Psychiatry, 31*, 87–101.

Mindus, P., Edman, G., & Andreewitch, S. (1999). A prospective, long-term study of personality traits in patients with intractable obsessional illness treated by capsulotomy. *Acta Psychiatrica Scandinavica, 99*, 40–50.

Mohamed, S., Fleming, S., Penn, D., & Spaulding, W. (1999). Insight in schizophrenia: Its relationship to measures of executive functions. *Journal of Nervous and Mental Disease, 187*, 525–531.

Monahan, J., Bonnie, R., Appelbaum, P., Hyde, P., Steadman, H., & Swartz, M. (2001). Mandated community treatment: Beyond outpatient commitment. *Psychiatric Services, 52*, 1198–1205.

Monroe-DeVita, M., & Mohatt, D. (1999). The state hospital and the community: An essential continuum for persons with severe and persistent mental illness. In W. Spaulding (Ed.), *The role of the state hospital in the 21st century* (Vol. 84, pp. 85–98). San Francisco: Jossey-Bass.

Morgan, J., & Crisp, A. (2000). Use of leukotomy for intractable anorexia nervosa: A long-term follow-up study. *International Journal of Eating Disorders, 27,* 249–258.

Morgan, K., Orr, K., Hutchinson, G., Vearnals, S., Greenwood, K., Sharpley, R., Mallet, R., Morris, R., David, A., Leff, J., & Murray, R. (1999). Insight and neuropsychology in first-onset schizophrenia and other psychoses. *Schizophrenia Research, 36,* 145.

Morgan, K., Vearnals, S., Hutchinson, G., Orr, K., Greenwood, K., Sharpley, R., Mallet, R., David, A., Leff, J., & Murray, R. (1999). Insight, ethnicity and neuropsychology in first-onset psychosis. *Schizophrenia Research, 36,* 144.

Morin, C. (2001). Combined treatments of insomnia. In M. T. Sammons & N. B. Schmidt (Eds.), *Combined treatments for mental disorders: A guide to psychological and pharmacological interventions.* Washington, DC: American Psychological Association.

Morisse, D., Batra, L., Hess, L., Silverman, R., & Corrigan, P. (1996). A demonstration of a token economy for the real world. *Applied and Preventive Psychology, 5,* 41–46.

Morrison, A. (1998). Cognitive behavior therapy for psychotic symptoms in schizophrenia. In N. Tarrier & A. Wells (Eds.), *Treating complex cases: The cognitive behavioral therapy approach* (pp. 195–216). Chichester, England: Wiley.

Mosher, L. (1999). Soteria and other alternatives to acute psychiatric hospitalization: A personal and professional review. *Journal of Nervous and Mental Disease, 187,* 142–149.

Mosher, L. R., & Burti, L. (1989). *Community mental health: Principles and practice.* New York: Norton.

Mosher, L. R., & Menn, A. Z. (1978). Community residential treatment for schizophrenia: A two-year follow-up. *Hospital and Community Psychiatry, 29,* 715–723.

Mueser, K., Bond, G., Drake, R., & Resnick, S. (1998). Models of community care for severe mental illness: A review of research on case management. *Schizophrenia Bulletin, 24,* 37–73.

Mueser, T., & Glynn, S. (1995). *Behavioral family therapy for psychiatric disorders.* Boston: Allyn & Bacon.

Mullins, L., Keller, J., & Chaney, J. (1994). A systems and social cognitive approach to team functioning in physical rehabilitation settings. *Rehabilitation Psychology, 39,* 161–178.

Mumma, G. (1998). Improving cognitive case formulation and treatment planning in clinical practice and research. *Journal of Cognitive Psychotherapy, 12,* 251–274.

Musselman, D., Nathan, K., DeBattista, C., Kilts, C., Schatzberg, A., & Nemeroff, C. (1998). Biology of mood disorders. In A. F. Schatzberg & C. B. Nemeroff (Eds.), *Textbook of psychopharmacology* (2nd ed., pp. 549–588). Washington, DC: American Psychiatric Press.

Nelson, D. L., Schreiber, T. A., & McEvoy, C. L. (1992). Processing implicit and explicit representations. *Psychological Review, 99,* 322–348.

Nelson, R., & Hayes, S. (1981). Nature of behavioral assessment. In M. Herson & A.

Bellack (Eds.), *Behavior assessment: A practical handbook* (2nd ed., pp. 3–37). New York: Pergamon.

Neuchterlein, K. H. (1991). Vigilance in schizophrenia and related disorders. In S. R. Steinhauer, J. H. Gruzelier, & J. Zubin (Eds.), *Handbook of schizophrenia. Vol. 5: Neuropsychology, psychopathology and information processing* (pp. 397–433). Amsterdam: Elsevier Science.

Neuchterlein, K. H., & Dawson, M. E. (1984). Information processing and attentional functioning in the developmental course of schizophrenic disorders. *Schizophrenia Bulletin, 10,* 106–203.

Neuchterlein, K. H., Dawson, M. E., Gitlin, M., Ventura, J., Goldstein, M. J., Snyder, K. S., Yee, C. M., & Mintz, J. (1992). Developmental processes in schizophrenic disorders: Longitudinal studies of vulnerability and stress. *Schizophrenia Bulletin, 18*(3), 387–425.

Newman, L. (2001). What is "social cognition"? Four basic approaches and their implication for schizophrenia research. In P. Corrigan & D. Penn (Eds.), *Social cognition and schizophrenia* (pp. 41–72). Washington, DC: American Psychological Association.

Nezu, A. M., Nezu, C. M., Friedman, S. H., & Haynes, S. N. (1997). Case formulation in behavior therapy: Problem-solving and functional analytic strategies. In T. D. Eells (Ed.), *Handbook of psychotherapy case formulation* (pp. 368–401). New York: Guilford Press.

Nydegger, R. (1972). The elimination of hallucinatory and delusional behavior by verbal conditioning and assertive training: A case study. *Journal of Behavior Therapy and Experimental Psychiatry, 3,* 225–227.

O'Brian, W. (1993). Behavioral assessment in the psychiatric setting. In A. Bellak & M. Hersen (Eds.), *Handbook of behavior therapy in the psychiatric setting* (pp. 39–71). New York: Plenum Press.

O'Connor, F. (1991). Symptom monitoring for relapse prevention in schizophrenia. *Archives of Psychiatric Nursing, 5*(4), 193–201.

Olbrich, R., Kirsch, P., Pfeiffer, H., & Mussgay, L. (2001). Patterns of recovery of autonomic dysfunctions and neurocognitive deficits in schizophrenics after acute psychotic episodes. *Journal of Abnormal Psychology, 110,* 142–150.

Oltmanns, T., & Maher, B. (Eds.). (1988). *Delusional beliefs.* New York: Wiley.

Ottenbacher, K., & Cusick, A. (1990). Goal attainment as a method of clinical service evaluation. *American Journal of Occupational Therapy, 44,* 519–525.

Patrick, D., & Riggar, R. (1985). Organizational behavior management: Applications for program evaluation. *Journal of Rehabilitation Administration, 9,* 100–105.

Patterson, R. L., & Teigen, J. R. (1973). Conditioning and post-hospital generalization of non-delusional responses in a chronic psychotic patient. *Journal of Applied Behavior Analysis, 6,* 65–70.

Paul, G. L. (Ed.). (1986a). *Principles and methods to support cost-effective quality operations: Assessment in residential treatment settings. Part I.* Champaign, IL: Research Press.

Paul, G. L. (1986b). Rational operations in residential treatment settings through ongoing assessment of resident and staff functioning. In D. B. Fishman (Ed.), *Assessment for decision.* New Brunswick, NJ: Rutgers University Press.

Paul, G. L. (Ed.). (1988a). *Observational assessment instrumentation for service and research the computerized TSBC/SRIC planned access observational informa* - *tion system: Assessment in residential treatment settings. Part 4.* Champaign, IL: Research Press.

Paul, G. L. (Ed.). (1988b). *Observational assessment instrumentation for service and research the Staff-Resident Interaction Chronograph: Assessment in residen* - *tial treatment settings. Part 3.* Champaign, IL: Research Press.

Paul, G. L. (Ed.). (1988c). *Observational assessment instrumentation for service and research the Time-Sample Behavioral Checklist: Assessment in residential treatment settings. Part 2.* Champaign, IL: Research Press.

Paul, G. L., & Lentz, R. J. (1977). *Psychosocial treatment of chronic mental patients: Milieu vs. social learning programs.* Cambridge, MA: Harvard University Press.

Paul, G. L., & Menditto, A. (1992). Effectiveness of inpatient treatment programs for mentally ill adults in public psychiatric facilities. *Applied and Preventive Psychology, 1*(1), 41–63.

Paul, G. L., Stuve, P., & Cross, J. (1997). Real-world inpatient programs: Shedding some light: A critique. *Applied and Preventive Psychology, 6,* 193–204.

Penn, D. (1991). Cognitive rehabilitation of social deficits in schizophrenia: A direction of promise or following a primrose path? *Psychosocial Rehabilitation Journal, 15,* 27–41.

Penn, D., Combs, D., & Mohamed, S. (2001). Theory of mind and schizophrenia. In P. Corrigan & D. Penn (Eds.), *Social cognition and schizophrenia* (pp. 97–121). Washington, DC: American Psychological Association.

Penn, D., Corrigan, P., Bentall, R., & Racenstein, J. (1997). Social cognition in schizophrenia. *Psychological Bulletin, 121,* 114–132.

Penn, D., Hope, D., Spaulding, W., & Kucera, J. (1994). Social anxiety in schizophrenia. *Schizophrenia Research, 11,* 277–284.

Penn, D., vander Does, J., Spaulding, W., Garbin, C., Linzen, D., & Dingamans, P. (1993). Information processing and social-cognitive problem solving in schizophrenia. *Journal of Nervous and Mental Disease, 181,* 13–20.

Pestle, K., Card, J., & Menditto, A. (1998). Therapeutic recreation in a social-learning program: Effect over time on appropriate behaviors of residents with schizophrenia. *Therapeutic Recreation Journal, 32*(1), 28–41.

Pettit, J., Voelz, Z., & Joiner, T. (2001). Combined treatments for depression. In M. T. Sammons & N. B. Schmidt (Eds.), *Combined treatments for mental disorders: A guide to psychological and pharmacological interventions* (pp. 131–160). Washington, DC: American Psychological Association.

Petty, R. (1999). Structural asymmetries of the human brain and their disturbance in schizophrenia. *Schizophrenia Bulletin, 25,* 121–139.

Peveler, R., & Fairburn, C. (1990). Measurement of neurotic symptoms by self-report questionnaire: Validity of the SCL-90R. *Psychological Medicine, 20,* 873–879.

Phillips, D. (1972). Medical records: The problem-oriented system. *Hospitals, 46,* 84–88.

Piasecki, J., & Hollon, S. D. (1987). Cognitive therapy for depression: Unexplicated schemata and scripts. In N. S. Jacobson (Ed.), *Psychotherapists in clinical practice: Cognitive and behavioral perspectives.* New York: Guilford Press.

Platt, J., & Siegel, J. (1976). MMPI characteristics of good and poor social problem-solvers among psychiatric patients. *Journal of Psychology, 94,* 245–251.

Platt, J., & Spivack, G. (1975). Unidimensionality of the means-ends problem-solving (MEPS) procedure. *Journal of Clinical Psychology, 31,* 15–16.

Poland, J., VonEckardt, B., & Spaulding, W. (1994). Problems with the DSM approach to classifying psychopathology. In G. Graham & L. Stevens (Eds.), *Philosophical issues in psychopathology*. Boston: MIT Press.

Pressman, J. (1998). *Last resort: Psychosurgery and the limits of medicine*. New York: Cambridge University Press.

Price, B., Baral, I., Cosgrove, G., Rauch, S., Nierenberg, A., Jenike, M., & Cassem, E. (2001). Improvement in severe self-mutilation following limbic leucotomy: A series of 5 consecutive cases. *Journal of Clinical Psychiatry, 62*, 925–932.

Randolph, C., Goldberg, T., & Weinberger, D. (1993). The neuropsychology of schizophrenia. In K. Heilman & E. Valenstein (Eds.), *Clinical neuropsychology* (3rd ed., pp. 499–522). London: Oxford University Press.

Reed, D., Sullivan, M., Penn, D., Stuve, P., & Spaulding, W. (1992). Assessment and treatment of cognitive impairments. In R. P. Liberman (Ed.), *Effective psychiatric rehabilitation* (Vol. 53, pp. 7–20). San Francisco: Jossey-Bass.

Rehm, L. P., Kaslow, N. J., & Rabin, A. S. (1987). Cognitive and behavioral targets in a self-control therapy program for depression. *Journal of Consulting and Clinical Psychology, 55*, 60–67.

Reid, D., & Parsons, M. (2000). Organizational behavior management in human service settings. In J. Austin & J. Carr (Eds.), *Handbook of applied behavior analysis* (pp. 275–294). Reno, NV: Context Press.

Rickard, H., Collier, J., McCoy, A., & Crist, D. (1993). Relaxation training for psychiatric inpatients. *Psychological Reports, 72*, 1267–1274.

Ridgely, M., Borum, R., & Petrila, J. (2001). *The effectiveness of involuntary outpatient treatment: Empirical evidence and the experience of eight states*. Santa Monica, CA: Rand.

Roder, V., Jenull, B., & Brenner, H. (1998). Teaching schizophrenic patients recreational, residential and vocational skills. *International Review of Psychiatry, 10*(1), 35–41.

Roos, P. (1974). Human rights and behavior modification. *Mental Retardation, 12*, 3–6.

Rosvold, H. E., Mirsky, A. F., Sarason, I., Bransome, E. D., Jr., & Beck, L. H. (1956). A continuous performance test of brain damage. *Journal of Consulting Psychology, 20*, 343–350.

Salzinger, K. (1973). *Schizophrenia: Behavioral aspects*. New York: Wiley.

Salzinger, K. (1984). The immediacy hypothesis in a theory of schizophrenia. In W. Spaulding & J. Cole (Eds.), *Theories of schizophrenia and psychosis: The Nebraska symposium on motivation* (Vol. 31). Lincoln: University of Nebraska Press.

Sameroff, A. (1995). General systems theories and developmental psychopathology. In D. Cicchetti & D. Cohen (Eds.), *Developmental psychopathology: Vol 1. Theory and methods* (pp. 659–695). New York: Wiley.

Saugstad, L. (1999). A lack of cerebral lateralization in schizophrenia is within the normal variation in brain maturation but indicates late, slow maturation. *Schizophrenia Research, 39*, 183–196.

Schaub, A., & Liberman, P. (1999). Training individuals with schizophrenia to manage their illness: Experiences from Germany and Switzerland. *Psychiatric Rehabilitation Skills, 3*, 246–267.

Schmidt, N.B., Koselka, M., & Woolaway-Bickel, K. (2001). Combined treatments for phobic anxiety disorders. In M. T. Sammons & N. B. Schmidt (Eds.), *Com-

*bined treatments for mental disorders: A guide to psychological and pharmacological interventions* (pp. 81–110). Washington, DC: American Psychological Association.

Schotte, D. E., & Clum, G. A. (1987). Problem-solving skills in suicidal psychiatric patients. *Journal of Consulting and Clinical Psychology, 55*, 49–54.

Schuster, J., & Lovell, M. (1997). *Training behavioral health care professionals: Higher learning in the era of managed care.* San Francisco: Jossey-Bass.

Searles, R., & Fox, R. (1998). Behavioral health: A view from the industry. In D. Mechanic (Ed.), *Managed behavioral healthcare: Current realities and future potential. New direction in mental health services* (No. 78, pp. 25–30). San Francisco: Jossey-Bass.

Seligman, M. (1975). *Helplessness: On depression, development, and death.* San Francisco: Freeman.

Shagass, C. (1991). EEG studies of schizophrenia. In S. R. Steinhauer, J. H. Gruzelier, & J. Zubin (Eds.), *Handbook of schizophrenia. Vol. 5: Neuropsychology, psychopathology and information processing* (pp. 39–69). Amsterdam: Elsevier Science.

Sheils, R., & Rolfe, T. (2000). Towards an integrated approach to a family intervention for co-occuring substance abuse and schizophrenia. *Australian and New Zealand Journal of Family Therapy, 21*, 81–87.

Sheldon, K., & Elliot, A. (1998). Not all personal goals are personal: Comparing autonomous and controlled reasons for goals as predictors of effort and attainment. *Personality and Social Psychology Bulletin, 24*, 546–557.

Shelly, C., & Goldstein, G. (1983). Discrimination of chronic schizophrenia and brain damage with the Luria–Nebraska battery: A partially successful replication. *Clinical Neuropsychology, 5*, 82–85.

Shutty, M., & Song, Y. (1997). Behavioral analysis of drinking behaviors in polydipsic patients with chronic schizophrenia. *Journal of Abnormal Psychology, 106*, 483–485.

Sigmon, S., Steingard, S., Badges, G., Anthony, S., & Higgins, S. (2000). Contingent reinforcement of marijuana abstinence among individuals with serious mental illness: A feasibility study. *Experimental and Clinical Psychopharmacology, 8*, 509–517.

Silbergeld, S., & Noble, E. (1973). Corticosteroids in psychiatric patients: Subacute and diurnal effects of free fatty acids and catecholamine metabolism. *Journal of Psychiatric Research, 10*, 59–71.

Silverstein, S., Bowman, J., & McHugh, D. (1997). Strategies for hospital-wide dissemination of psychiatric rehabilitation interventions. *Psychiatric Rehabilitation Skills, 2*, 1–23.

Silverstein, S., Menditto, A., & Stuve, P. (2000). Shaping procedures as cognitive retraining techniques in individuals with severe and persistent mental illness. *Psychiatric Rehabilitation Skills, 3*, 59–76.

Simons, A. D., Garfield, S. L., & Murphy, G. E. (1984). The process of change in cognitive therapy and pharmacotherapy: Changes in mood and cognition. *Archives of General Psychiatry, 41*, 45–51.

Sirota, P., Epstein, B., Benatov, R., Sousnostzky, M., & Kindler, S. (2001). An open study of buspirone augmentation of neuroleptics in patients with schizophrenia. *Journal of Clinical Psychopharmacology, 21*, 454–455.

Slaton, K., & Westphal, J. (1999). The Slaton-Westphal Functional Assessment Inventory for adults with psychiatric disability: Development of an instrument to measure functional status and psychiatric rehabilitation outcome. *Psychiatric Rehabilitation Journal, 23,* 119–126.

Sluyter, G. (1998). *Improving organizational performance: A practical guidebook for the human services field.* Thousand Oaks, CA: Sage.

Smith, T. (1990). *Program evaluation in human services.* New York: Springer.

Smith, T., & Docherty, J. (1998). Standards of care and clinical algorithms for treating schizophrenia. *Psychiatric Clinics of North America, 21*(1), 203–220.

Snyder, K. S., & Liberman, R. P. (1981). Family assessment and intervention with schizophrenics at risk for relapse. In M. Goldstein (Ed.), *New directions for mental health services* (No. 2). San Francisco: Jossey-Bass.

Sohlberg, M. M., & Mateer, C. A. (1989). *Introduction to cognitive rehabilitation theory and practice.* New York: Guilford Press.

Sommer, I., Aleman, A., Ramsey, N., Bouma, A., & Kahn, R. (2001). Handedness, language lateralization and anatomical asymmetry in schizophrenia. *British Journal of Psychiatry, 178,* 344–351.

Sorenson, D. J., Paul, G. L., & Mariotto, M. J. (1988). Inconsistencies in paranoid functioning, premorbid adjustment, and chronicity: Question of diagnostic criteria. *Schizophrenia Bulletin, 14*(2), 323–336.

Spaulding, W. (1992). Design prerequisites for research on cognitive therapy for schizophrenia. *Schizophrenia Bulletin, 18*(1), 39–42.

Spaulding, W. (Ed.). (1994). *Integrated theories of motivation, cognition and emotion* (Vol. 41). Lincoln: University of Nebraska Press.

Spaulding, W., & Cole, J. (Eds.). (1984). *Theories of schizophrenia and psychosis* (Vol. 31). Lincoln: University of Nebraska Press.

Spaulding, W., Fleming, S., Reed, D., Sullivan, M., Storzbach, D., & Lam, M. (1999). Cognitive functioning in schizophrenia: Implications for psychiatric rehabilitation. *Schizophrenia Bulletin, 25*(2), 275–289.

Spaulding, W., Johnson, D., & Coursey, R. (2001). Combined treatments and rehabilitation of schizophrenia. In M. T. Sammons & N. B. Schmidt (Eds.), *Combined treatments for mental disorders: A guide to psychological and pharmacological interventions* . Washington, DC: American Psychological Association.

Spaulding, W., Poland, J., Elbogen, E., & Ritchie, J. (2000). Therapeutic jurisprudence in psychiatric rehabilitation. *Thomas M. Cooley Law Review, 17,* 135–170.

Spaulding, W., Sullivan, M., Weiler, M., Reed, D., Richardson, C., & Storzbach, D. (1994). Changing cognitive functioning in rehabilitation of schizophrenia. *Acta Psychiatrica Scandinavica, 90*(Suppl. 384), 116–124.

Spaulding, W., Wyss, H., & Littrell, R. (1990). Training psychophysiological self-regulation skills in psychiatric rehabilitation. *Psychosocial Rehabilitation Journal, 13,* 37–39.

Spaulding, W. D., Reed, D., Sullivan, M., Richardson, C., & Weiler, M. (1999). Effects of cognitive treatment in psychiatric rehabilitation. *Schizophrenia Bulletin, 25*(4), 657–676.

Spaulding, W. D., Storms, L., Goodrich, V., & Sullivan, M. (1986). Applications of experimental psychopathology in psychiatric rehabilitation. *Schizophrenia Bulletin, 12*(4), 560–577.

Spohn, H., & Strauss, M. (1989). Relation of neuroleptic and anticholinergic medication to cognitive functions in schizophrenia. *Journal of Abnormal Psychology, 98,* 367–380.

Stark, F., & Stutte, K. (1990). Behavioral rehabilitation in West Germany: Patient care, staff training and administrative obstacles. *Psychosocial Rehabilitation Journal, 13,* 23–26.

Starkey, D., Deleone, H., & Flannery, R. (1995). Stress management for psychiatric patients in a state hospital setting. *American Journal of Orthopsychiatry, 65,* 446–450.

Steadman, H. J., Gounis, K., Dennis, D., Hopper, K., Roche, B., Swartz, M., & Robbins, P. C. (1999). Assessing the New York City involuntary outpatient commitment pilot program. *Psychiatric Services, 52,* 330–336.

Stein, M., & Uhde, T. (1998). Biology of anxiety disorders. In A. F. Schatzberg & C. B. Nemeroff (Eds.), *Textbook of psychopharmacology* (2nd ed., pp. 608–628). Washington, DC: American Psychiatric Press.

Steinhauer, S. R., Gruzelier, J. H., & Zubin, J. (Eds.). (1991). *Handbook of schizophrenia. Vol. 5: Neuropsychology, psychopathology and information processing.* Amsterdam: Elsevier Science.

Steinwachs, D. (1997). Experiences with managed care and PACT. *Community Support Network News, 11,* 14–16.

Stepleton, J. (1975). Legal issues confronting behavior modification. *Behavioral Engineering, 2,* 35–43.

Storms, L., & Broen, W. (1969). A theory of schizophrenic behavioral disorganization. *Archives of General Psychiatry, 20,* 129–144.

Storzbach, D., & Corrigan, P. (1996). Cognitive rehabilitation for schizophrenia. In P. Corrigan & S. Yudofsky (Eds.), *Cognitive rehabilitation for neuropsychiatric disorders* (pp. 299–328). Washington, DC: American Psychiatric Press.

Stoudemire, A. (1990). Biopsychosocial assessment and case formulation. In A. Stoudemire (Ed.), *Clinical psychiatry for medical students* (pp. 58–71). Philadelphia: Williams & Wilkins.

Strauss, J., & Carpenter, W. (1977). The treatment of acute schizophrenia without drugs: An investigation of some current assumptions. *American Journal of Psychiatry, 134,* 14–20.

Strauss, J., Carpenter, W., & Bartko, J. (1974). Speculations on the processes that underlie schizophrenic symptoms and signs. *Schizophrenia Bulletin, 11,* 61–75.

Sullivan, M., Richardson, C., & Spaulding, W. (1991). University-state hospital collaboration in an inpatient psychiatric rehabilitation program. *Community Mental Health Journal, 27*(6), 441–453.

Swartz, M. S., Swanson, J. W., Hiday, V. A., Wagner, H. R., Burns, B. J., & Borum, R. (2001). A randomized controlled trial of outpatient commitment in North Carolina. *Psychiatric Services, 52,* 325–329.

Sweeney, P. D., Anderson, A., & Bailey, S. (1986). Attributional style in depression: A meta-analytic review. *Journal of Personality and Social Psychology, 50,* 974–999.

Swett, C., & Mills, T. (1997). Use of the NOSIE to predict assaults among acute psychiatric patients. *Psychiatric Services, 48,* 1177–1180.

Szasz, T. S. (1961). *The myth of mental illness.* New York: Harper & Row.

Tarrier, N., Sharpe, L., Beckett, R., Harwood, R., Baker, & Yusopoff, L. (1993). A trial of two cognitive behavioural methods of treating drug-resistant residual psychotic symptoms in schizophrenic patients: II. Treatment-specific changes in coping and problem-solving skills. *Social Psychiatry and Psychiatric Epidemiology, 28*(1), 5–10.

Taube, C., Eun, S., & Forthofer, R. (1984). Diagnosis-related groups for mental disorders, alcoholism and drug abuse: Evaluation and alternatives. *Hospital and Community Psychiatry, 35,* 452–455.

Taylor, C. B. (1998). Treatment of anxiety disorders. In A. F. Schatzberg & C. B. Nemeroff (Eds.), *Textbook of psychopharmacology* (2nd ed., pp. 775–790). Washington, DC: American Psychiatric Press.

Toomey, R., Schuldberg, D., Green, M., & Corrigan, P. (1993). *Social perception of nonverbal cues in schizophrenia: Relationship with deficits in cognition and social problem solving.* Paper presented at the Association for Advancement of Behavior Therapy, Atlanta, GA.

Tryon, W. (1976). Behavior modification therapy and the law. *Professional Psychology: Research and Practice, 7,* 468–474.

Tsuang, M., Eckman, T., Shaner, A., & Marder, S. (1999). Clozapine for substance abusing schizophrenia patients. *American Journal of Psychiatry, 156,* 1119–1120.

Ullman, L., & Krasner, L. (1965). *Case studies in behavior modification.* New York: Holt, Rinehart & Winston.

Upper, D., & Flowers, J. V. (1994). Behavioral group therapy in rehabilitation settings. In J. Bedell (Ed.), *Psychological assessment and treatment of persons with severe mental disorders* (pp. 31–56). Philadelphia: Taylor & Francis.

Vacarro, J., Liberman, R., Wallace, C., & Blackwell, G. (1992). Combining social skills training and assertive case management: The social and independent living skills program of the Brentwood Veterans Affairs Medical Center. In R. Liberman (Ed.), *Effective psychiatric rehabilitation* (Vol. 53, pp. 33–42). San Francisco: Jossey-Bass.

vanderGaag, M. (1992). *The results of cognitive training in schizophrenic patients.* Delft, Netherlands: Eburon.

vanderGaag, M., Woonings, F., vandenBosch, R., Appelo, M., Sloof, C., & Louwerens, J. (1994). Cognitive training of schizophrenic patients: A behavioral approach based on experimental psychopathology. In W. Spaulding (Ed.), *Cognitive technology in psychiatric rehabilitation* (pp. 139–158). Lincoln: University of Nebraska Press.

Velligan, D., Bow-Thomas, L., Huntzinger, C., Ritch, J., Ledbetter, N., Prihoda, T., & Miller, A. (2000). Randomized controlled trial of the use of compensating strategies to enhance adaptive functioning in outpatients with schizophrenia. *American Journal of Psychiatry, 157,* 1317–1323.

Ventura, J., Green, M., Shaner, A., & Liberman, R. (1993). Training and quality assurance with the BPRS. *International Journal of Methods in Psychiatric Research, 3,* 221–244.

Ventura, J., Liberman, R., Green, M., Shaner, A., & Mintz, J. (1998). Training and quality assurance with structured clinical interview for DSM-IV (SCID I/P). *Psychiatry Research, 79*(2), 163–173.

Verghese, C., De Leon, J., & Josiassen, R. (1996). Problems and progress in the diagnosis and treatment of polydipsia and hyponatremia. *Schizophrenia Bulletin, 22,* 455–464.

von Bertalanffy, L. (1965). *General systems theory: Foundation, development applications.* New York: Braziller.

von Bertalanffy, L. (1966). General systems theory in psychiatry. In S. Arieti (Ed.), *American handbook of psychiatry* (Vol. 3). New York: Basic Books.

Waddington, L. (1997). Clinical judgement and case formulation. *British Journal of Clinical Psychology, 36,* 309–311.

Wakefield, J. C. (1992). Disorder as harmful dysfunction: A conceptual critique of DSM-III-R's definition of mental disorder. *Psychological Review, 99,* 232–247.

Walker, E. (1994). Developmentally moderated expressions of the neuropathology underlying schizophrenia. *Schizophrenia Bulletin, 20*(3), 453–480.

Wallace, C. J. (1982). The social skills training project of the Mental Health Clinical Research Center for the Study of Schizophrenia. In J. P. Curran & P. M. Monti (Eds.), *Social skills training: A practical handbook for assessment and treatment.* New York: Guilford Press.

Wallace, C. J., & Boone, S. E. (1984). Cognitive factors in the social skill of schizophrenic patients. In W. D. Spaulding & J. K. Cole (Eds.), *Theories of schizophrenia and psychosis.* Lincoln: University of Nebraska Press.

Wallace, C. J., Boone, S. E., Donahoe, C. P., & Foy, D. W. (1985). The chronic mentally disabled: Independent living skills training. In D. H. Barlow (Ed.), *Clinical handbook of psychological disorders: A step-by-step treatment manual.* New York: Guilford Press.

Wallace, C. J., Nelson, C., Liberman, R. P., Hitchison, R., Lukoff, D., Elder, J., & Ferris, C. (1980). A review and critique of social skills training for schizophrenics. *Schizophrenia Bulletin, 6,* 42–60.

Waller, G., Hypde, C., & Thomas, C. (1994). A "biofeedback" approach to the treatment of chronic polydipsia. *Journal of Behavior Therapy and Experimental Psychiatry, 24,* 255–259.

Watson, A., Luchins, D., Hanrahan, P., Heyman, M., & Lurigio, A. (2000). Mental health court: Promises and limitations. *Journal of the American Academy of Psychiatry and the Law, 28,* 476–482.

Weinberger, D. (1987). Implications of normal brain development for the pathogenesis of schizophrenia. *Archives of General Psychiatry, 44,* 660–669.

Weinberger, D. (1994). Biological basis of schizophrenia: Structural/functional considerations relevant to potential for antipsychotic drug response. *Journal of Clinical Psychiatry Monograph Series, 12*(2), 4–9.

Weinberger, D. (1996). On the plausibility of "the neurodevelopmental hypothesis" of schizophrenia. A new understanding: Neurological basis and long-term outcome of schizophrenia. *Neuropsychopharmacology, 14*(3, Suppl.), 1–11.

Weinberger, D., & Lipska, B. (1995). Cortical maldevelopment, antipsychotic drugs and schizophrenia: A search for common ground. *Schizophrenia Research, 16,* 87–110.

Weiner, B., Frieze, I., Kukla, A., Reed, L., Rest, S., & Rosenbaum, R. M. (1971). *Perceiving the causes of success and failure.* New York: General Learning Press.

Weiner, M. (1982). *Human services management: Analysis and applications.* Homewood, IL: Dorsey Press.

Wexler, B., Hawkins, K., Rounsaville, B., Anderson, M., Sernyak, M., & Green, M.

(1997). Normal neurocognitive performance after extended practice in patients with schizophrenia. *Schizophrenia Research, 26,* 173–180.

Wexler, D. (1973). Token and taboo: Behavior modification, token economies, and the law. *California Law Review, 61,* 81–109.

Wexler, D., & Winick, B. (1991). *Essays in therapeutic jurisprudence.* Durham, NC: Carolina Academic Press.

White, L., & Morse, L. (1988). Behavior modification in institutions: The development of legal protections of patients' rights. *Behavioral Residential Treatment, 3,* 287–314.

Wilkerson, D., Migas, N., & Slaven, T. (2000). Outcome-oriented standards and performance indicators for substance dependency rehabilitation programs. *Substance Use and Misuse, 35,* 1679–1703.

Willerman, L., & Cohen, D. (1990). *Psychopathology.* New York: McGraw Hill.

Williams, J. M. G. (1984). Cognitive-behavior therapy for depression: Problems and perspectives. *British Journal of Psychiatry, 145,* 254–262.

Wincze, J. P., Leitenberg, H., & Agras, W. S. (1972). The effects of token reinforcement and feedback on delusional verbal behavior of chronic paranoid schizophrenics. *Journal of Applied Behavior Analysis, 5,* 247–262.

Wong, S. E., & Woolsey, J. E. (1989). Re-establishing conversational skills in overtly psychotic, chronic schizophrenic patients: Discrete trials training on the psychiatric ward. *Behavior Modification, 13,* 415–430.

Woolfolk, R. L., & Lehrer, P. M. (Eds.). (1984). *Principles and practice of stress management.* New York: Guilford Press.

Wykes, T., Reeder, C., Corner, J., Williams, C., & Everitt, B. (1999). The effects of neurocognitive remediation on executive processing in patients with schizophrenia. *Schizophrenia Bulletin, 25*(2), 291–307.

Yates, B. (1996). *Analyzing costs, procedures, processes and outcomes in human services.* Thousand Oaks, CA: Sage.

Yoman, J., & Edelstein, B. (1994). Functional assessment in psychiatric disability. In J. Bedell (Ed.), *Psychological assessment and treatment of persons with severe mental disorders* (pp. 31–56). Philadelphia: Taylor & Francis.

Yudofsky, S. (1991). Psychoanalysis, psychopharmacology and the influence of neuropsychiatry. *Journal of Neuropsychiatry and Clinical Neuroscience, 3,* 1–5.

Yudofsky, S., Silver, J., & Hales, R. (1998). Treatment of agitation and aggression. In A. F. Schatzberg & C. B. Nemeroff (Eds.), *Textbook of psychopharmacology* (2nd ed., pp. 881–900). Washington, DC: American Psychiatric Press.

Zahn, T. P., Frith, C. D., & Steinhauer, S. R. (1991). Autonomic functioning in schizophrenia: Electrodermal activity, heart rate, pupillography. In S. R. Steinhauer, J. H. Gruzelier, & J. Zubin (Eds.), *Handbook of schizophrenia. Vol. 5: Neuropsychology, psychopathology and information processing* (pp. 185–224). Amsterdam: Elsevier Science.

Zelitch, S. (1980). Helping the family cope: Workshops for families of schizophrenics. *Health and Social Work, 5,* 47–52.

Zubin, J., & Spring, B. (1977). Vulnerability: A new view of schizophrenia. *Journal of Abnormal Psychology, 86,* 103–126.

# Index